Methods in Molecular Biology

Series Editor
John M. Walker
School of Life Sciences
University of Hertfordshire
Hatfield, Hertfordshire, AL10 9AB, UK

For further volumes:
http://www.springer.com/series/7651

Cytotoxic T-Cells

Methods and Protocols

Edited by

Elena Ranieri

Department of Medical and Surgical Sciences, University of Foggia, Foggia, Italy

Humana Press

Editor
Elena Ranieri
Department of Medical and Surgical Sciences
University of Foggia
Foggia, Italy

ISSN 1064-3745 ISSN 1940-6029 (electronic)
ISBN 978-1-4939-1157-8 ISBN 978-1-4939-1158-5 (eBook)
DOI 10.1007/978-1-4939-1158-5
Springer New York Heidelberg Dordrecht London

Library of Congress Control Number: 2014944379

Printed on acid-free paper

Humana Press is a brand of Springer
Springer is part of Springer Science+Business Media (www.springer.com)

Preface

My memories trace back to when I was an 8-year-old girl, busy searching for information and illustrations about animals in natural science books; eager to search and continually learn. Books have been my world, and my thoughts and wishes have originated from them.

Today, that girl has become a researcher who has edited the present textbook of molecular biology which is expected to stand as a *primum movens* that researchers may use while conducting a research activity applied to immunology; a textbook that can be used to start research for the characterization of Cytotoxic T Lymphocytes (CTL) by employing a systemic approach. The text is intended to outline basic and advanced laboratory methods in a way that will render straightforward and clear results.

This book aims to be an introductory course to Systems Biology in Cytotoxic T Cells. The emerging area of Systems Biology is a holistic approach that strives for a system-level understanding of biology. This means assessing the complex dynamics of how the structure of cells and organisms functions together, rather than the characteristics of isolated parts of a cell or organism.

One problem with this approach is that so far, no book has placed enough emphasis on laboratory methods applied to immunology. Our idea is to provide a book that introduces the concepts of Systems Biology along with the lab protocols that have generated such concepts. We stress the importance of offering clear explanations in order to show both students and researchers the relationship between experiments and concepts. The efforts and enthusiasm of all the contributing authors are apparent in this textbook that treats the main topic as an adventure in discovery. I personally thank all of them for taking part in this challenging project and for sharing their laboratory protocols.

The text is written in a clear-cut manner and elegantly illustrated in full color. It comprises 16 chapters. In the first part the book focuses on the isolation of T cells (Chapter 1), their expansion and characterization according to different methods (Chapters 2 and 3). The required techniques for intracellular signaling, monitoring of antigen T cell specific responses, and CTL exosomes are reported in Chapters 4–7. Microscopy and in vivo imaging applied to CTL studies are found in Chapters 8 and 9. "Omics" approaches are described in Chapters 10–13. Finally, the last three chapters include a specialist application of molecular methods into the study of CTL (Chapters 14–16) such as next generation sequencing of the Jack/stat pathway and CTL involvement in bone remodeling and transplantation.

Foggia, Italy — ***Elena Ranieri***

Acknowledgement

We thank the Section of Pathological Anatomy, Department of Emergency and Organ Transplantation, University of Bari "Aldo Moro," Bari, Italy for kindly providing the cover image.

Contents

Contributors

MATTEO ACCETTURO, PH.D. • *Nephrology, Dialysis and Transplantation Unit, Department of Emergency and Organ Transplantation, Policlinico, University of Bari "A. Moro", Bari, Italy*

JASON AKULIAN, M.D. M.P.H. • *Interventional Pulmonary, Division of Pulmonary and Critical Care, University of North Carolina School of Medicine, Chapel Hill, NC, USA*

PER-OLOF BERGGREN, PH.D. • *Hospital Stockholm, Karolinska Institutet, Stockholm, Sweden; Diabetes Research Institute, Miller School of Medicine, University of Miami, Miami, FL, USA*

GIACOMINA BRUNETTI, PH.D. • *Section of Human Anatomy and Histology, Department of Basic Medical Sciences, Neurosciences and Sense Organs, Policlinico, University of Bari, Bari, Italy*

SILVIA COLUCCI, PH.D. • *Section of Human Anatomy and Histology, Department of Basic Medical Sciences, Neurosciences and Sense Organs, Policlinico, University of Bari, Bari, Italy*

SHARON NATASHA COX, PH.D. • *Department of Emergency and Organ Transplantation, Policlinico, University of Bari, Bari, Italy*

STERPETA DIELLA • *Department of Medical and Surgical Sciences, University of Foggia, Foggia, Italy; Ospedali Riuniti, Foggia, Italy*

CHIARA DIVELLA, PH.D. • *Nephrology, Dialysis and Transplantation Unit, Department of Emergency and Organ Transplantation, Policlinico, University of Bari "A. Moro", Bari, Italy*

GAETANO FALEO, PH.D. • *Transplantation Research Laboratory, Department of Surgery, University of California San Francisco, San Francisco, CA, USA*

LORETO GESUALDO, M.D. • *Nephrology, Dialysis and Transplantation Unit, Department of Emergency and Organ Transplantation, Policlinico, University of Bari "A. Moro", Bari, Italy*

MARGHERITA GIGANTE, PH.D. • *Nephrology, Dialysis and Transplantation Unit, Department of Emergency and Organ Transplantation, Policlinico, University of Bari "A. Moro", Bari, Italy*

MADDALENA GIGANTE, PH.D. • *Department of Medical and Surgical Sciences, University of Foggia, Foggia, Italy; Ospedali Riuniti, Foggia, Italy*

GIUSEPPE GRANDALIANO, M.D. • *Nephrology, Dialysis and Transplantation Unit, Department of Surgery and Medical Sciences, University of Foggia, Foggia, Italy; Ospedali Riuniti, Foggia, Italy*

MARIA GRANO, PH.D. • *Section of Human Anatomy and Histology, Department of Basic Medical Sciences, Neurosciences and Sense Organs, Policlinico, University of Bari, Bari, Italy*

ADRIANA T. LARREGINA, M.D., PH.D. • *Department of Immunology, Dermatology, University of Pittsburgh Medical Center, Pittsburgh, PA, USA*

DEVIN B. LOWE, PH.D. • *Department of Dermatology, University of Pittsburgh School of Medicine, Pittsburgh, PA, USA*

JOHN MCDYER, M.D. • *Division of Pulmonary, Allergy and Critical Care Medicine, Department of Medicine, Thomas E. Starzl Transplantation Institute Associate Member, University of Pittsburgh School of Medicine, Pittsburgh, PA, USA*
ANGELA MONTECALVO, PH.D. • *Department of Immunology, University of Pittsburgh School of Medicine, Pittsburgh, PA, USA*
ADRIAN E. MORELLI, M.D., PH.D. • *Department of Surgery and Thomas E. Starzl Transplantation Institute, University of Pittsburgh Medical Center, Pittsburgh, PA, USA*
GIUSEPPE STEFANO NETTI, M.D., PH.D. • *Department of Medical and Surgical Sciences, University of Foggia, Foggia, Italy; Ospedali Riuniti, Foggia, Italy*
ANGELA ORANGER, PH.D. • *Section of Human Anatomy and Histology, Department of Basic Medical Sciences, Neurosciences and Sense Organs, Policlinico, University of Bari, Bari, Italy*
MASSIMO PAPALE, PH.D. • *Core Facility of Proteomics and Mass Spectrometry, Department of Surgery and Medical Sciences, University of Foggia, Foggia, Italy*
ANTONELLO PILEGGI, M.D., PH.D. • *Professor of Surgery, Microbiology and Immunology, and Biomedical Engineering, Cell Transplant Center, Diabetes Research Institute, Miller School of Medicine, University of Miami, Miami, FL, USA*
MATTHEW PIPELING, M.D. • *Division of Pulmonary, Allergy and Critical Care Medicine, Department of Medicine, University of Pittsburgh School of Medicine, Pittsburgh, PA, USA*
PAOLA PONTRELLI, PH.D. • *Nephrology, Dialysis and Transplantation Unit, Department of Emergency and Organ Transplantation, Policlinico, University of Bari "A. Moro", Bari, Italy*
IULIA POPESCU, PH.D. • *Division of Pulmonary Allergy and Critical Care Medicine, Department of Medicine, BST, University of Pittsburgh School of Medicine, Pittsburgh, PA, USA*
ELENA RANIERI, PH.D. • *Department of Surgical and Medical Sciences, School of Medicine, University of Foggia, Foggia, Italy; Ospedali Riuniti, Foggia, Italy*
FEDERICA RASCIO, PH.D. • *Nephrology, Dialysis and Transplantation Unit, Department of Surgery and Medical Sciences, University of Foggia, Foggia, Italy*
MARIA TERESA ROCCHETTI, PH.D. • *Department of Emergency and Organ Transplantation, University of Bari, Bari, Italy; Core Facility of Proteomics and Mass Spectrometry, University of Foggia, Foggia, Italy*
WALTER J. STORKUS, PH.D. • *Cancer Institute, University of Pittsburgh School of Medicine, University of Pittsburgh, Pittsburgh, PA, USA*
JENNIFER L. TAYLOR, PH.D. • *Department of Dermatology, University of Pittsburgh School of Medicine, Pittsburgh, PA, USA*

Chapter 1

Negative and Positive Separation Techniques for the Isolation of Antigen-Specific CD8$^+$ T Cells from Blood and Tumor Tissue

Margherita Gigante, Sharon Natasha Cox, and Elena Ranieri

Abstract

Adoptive transfer of tumor-reactive cytotoxic T cells (CTLs) is a promising therapeutic approach for the treatment of solid tumors. To develop these strategies, it is necessary to isolate specific leukocyte subpopulations from peripheral blood or tumor tissue (referred to as tumor-infiltrating lymphocytes (TIL)) that will be reinfused into the patient after expansion in vitro. The ideal cell isolation approach should be performed rapidly, thereby maximizing the recovery and viability of the purified cells. Here, we describe the negative or the positive separation procedures to isolate CD8$^+$ T cells from whole blood, from peripheral blood mononuclear cells (PBMCs), or from cancer tissue. Purified CD8$^+$ cells will be used for different downstream applications such as protein and gene expression profile analysis in order to assess their intrinsic cytotoxic ability.

Key words Tumor-infiltrating lymphocytes (TIL), CD8$^+$ T cells, Microbeads, Rosettes, Cancer

1 Introduction

Antigen-specific CD8$^+$ T cells are crucial for the elimination of intracellular pathogens, such as viruses, intracellular bacteria, or certain tumors, as well as for the development of long-term protection [1]. During an immune response, naïve CD8$^+$ T cells can differentiate into distinct memory subsets, effector memory or central memory cells, based on their differentiation state [2]. CD8 antigen is highly expressed on human cytotoxic T cells and dimly on a subset of natural killer (NK) cells. To become activated, naive CD8$^+$ T cells require two signals provided by the ligation of T-cell receptor (TCR) with specific MHC class I–peptide complex, followed by the interaction of costimulatory molecules expressed on antigen-presenting cell (APCs) surface with their respective ligands on T cells. Following their activation and clonal expansion, CD8$^+$ T cells acquire cytotoxic activity through the release of lytic granules

Elena Ranieri (ed.), *Cytotoxic T-Cells: Methods and Protocols*, Methods in Molecular Biology, vol. 1186,
DOI 10.1007/978-1-4939-1158-5_1, © Springer Science+Business Media New York 2014

containing perforin and granzymes which kill target cells activating various lytic pathways [3].

The isolation of $CD8^+$ T cells is a prerequisite in order to study them both phenotypically and functionally after in vitro stimulation with antigen-presenting cells (APC), obtained from freshly isolated PBMCs or from tumor tissues. There are a variety of available procedures, many of which are based on antibody-mediated separation such as immunomagnetic selection and cell sorting of fluorescence-labeled cells. The cell sorting by flow cytometry represents the most refined method; however the yield of cells is low making this technique severely limiting. In this chapter we describe two procedures for isolating antigen-specific $CD8^+$ T cells with negative or positive selection techniques from PBMCs and from cancer tissue. The choice of negative or positive selection method depends on the application that we intend to perform on the purified $CD8^+$ T cells, as explained below.

1.1 Isolation of Tumour-Infiltrating Lymphocytes (TIL)

The method described is referred to the isolation of TIL from renal cell carcinoma (RCC) [4] but could be applied to other solid tumors with some change depending on the tumor type and the leukocyte subset we intend to isolate. The protocol usually includes tissue disaggregation and cell enrichment. We recommend density centrifugation for initial enrichment, followed by specific magnetic bead negative or positive panning with $CD8^+$ T cell selective antibodies. The flow chart of experiment is showed in Fig. 1.

1.2 The Positive Selection of CTL from PBMC Using Microbeads

$CD8^+$ cells are labeled with CD8 Microbeads that are 50 nm magnetic particles conjugated to highly specific antibody against CD8 antigen on T cell surface (Fig. 2). Due to the small size, the microbeads do not activate cells and, unlike larger beads, they do not have to be removed for any downstream application. Microbeads are nontoxic and biodegradable. The positive selection will be used to isolate $CD8^+$ T cells after in vitro stimulation (IVS) of T cells with APCs in order to test their cytotoxic ability (i.e., by IFN-γ ELISPOT assay) [5, 6] and cytokine expression or could be isolated before activation and clonal expansion, from fresh PBMCs or whole blood.

1.3 Negative Selection of CTLs from Whole Blood Using the Rosette Procedure

The negative selection of CTLs using rosette procedure isolates untouched and highly purified $CD8^+$ T cells from whole blood in a single step without columns or magnets, avoiding the risk of activating or damaging cells [7]. The unwanted cells are targeted for removal with tetrameric antibody complexes recognizing known markers for mature hematopoietic cells (CD4, CD16, CD19, CD36, CD56, CD66b, CD123, TCRγ/δ, and glycophorin A). As illustrated in Fig. 3, after standard density gradient centrifugation, the unwanted cell pellet along with the red blood cells while highly enriched with $CD8^+$ T cell population is collected at the interface

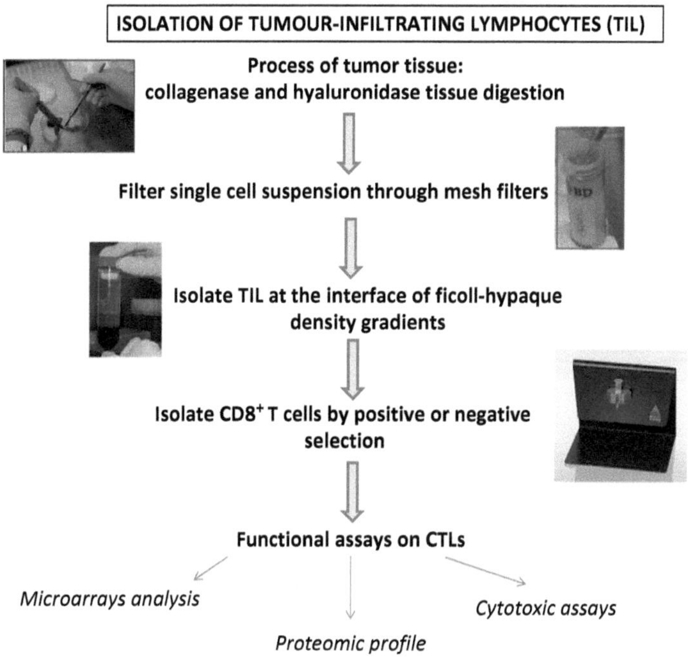

Fig. 1 Flow chart of TIL isolation experiment. The isolation of tumor-infiltrating lymphocytes requires a first tissue dissociation by enzymatic and mechanical method that will be optimized according to the specific needs of a given tumor tissue or cell type. The cell suspension obtained passes through a 70 μm cell strainer and will be pre-enriched using density gradient centrifugation. TIL will be collected at interphase layer and $CD8^+$ T cells will be then isolated by negative or positive selection techniques

between the plasma and the buoyant density medium. The isolated $CD8^+$ T cells are bead and antibody free and suitable straightway for any downstream application that requires viable, functional cells with minimal manipulation, such as microarray analyses or immune reconstitution in SCID mice. This procedure is fast and easy and does not require special equipment such as columns or magnets.

2 Materials

2.1 Isolation of Tumor-Infiltrating Lymphocytes (TIL)

1. Dissociation buffer: Collagenase type I-IV (GIBCO by Life Technologies; *see* **Note 1**), Hyaluronidase (GIBCO), DNase (Calbiochem) in RPMI + 10 % heat-inactivated fetal calf serum (FCS).
2. Ficoll-Hypaque.
3. Petri dishes.
4. Autoclaved sterile surgical scissors.
5. 50 ml Conical tubes.

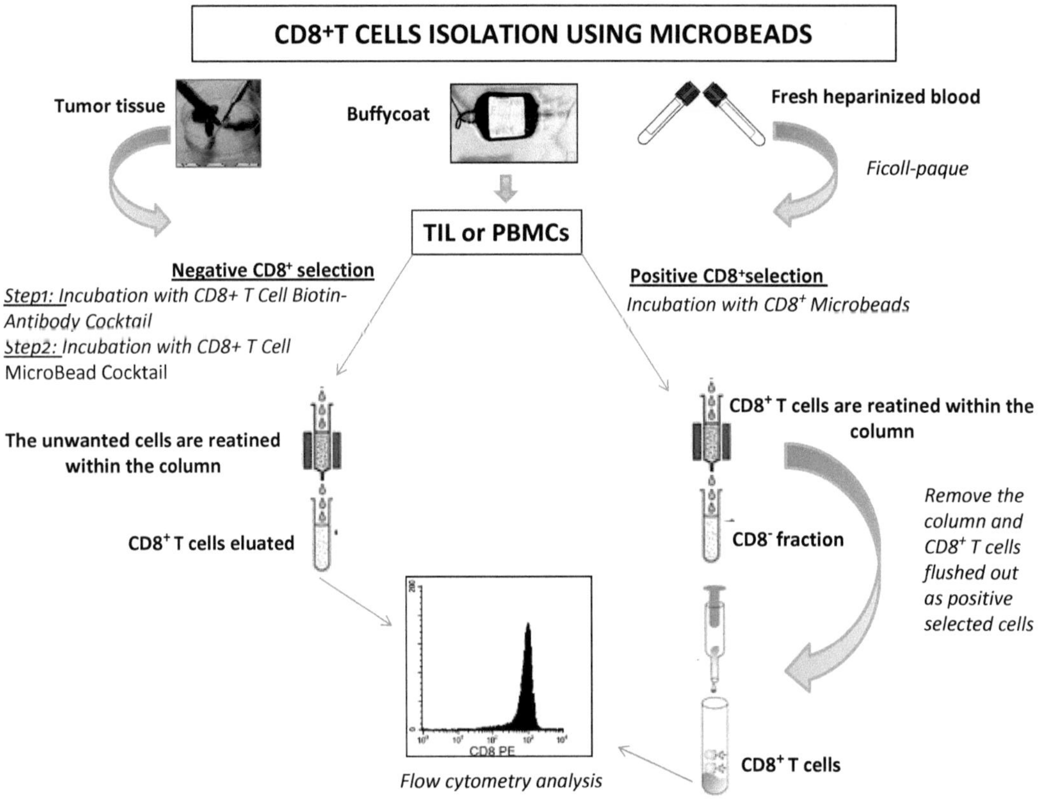

Fig. 2 Magnetic bead-based CD8+ T cell separation method. Human CD8+ T cells could be isolated from any sample including whole blood, buffy coat, mononuclear cells (PBMCs), and tissue digests. During CD8+ positive selection, TIL or PBMCs are incubated with CD8+ Microbeads that are coated with a primary monoclonal antibody specific for the CD8 membrane antigen largely expressed on human CTLs. The CD8+ T cells are retained into the column and the unwanted cells flow through. Then, the column is removed from the magnetic field and the retained CD8+ T cells are ejected by plugging the plunger on the column. The negative selection is performed by a first incubation with a biotin-antibody mix towards the non-CD8+ T cells followed by a second incubation with microbeads conjugated to anti-biotin and CD14 monoclonal antibodies. The magnetically labeled unwanted cells are retained within the column while the untouched CD8+ T cells run through the column

6. 10 and 3 ml syringes.
7. 70 μm Mesh filters.

2.2 Positive Selection of CTLs from PBMC Using Microbeads

1. Ficoll-Hypaque density gradient solution (GE Healthcare).
2. Phosphate-buffered saline (PBS).
3. Bovine serum albumin (BSA).
4. EDTA.
5. CD8+ Microbeads (Miltenyi Biotec).
6. MACS Columns and Separators (Miltenyi Biotec).
7. 50 and 15 ml conical tubes.

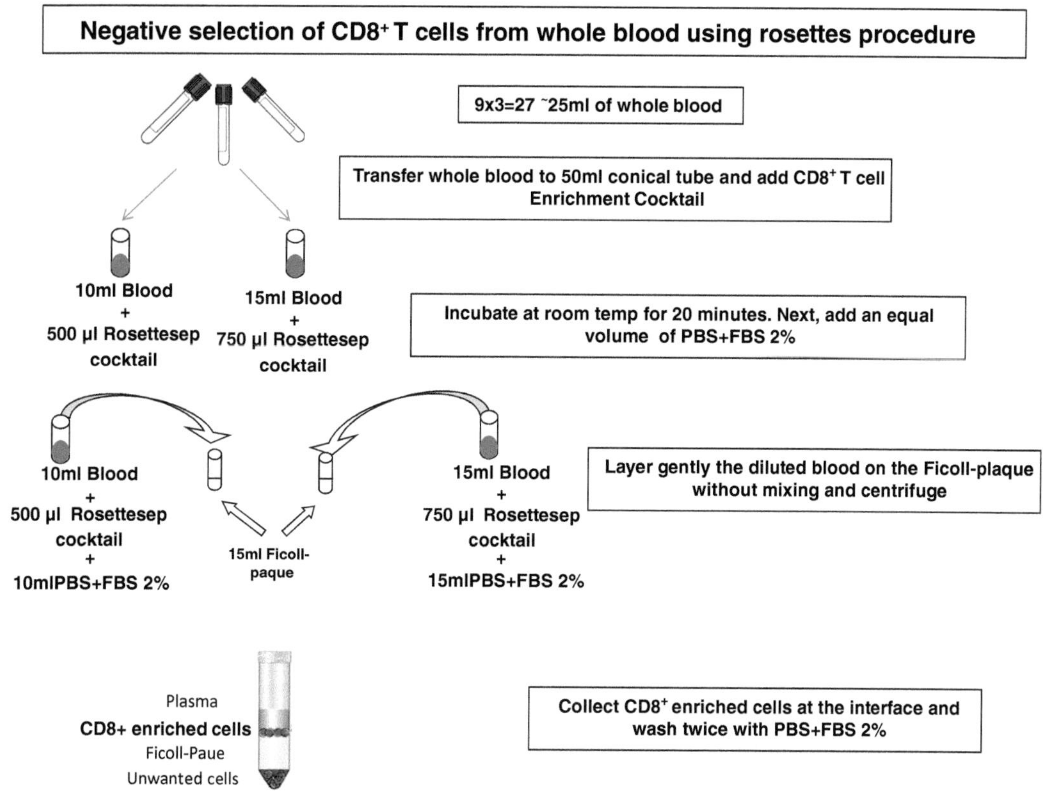

Fig. 3 Negative CD8+ T cell isolation from whole blood. The negative CD8+ T cell isolation procedure from whole blood requires a first incubation of whole blood with RosetteSep CD8+ T cell Enrichment Cocktail for 20 min at room temperature. The blood collected in the standard collection tubes will be then diluted 1:1 with PBS plus 2 % FBS and layered over Ficoll-Paque. Post-centrifugation, the enriched CD8+ T cells will be collected at the interface while unwanted cells will pellet along with red blood cells

2.3 Negative Selection of CTLs from Whole Blood Using the Rosette Procedure

1. Ficoll-Hypaque density gradient solution (GE Healthcare).
2. Phosphate-buffered saline (PBS).
3. Fetal calf serum (FCS, heat inactivated for 1 h at 56 °C).
4. Bovine serum albumin.
5. RosetteSep™ Human CD8+ T Cell Enrichment Cocktail (Qiagen).
6. 50 ml Conical tubes.

3 Methods

3.1 Isolation of Tumor-Infiltrating Lymphocytes (TIL)

Tumor tissue will be obtained from cancer patient's previous consent under an institutional review board (IRB)-approved protocol.

1. Place tumor explant intro petri dish with a small amount of RPMI (*see* **Note 2**).
2. Harvest media from tissue and centrifuge at 800 × *g* for 10 min (some lymphocytes are present). Later, it will be added to the digested tumor tissue.
3. Mince the tumor tissue using sterile dissection scissors to obtain pieces of about 10–20 mm in diameter.
4. Using the back end of 10 ml syringe, mash the tissue to further mechanically disaggregate the tumor tissue and add the pellet obtained from **step 2**.
5. Total volume/dish = 25 ml (up to 3 g tumor/dish); add dissociation buffer (*see* **Note 3**) to achieve proper final concentration (*see* **Note 4**).
6. Place dish on rotary shaker for 30–60 min at room temperature.
7. Mash the tumor tissue further with the back end of 3 ml syringe.
8. Harvest the digested tumor tissue into two 50 ml tubes and filter it through 75 μm mesh filters. Wash dish three times with 25 ml RPMI or PBS and let this washout also pass through the same mesh into 50 ml tubes.
9. Centrifuge the two tubes for 10 min at 600 × *g*.
10. Discard the supernatant, resuspend the pellet, and add 25 ml of RPMI for each tube.
11. Slowly add 12 ml Ficoll-Hypaque at the bottom of the tube so that the cell suspension overlays the density gradient solution.
12. Spin for 20 min at 800 × *g* without breaks, at room temperature.
13. Carefully isolate interface with a 10 ml pipette.
14. Wash TIL twice with PBS/1 % FBS or media up to 50 ml and centrifuge for 10 min at 250 × *g* (4 °C).
15. Resuspend TIL in 10 ml of cold buffer (PBS/EDTA/BSA) in order to proceed with $CD8^+$ T cell isolation (*see* step 6 of Subheading 3.2.1.) and count the cells with trypan blue to check viability (*see* **Note 5**).
16. Stain a small aliquot of the cells for flow cytometry analyses (*see* **Note 6**).

3.2 Positive Selection of CTLs from PBMCs Using Microbeads

All solutions and equipment coming into contact with cells and human blood must be sterile and aseptic procedures should be used accordingly.

3.2.1 Human Peripheral Blood Mononuclear Cell (PBMC) Isolation

1. Dilute fresh heparinized blood with PBS 1× pH 7.4 plus 1 mM EDTA in ratio 1:2 and mix well (*see* **Notes 7** and **8**).
2. Place 15 ml of Ficoll-Hypaque into three 50 ml conical centrifuge tubes and gently transfer 25 ml of the diluted blood onto the Ficoll so that they form two separate layers.

3. Centrifuge in room temperature at 800×*g* for 25 min with brake off.
4. Using a sterile pipet, collect the leukocytes at the interphase layer and transfer them to another 50 ml tubes up to 25 ml. Try to avoid aspirating the plasma and Ficoll-Hypaque.
5. Wash twice the cell suspensions with PBS up to 50 ml in each tube and centrifuge for 12 min at 500×*g* at 4 °C.
6. Remove the supernatant, resuspend the cells in 10 ml of cold buffer (PBS/EDTA/BSA), and count the cells as described in **Note 5**.
7. Centrifuge cell suspension at 300×*g* for 10 min (4 °C) while you are counting (*see* **Note 9**).

3.2.2 Magnetic Labeling with CD8 Microbeads from PBMC

1. Pipette off supernatant completely.
2. Resuspend cell pellet in 80 μl of buffer for 10^7 total cells. For higher cell number, scale up all reagent volumes (*see* **Note 10**).
3. Add 20 μl of CD8 Microbeads for 10^7 total cells (*see* **Note 11**).
4. Mix well and incubate for 15 min at 4–8 °C
5. Wash cells by adding 1–2 ml of buffer for 10^7 total cells, and centrifuge at 300×*g* for 10 min at 4 °C.
6. Pipette off supernatant completely and resuspend up to 10^8 cells in 500 μl of buffer (take 50 μl aliquot for flow cytometric analysis).
7. Proceed to magnetic separation with MS columns.
8. Place fresh MS column on the magnetic field of a MiniMacs Separator and label two 15 ml tubes as "$CD8^+$ T cells" and "$CD8^-$ T cells".
9. Rinse the column with cold buffer (for LC MS columns use 500 μl, for LS columns use 1 ml).
10. Apply cell suspension onto the column (*see* **Note 12**).
11. Collect the negative fraction of cells ($CD8^-$ T cells) which pass through the column and wash three times with 0.5 ml of buffer (*see* **Note 13**). As soon as the column drips the last drop, add more buffer. Do not let column stand without flow or allow it to run dry (drying of the column can affect purity and lead to significant loss of cell viability.)
12. Remove column from the separator and place it on "$CD8^+$ T cells" tube.
13. Pipette 1.2 ml of buffer onto column and immediately apply the plunger supplied with the column (*see* **Note 14**).
14. Proceed for flow cytometric analyses of samples before and after enrichment in order to determine the purity and recovery (*see* **Note 15**).

15. Cryopreserve cells or use immediately for functional studies, such as cytotoxicity assays or analysis of in vitro cytokine production following the procedures described in the previous chapter.

3.3 Negative Selection of $CD8^+$ T Cells from Whole Blood Using the Rosette Procedure

1. Transfer human whole blood from heparinized tubes to 50 ml conical tube (do not exceed 15 ml).
2. Add 50 μl/ml $CD8^+$ T cell Enrichment Cocktail, mix well by inversion, and incubate the tubes at room temperature for 20 min.
3. Dilute the sample with an equal volume of PBS + FBS 2 %.
4. Place 15 ml of Ficoll-Paque PLUS in a labeled 50 ml conical tube.
5. Layer gently the diluted blood on the Ficoll-Paque without mixing.
6. Centrifuge immediately for 20 min at 1,200 × *g* at room temp with brake off.
7. Carefully suck up the interphase containing the enriched cells and transfer it into new labeled tube. *From this point onwards the tubes must be kept cold!*
8. Fill the centrifuge tube to a volume of 50 ml with PBS + FBS 2%, and invert gently several times.
9. Centrifuge at 250 × *g* for 12 min at 4 °C (acc.9–dec9).
10. Gently decant the supernatant, release the pellet by flicking, and resuspend the cells with 50 ml of ice-cold PBS + FBS 2 %.
11. Centrifuge at 180 × *g* for 12 min at 4 °C.
12. Gently decant the supernatant, release the pellet by flicking, and resuspend the cells with 5 ml of ice-cold PBS + FBS 2 %.
13. Mix the cells by gently aspirating and releasing with the 5 ml pipette; the end part must be put away in a 1.5 ml Eppendorf ready for the cell count.
14. After that, resuspend the cells to a density of 2×10^6 cells/ml. Take out samples of 0.5×10^6 cells (=250 μl) and add to three tubes ("FACS tubes").

4 Notes

1. The grade of collagenase (I–IV) depends on the cell population we intend to isolate; to isolate myeloid cell it is suggested to use collagenase type IV, whereas lymphocyte yield is higher using type I.
2. For every processed tumor, it is important to have paraffin-embedded sections of the same tissue ready for immunohistochemical analysis.

3. Each tumor may require unique dissociation conditions.
4. Prepare in advance in 5 ml aliquots 10× stocks in RPMI stored at −20 °C of:

   0.1 % w/v Collagenase (to be used at final concentration of 0.01 %); add 2.5 ml of this solution.

   0.01 w/v Hyaluronidase (to be used at final concentration of 0.001 %); add 2.5 ml of this solution.

   0.1 % w/v DNase (to be used at final concentration of 0.01 % of 0.01 %); add 2.5 ml of this solution.
5. In an Eppendorf put 10 µl of trypan blue and 10 µl of cell suspension, mix well, and apply 10 µl of the colored suspension on the counting chamber ($Fd = 2$). Apply the following formula:

$$n \text{ cells} = M / 4 \times Fd \times V \times 10^4.$$

   M = Total no. of cells after counting the four squares.

   Fd = Dilution factor with trypan blue (2 in our case).

   10^4 = Dilution factor of the chamber.

   V = Resuspension volume in which the cells are found in (10 ml in our case).
6. Take out three aliquots of sample (corresponding to 0.3×10^6 cells), transfer them to three different 5 ml tubes ("FACS tubes"), and label with 1, 2, and 3. The staining of the cell is performed in a total of 100 µl where 70 µl is cell suspension and 30 µl is the fluorochrome-conjugated antibody cocktail. Add antibody cocktail or isotype control to the cell suspension as follows:

   Tube 1: Unstained cells (100 µl of cell suspension).

   Tube 2: Isotype control (90 µl is cell suspension and 10 µl of isotype control).

   Tube 3: Anti-human CD3FITC/CD4 FITC/CD8 Pc5 (70 µl is cell suspension and 30 µl of antibody cocktail).

   Incubate the cells on ice in the dark for 15 min, then add 1 ml of ice-cold FACS buffer (PBS, BSA 0.5 %, sodium azide 0.02 %) for each tube, and centrifuge the tubes at 500×g for 5 min at 4 °C (two times). Discard the supernatant, resuspend the cells in 0.5 ml of FACS buffer, and keep in the dark at 4 °C until it can be run on the flow cytometer.
7. If you start from buffy coat, blood should be diluted at a 1:3 ratio with PBS/1 mM EDTA.
8. Although freshly harvested PBMCs are recommended, we have successfully isolated CD8+ T cell from cryopreserved PBMCs (in 90 % FCS/10 % DMSO) in liquid nitrogen. The cells must

be frozen in 1–2 ml vials containing 10^7–10^8 cells/vial. When needed, thaw frozen PBMCs in a 37–40 °C water bath by shaking the cryovial. Take the vial from the water bath when there is still a very small piece of ice in the suspension. Wipe outside of vial with alcohol (for asepsis) and place in hood. The PBMCs should be transferred in a 15 ml conical tube containing 10 ml of RPMI medium supplemented with 10 % fetal bovine serum (FBS heat inactivated at 56 °C for 30 min) and 100 U/ml of benzonase which dramatically reduces cell clumping. The transfer of the cells from the cryovial to the canonical tube should be done in a dropwise manner over a period of 2 min, shaking the tube frequently. Then centrifuge cell suspension at 200×*g* for 10 min at 4 °C and carefully remove supernatant. Follow directly Subheading 3.2.2, **step 2**.

9. Always keep the cells and buffer on ice after this point to avoid that cells form "clumps" and nonspecific cell labeling. Do not pipette quickly, work gently with the cells in particular lymphocytes, and assume that they are small living creatures.
10. 80 μl Should be the final volume where microbeads will be added. So, when discarding the supernatant, it is recommended to measure the volume of cell resuspension that remains in the tube and add the buffer up to 80 μl.
11. The amount of microbeads required may vary depending upon the frequency/number of cells of the desired population; therefore, this step may require optimization. We can use up to half the amount of recommended beads: if we use a smaller amount of beads the recovery is less but we will obtain a $CD8^+$ T cell population characterized by a higher purity.
12. Check that there is no cell clumps that may occlude the column. If they are evident, remove them with a tip of 200 μl Pasteur pipette or pass cells through 30 μm nylon mesh.
13. If the column becomes clogged, you can grope to unlock it, pipetting up and down with a 200 μl Pasteur in order to remove the cell clumps or harvest the cell suspension in the column and transfer it in a new column after rinse with cold buffer.
14. It is possible to isolate untouched $CD8^+$ T cells using the "$CD8^+$ T Cell Isolation Kit"(Miltenyi Biotec) as illustrated in the Fig. 2. The kit provides a first incubation for 10 min with biotin-conjugated monoclonal antibodies against CD4, CD15, CD16, CD19, CD34, CD36, CD56, CD123, TCR γ/δ, and glycophorin A, followed by incubation with microbeads conjugated to antibodies against CD14 and biotin. The unwanted cells are depleted by retaining within column, while the unlabeled $CD8^+$ T cells elute through the column.

15. Suboptimal purity may result from inadequate coating of the cells with microbeads or inadequate removal of CD8+ T cells. If the recovery or the purity is not satisfactory, repeat the separation.

Acknowledgments

This work was supported by Ministero dell'Istruzione, dell'Università e della Ricerca (MIUR) PROGRAMMA OPERATIVO NAZIONALE (PON) RICERCA E COMPETITIVITÀ 2007–2013 PONa3_00395 "BIOSCIENCES AND HEALTH" (B&H). The authors declare no conflicts of interest.

References

1. Kershaw MH, Trapani JA, Smyth MJ (1995) Cytotoxic lymphocytes: redirecting the cell-mediated immune response for the therapy of cancer. Ther Immunol 2:173–181
2. Klebanoff CA, Gattinoni L, Torabi-Parizi P et al (2005) Central memory self/tumor-reactive CD8+ T cells confer superior antitumor immunity compared with effector memory T cells. Proc Natl Acad Sci U S A 5:9571–9576
3. Anikeeva N, Sykulev Y (2011) Mechanisms controlling granule-mediated cytolytic activity of cytotoxic T lymphocytes. Immunol Res. doi:10.1007/s12026-011-8252-8
4. Shablak A, Hawkins RE, Rothwell DG, Elkord E (2009) T cell-based immunotherapy of metastatic renal cell carcinoma: modest success and future perspective. Clin Cancer Res. doi:10.1158/1078-0432
5. Cavalcanti E, Gigante M, Mancini V et al (2010) JAK3/STAT5/6 pathway alterations are associated with immune deviation in CD8 T cells in renal cell carcinoma patients. J Biomed Biotechnol. doi:10.1155/2010/935764
6. Gigante M, Mandic M, Wesa AK et al (2008) Interferon-alpha (IFN-alpha)-conditioned DC preferentially stimulate type-1 and limit Treg-type in vitro T-cell responses from RCC patients. J Immunother. doi:10.1097/CJI.0b013e318167b023
7. Groh V, Rhinehart R, Randolph-Habecker J et al (2001) Costimulation of CD8alphabeta T cells by NKG2D via engagement by MIC induced on virus-infected cells. Nat Immunol 2:255–260

Chapter 2

In Vitro\Ex Vivo Generation of Cytotoxic T Lymphocytes

Margherita Gigante and Elena Ranieri

Abstract

The in vitro generation of human cytotoxic T lymphocytes (CTL) is a reliably approach useful not only to assess intrinsic CD8+ T cell responses in individuals but also to screen immunogenic antigens that could be considered as candidates for adoptive immunotherapeutic approaches. In vitro methods to expand CTL require culturing naïve T cells with antigen-presenting cells (APC) as stimulator cells that express specific antigens. Here, we describe the protocol for generating CTL against target antigens presented by monocyte-derived dendritic cells (DCs).

Key words CD8+ T cell, Cytotoxicity, Dendritic cells, Peptides, Cancer

1 Introduction

CTL are lymphocytes that kill target cells expressing target antigen in class I histocompatibility (MHC) restricted manner [1]. They are generally CD8+ T cells and play an effector role in the host response to virus-infected cells, organ transplants, and cancer cells. Effector CTLs generated from naive T cells which following stimulation by antigen presenting cells (APCs), differentiate into effector ("killer") cells. The in vitro expansion of CTLs could be performed using anti-CD3 antibody that allows a polyclonal stimulation of T cell populations mediated by binding to T cell receptor complex [2]. However, this approach measures the cytotoxic activity of effector T cells but it is not antigen specific. Here, we describe a protocol to expand antigen-specific CTL in vitro by stimulation with monocyte-derived dendritic cells (DCs) loaded with the target antigen. This procedure is useful both to measure cytolytic capacity of effector T cells in a physiological fashion and to evaluate the immunogenic potential of target antigens that could be envisioned for immunotherapeutic approach [3–5].

To date, a number of protocols for generating monocyte-derived DC have been described, using various types of media, serum, and cytokine combination [5]. Here, we reported the

Elena Ranieri (ed.), *Cytotoxic T-Cells: Methods and Protocols*, Methods in Molecular Biology, vol. 1186,
DOI 10.1007/978-1-4939-1158-5_2, © Springer Science+Business Media New York 2014

traditional protocol which requires the culture of monocytes with rGM-CSF and rIL-4 for 6 days, followed by application of cytokine maturation cocktail (i.e., IL-1β, TNF-α, IL-6, and PGE_2) for 2 additional days [6]. The so generated DCs exhibited a fully mature surface phenotype expressing the maturation markers (CD80, CD83, CD86, and CCR7). To be effective as APCs, DCs must be loaded with different antigenic formats such as peptide antigens, tumor lysates, apoptotic tumor cells, antigenic DNA, and mRNA [7]. In cancer setting, the loading of DCs with tumor lysate allows the processing of multiple immunogenic CTL epitopes, and the antigen-presenting cells present peptides fitting their own major histocompatibility complex (MHC) molecules [8, 9]. Here, we describe the procedure for pulsing DCs with HLA-A2 restricted peptides that will be used for multiple cycles of T cells stimulation taking 2–3 weeks, as illustrated in Fig. 1. The antigen-specific T cells

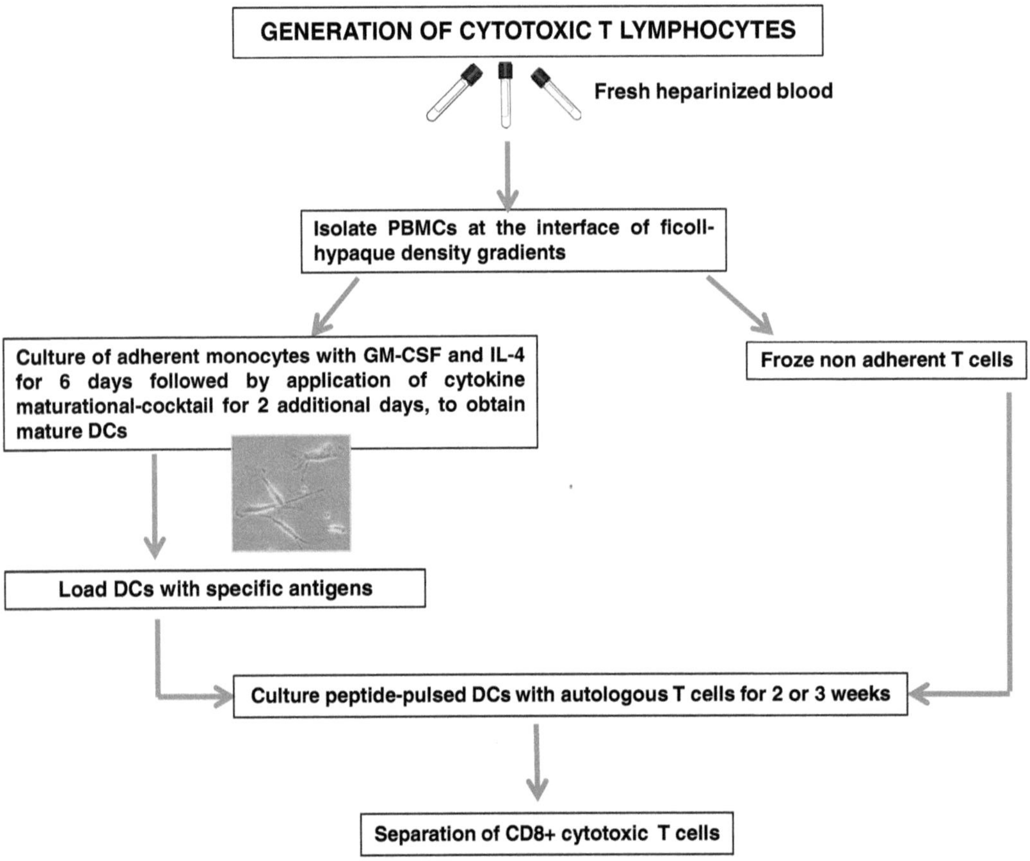

Fig. 1 Flow chart of CTLs generation experiment. The generation of $CD8^+$ CTLs requires first the isolation of PBMCs from peripheral blood. The adherent fraction of cells (monocytes) will be cultured for 8 days in order to generate mature DCs, while the non-adherent T cells will be frozen. After pulsing of DC with peptides, T cells will be thawed out and used for multiple rounds of stimulation with DCs. After 14 or 21 days of culture, $CD8^+$ T cells by immunomagnetic techniques will be separated and tested for cytotoxic functional status

generated by this protocol will be mainly $CD8^+$ cytotoxic T cells and will be used for different downstream applications such as protein and gene expression profile analysis.

2 Materials

1. Human blood or buffy coats.
2. Ficoll-Hypaque density gradient solution (GE Healthcare).
3. Phosphate Buffered Saline (PBS).
4. AIM V Medium (Life Technologies).
5. T cell medium (Iscove's Medium (IMDM), containing 10 % heat-inactivated normal human serum, 1 % Glutamine, 1 % Pen Strep, and nonessential amino acids).
6. Recombinant human (rh) GM-CSF (Sargramostim, Amgen, CA); IL4 (Schering-Plough); IL6 (Pepro-Tech), IL-1β (Strathman Biotech); PGE-2 (Sigma-Aldrich); TNF-α (Strathman Biotech).
7. HLA-A2 restricted peptides.
8. 50 ml centrifuge tubes.
9. T75 flask and 6-well plates.
10. Additional reagents and equipment for counting the cells, flow cytometry analysis, and cell isolation.

3 Methods

3.1 Isolation of Peripheral Blood Mononuclear Cell (PBMC)

All solutions and equipment coming into contact with cells and human blood must be sterile and aseptic procedures should be used accordingly.

1. Dilute fresh heparinized blood with PBS 1× pH 7.4 plus 1 mM EDTA in ratio 1:2 and mix well (*see* **Note 1**).
2. Place 12 ml of Ficoll-Hypaque into three 50 ml conical centrifuge tubes and gently transfer 30 ml of the diluted blood onto the Ficoll so that they form two separate layers.
3. Centrifuge in room temperature at 460 × *g* for 25 min without breaks.
4. Using a sterile pipet, collect the leukocytes at the interphase layer and transfer them to another 50 ml tubes up to 25 ml. Try to avoid to aspirate the plasma and Ficoll-Hypaque.
5. Wash the cell suspensions with PBS up to 50 ml in each tube and centrifuge 12 min at 250 × *g* at 4 °C (*see* **Note 2**).
6. Discard the supernatants, resuspend the cells with PBS, and repeat the wash centrifuging 10 min at 175 × *g*, at 4 °C (*see* **Note 3**).

7. Remove the supernatant, resuspend the cells in 10 ml of cold PBS, and count the cells with trypan blue (*see* **Note 4**). Centrifuge cell suspension at 450 × *g* for 5 min (4 °C) while you are counting.

3.2 Separation of Monocyte from Non-adherent T Cell

At this stage, the PBMCs collected comprehend two cell populations: lymphocytes and monocytes. Monocytes CD14⁺ could be separated from lymphocytes given their ability to adhere to plastic surfaces of the flask and they will be differentiated in DC. Non-adherent T cells will be frozen in order to be used for the next step that is in vitro stimulation.

1. Resuspend the cells in cell culture medium (AIMV) to a cell concentration of 10×10^6 cells/ml (*see* **Note 5**).
2. Transfer 90–100 × 10^6 in a final volume of 10 ml of AIMV to a T75 flask cells (*see* **Note 6**).
3. Incubate the cells at 37 °C for 1–2 h, avoid moving the flask during incubation to allow the adhesion of monocytes.
4. After incubation, take out the flasks and collect the supernatant containing T cells (*see* **Note 7**).
5. Wash the flask twice adding 10 ml of PBS at room temperature (*without EDTA*) (*see* **Note 8**).
6. Centrifuge at 450 × *g* for 5 min at 4 °C.
7. Discard the supernatant completely and freeze the cells in FBS/DMSO (*see* **Note 9**).

3.3 Generation of DCs from Monocytes

The following protocol represents the standard procedure for generating mature monocyte-derived DCs (mDCs). It is based on a widely used, two-step culture protocol. The first step involves the culture of monocytes with GM-CSF and IL4 for 5 days. The so generated immature DCs are induced to mature with additional cytokines cocktail including IL-6, IL-1β, TNF-α, and PGE-2 in order to acquire the characteristic typical of activated/mature DC. To be effective as APCs, DC must be loaded with an antigenic format.

1. Add 10 ml of immature DC medium (AIM-V medium supplemented with recombinant human GM-CSF (1,000 U/ml) and IL-4 (1,000 U/ml)) to adherent monocyte flask (*see* **Note 10**).
2. Incubate at 37 °C and 5 % CO_2 for 6 days.
3. After 3 days of incubation, add to the culture 3 ml/T75 flask of fresh DC medium.
4. At day 6, remove all the medium from the flask and perform two wash steps adding 10 ml of PBS at room temperature.
5. Add 10 ml of DC medium containing IL-1β (25 ng/ml), TNF-α (50 ng/ml), IL-6 (1,000 U/ml), and PGE2 (10^{-6} mol/l) and incubate for 48 h at 37 °C and 5 % CO_2 (*see* **Note 11**).

6. After 48 h, detach mDCs from the flask with cold PBS. Check that the mDCs have come off from the plastic surface. If not, try to hit the flask gently.
7. Transfer the cell suspension to a 50 ml tube and count the cells with trypan blue. Take out half a million of cells to perform cytometric analysis of DC generated (*see* **Note 12**).
8. Centrifuge at 450 × *g* for 5 min while you are counting and prepare three aliquots of DCs.
9. Freeze two aliquots for second and third stimulation (*see* **Note 13**).
10. Use the first aliquot for peptide loading.

3.4 Pulsing of mDCs with Peptides

Peptides should be 8–10 amino acids long and bind the HLA-A2 peptide domain in order to evaluate intrinsic CTL responses in HLA-A2$^+$ individuals. Thus, before starting, you need to identify HLA-A2$^+$ donors by flow cytometry analysis of PBMC using specific monoclonal antibody (mAb).

1. Wash twice mDCs in AIM-V, resuspend the cells in AIM-V at concentration of $0.5–1 \times 10^6$/1.5 ml/well in 6-well culture plate
2. Add the desired HLA-A2–restricted peptide at the final concentration of 10 μg/ml (*see* **Note 14**).
3. Add β2 microglobulin at the final concentration of 3 μg/ml (stock 1 mg/ml).
4. Incubate at 37 °C and 5 % CO_2 for an optimal period of time (generally 2–4 h), with occasional agitation.
5. Wash the cells twice with AIMV and resuspend in 2 ml of T cell medium.

3.5 In Vitro Generation of Antigen-Specific CTL

In vitro stimulation of mDCs can be performed using fresh or cryopreserved peripheral blood T lymphocytes.

1. Resuspend T cells in T cell medium and adjust to $10–20 \times 10^6$ cells/ml. The ratio of responder T cells to DCs ranges from 20:1 to 30:1 (*see* **Note 15**).
2. Add 3 ml of T cell suspension for well in the 6-well culture plate up to a max volume of 5 ml/well in a 6-well plate. Fill the empty wells with 5 ml of PBS to equilibrate the system.
3. Incubate for 1 week at 37 °C and 5 % CO_2 (*see* **Note 16**).
4. At day 7, thaw the second aliquot of mDCs and repeat the stimulation of T cells as described for first stimulation.
5. Add rhIL-7 [5 ng/ml] and rhIL-2 [20 U/ml].
6. At day 14, thaw the third aliquot of mDCs and repeat the stimulation of T cells in the same way of first and second stimulation.
7. Add IL-7 [5 ng/ml] e IL-2 [20 U/ml].

8. On day 21, isolate $CD8^+$ T cells from the bulk T cell cultures by negative selection using MACSTM magnetic beads (Miltenyi Biotec, Auburn, CA) on MiniMACS columns, according to the manufacturer's protocol described in the previous chapter and the cells are ready to be assessed for CTL activity or analysis of gene and protein expression.

4 Notes

1. Blood should be diluted at a 1:3 ratio with PBS/1 mM EDTA if you start from buffy coat.
2. Resuspend the cell pellet in a small volume of liquid first and then add more liquid. Otherwise the cells will form "clumps."
3. If the supernatant results still torbid, repeat this passage. You should be able to clearly watch the notches of the 50 ml tube from the opposite side.
4. In an Eppendorf put 10 μl of Trypan blue and 10 μl of cell suspension, mix well, and apply 10 μl of the colored suspension on the Counting Chamber ($Fd=2$). Apply the following formula:

$$n^{\circ}\text{ cells} = M\ /\ 4 \times Fd \times V \times 10^4.$$

   M= Total n° of cells after counting the four squares.

   Fd= Dilution Factor with Trypan blue (2 in our case).

   10^4= Dilution factor of the chamber.

   V= Resuspension volume in which the cells are found in (10 ml in our case).

5. Monocytes $CD14^+$ can also be obtained by negative selection using MACS system. Even if this system is certainly faster, however, purifying such cells may not be the most economical use of time.
6. In order to obtain a high yield and purity of DCs, it is important to plate the cells in the flask at optimal concentration. Please consider the following ratio:

   -90–100 × 10^6 PBMCs in 10 ml of AIMV in T75 flask.

   -25 × 30 × 10^6 PBMCs in 4 ml of AIMV in T25 flask.

   -180–200 × 10^6 PBMCs in 18 ml of AIMV in T150 flask.

   If more than the recommended number of cells are plated, there is the risk that not all monocytes can adhere to the flask. It will lead to have a low yield of DC and the non-adherent T cells population will also contain monocyte.

7. Before harvesting the supernatant, look at the cells in microscope. The adherent monocytes look like "flattened amoebas." If you cannot see this yet, incubate the cells for longer period of time and check them every half hour.
8. At this stage, it is recommended to take out a small aliquot of sample for flow cytometry analyses, for studying the functional and phenotypic profile of freshly isolated T cells.
9. Resuspend the cells at a maximum of 1×10^7 cell/ml in cryo fluid (90 % FBS/10 % DMSO). Label different cryo vials identifying the name of sample, the data, and the cell number. Transfer aliquots into cryo vials and place in freezing container in −80 °C freezer within 10 min of adding cryo fluid.
10. It is possible to use GM-CSF at the concentration of 500 U/ml.
11. Even if the most "traditional" protocols for monocyte-derived DCs generation involve 8 days of culture, we found that a faster protocol based on the culture of adherent monocytes with GM-CSF (1,000 U/ml) and natural IFN-α (Intron A-IFN-α2b, 8,000 U/ml) for only 3 days induces superior CTL activities. Such DCs express an "intermediate mature" phenotype and morphologically appear distinct from the more classical DC. The advantage of using "fast DC" would be relevant savings in time and cost (especially related to cytokine cost) for DC production.
12. Stain mDCs with fluorochrome-conjugated monoclonal antibodies (mAb) against human cell identification marker (CD14, CD123, CD11c); co-stimulatory marker (CD40, CD80, CD86); maturation and antigen-presenting molecules (CD1a, CD83, DC-LAMP, HLA-DR, HLA-ABC); and cytokine receptors (CCR7 and CCR5). Resuspend cells (1×10^5) in 90 μl of FACS buffer (PBS, 0.5 % BSA, and 0.02 % sodium azide) and incubate with appropriate fluorochrome-conjugated monoclonal antibodies (mAbs), for 15 min at 4 °C. After incubation, wash the cells twice with FACS buffer and resuspend in 0.5 ml PBS.
13. As this approach requires long-term cell culture and multiple manipulations, contamination represents a common problem with these culture. Therefore, it is highly recommended to cryopreserve different aliquots of each cell type (i.e., DC or freshly isolated non-adherent T cells).
14. Peptides are solubilized in DMSO at a concentration of 10 mg/ml and stored at −20 °C for a long period. Temporary peptide storage (<1 month) is recommended at 4 °C.
15. Generally, the ratio of T cells to mDCs ranges from 20:1 to 30:1. Titration of the ratio of DCs to T cells should ideally be

done for each strain. The optimal ratio may differ depending on the type of stimulation, e.g., antigen versus tumor lysate or anti-CD3 plus anti-CD28 stimulation.

16. During this incubation, check every day the eventual color change of the medium. In this case, start with a simple addition of fresh medium, for a maximum of 8 ml per well or slowly aspirate the medium from the side surface of well (without disturbing the cells on the bottom) and put it in the waste. If the cells have reached a high density, gently mix the cells in the well and split equally into two wells. In all cases, add fresh medium in the wells.

Acknowledgments

This work was supported by Progetto Strategico Regione Puglia grant (E.R., 2008), Ministero dell'Istruzione, dell'Università e della Ricerca (MiUR) FIRB, CAROMICS grant (E.R., 2011), and a Postdoctoral Fellowship by MiUR, PROGRAMMA OPERATIVO NAZIONALE (PON) RICERCA E COMPETITIVITÀ 2007–2013 PONa3_00395 "BIOSCIENCES AND HEALTH" (B&H) (M.G., 2013). The authors declare no conflicts of interest.

References

1. Williams MA, Bevan MJ (2007) Effector and memory CTL differentiation. Annu Rev Immunol 25:171–192
2. Biddison WE, Lichtenfels R, Adibzadeh M, Martin R (2001) Measurement of polyclonal and antigen-specific cytotoxic T cell function. Curr Protoc Immunol. Chapter 7: Unit 7.17. doi: 10.1002/0471142735.im0717s17
3. Gigante M, Mandic M, Wesa AK et al (2008) Interferon-alpha (IFN-alpha)-conditioned DC preferentially stimulate type-1 and limit Treg-type in vitro T-cell responses from RCC patients. J Immunother 31:254–262. doi:10.1097/CJI.0b013e318167b023
4. Ho WY, Nguyen HN, Wolfl M, Kuball J, Greenberg PD (2006) In vitro methods for generating CD8+ T-cell clones for immunotherapy from the naïve repertoire. J Immunol Methods 310:40–52
5. Santin AD, Hermonat PL, Ravaggi A et al (2000) In vitro induction of tumor-specific human lymphocyte antigen class I-restricted CD8 cytotoxic T lymphocytes by ovarian tumor antigen-pulsed autologous dendritic cells from patients with advanced ovarian cancer. Am J Obstet Gynecol 183:601–609
6. Buchler T, Hajek R, Bourkova L et al (2003) Generation of antigen-loaded dendritic cells in a serum-free medium using different cytokine combinations. Vaccine 21:877–882
7. de Vries IJ, Lesterhuis WJ, Scharenborg NM et al (2003) Maturation of dendritic cells is a prerequisite for inducing immune responses in advanced melanoma patients. Clin Cancer Res 9:5091–5100
8. Turtle CJ, Hart DN (2004) Dendritic cells in tumor immunology and immunotherapy. Curr Drug Targets 5:17–39
9. Gitlitz BJ, Belldegrun AS, Zisman A et al (2003) A pilot trial of tumor lysate-loaded dendritic cells for the treatment of metastatic renal cell carcinoma. J Immunother 26:412–419

Chapter 3

Phenotypic and Functional Characterization of Cytotoxic T Lymphocytes by Flow Cytometry

Iulia Popescu, Matthew Pipeling, Jason Akulian, and John McDyer

Abstract

Cytotoxic T lymphocytes (*CTLs*) are important constituents of the adaptive immune system. Development of CTLs are particularly important for bacterial and viral infections, in addition to tumor surveillance. Measuring T cell immune function is important in evaluating host defense, allergy, autoimmunity, transplant rejection, and tumor immunity. In these recent years it has become possible to measure multiple effector functions in a single cell such as cytokine, transcription factors, and cytolytic function. In addition these parameters can be evaluated in conjunction with cellular proliferation. In this chapter we detail these cellular based assays and the methods used to characterize and quantify both phenotype and function of CTL.

Key words $CD8^+$ T cells, CTL, Flow cytometry, Cellular assay

1 Cytotoxic T Cell (CTL)

Cytotoxic T lymphocytes (CTLs) are important constituents of the adaptive immune system. CTLs are frequently αβ T lymphocytes that often express the $CD8^+$ co-receptor and an antigen-specific T cell receptor (TCR), though subsets of $CD4^+$ T cells can also exhibit CTL features. $CD8^+$ CTLs recognize *endogenous* antigen (Ag) presented in the context of MHC class I molecules on professional antigen-presenting cells (APC), whereas $CD4^+$ CTLs can recognize *exogenous* Ag presented to the TCR in the context of MHC class II molecules. In the case of endogenous Ag, peptide fragments are transported to the cell surface and 8–13-mer peptides derived from viruses or tumor are expressed in the context of MHC class I molecules and recognized by antigen-specific CTL. Once CTLs are activated these cells can kill Ag-bearing cells. Developments of CTLs are particularly important for bacterial and viral infections, in addition to tumor surveillance. In the case of active infection, $CD8^+$ cells traffic to and target infected cells via the systemic circulation and at end-organ sites of infection.

Elena Ranieri (ed.), *Cytotoxic T-Cells: Methods and Protocols*, Methods in Molecular Biology, vol. 1186,
DOI 10.1007/978-1-4939-1158-5_3, © Springer Science+Business Media New York 2014

The immune response that is triggered by CTL in response to acute or chronic infection [1] is divided into four phases: (a) *the effector phase*, where Ag-specific CTLs are primed from a population of naïve precursor CTL; these cells proliferate, acquire effector function(s), migrate to sites of infection, and clear pathogen via the elaboration of effector cytokines (e.g., IFN-γ, TNF-α) or killing target cells via cytotoxic molecules (e.g., granzyme B (GrzB), perforin); (b) the *contraction phase*, in which the effector CTL population undergoes massive apoptotic contraction, yet marked by the persistence of an approximate 5–10 % population of memory cells; (c) the *memory maintenance phase*: where memory CTLs are maintained (frequently for years in humans); and, finally, (d) the *recall response phase,* where following re-challenge with Ag, memory CTLs have the capacity for rapid re-expansion and effector function, providing durable protection for the host [1, 2].

Generation of effector CTL requires three signals: Signal 1, via cognate TCR/MHC interactions, that provides specificity to the response; Signal 2, via a variety of co-stimulatory molecules expressed by activated DCs and T cells, that provides mechanisms for regulating a given response; and Signal 3, which is derived from local cytokines produced, such as interleukin 12 (IL-12) or the type 1 interferons (IFN-α, IFN-β) as inflammatory signals generated in response to toll-like receptor (TLR) activation, and that are necessary for the induction of optimal CTL responses [3, 4].

$CD4^+$ T cells, or "helper" T cells (Th), play an important role in generation of the effector CTL. Signals from $CD4^+$ T cells have been shown in vitro and in vivo to prime CTL via professional APC, such as dendritic cells (DCs). $CD4^+$ T cells interact with DCs via co-stimulatory molecules, such as CD154 (CD40L)/CD40 interactions, enabling activated DC to prime CTL responses. In addition, this pathway can lead to the induction of important regulatory cytokines, such as IL-12. In addition, $CD4^+$ T cells are important in maintaining long-lived $CD8^+$ memory T cell function [2–4].

Upon activation of CTL releases cytotoxic granules and cytokines. Cytotoxic granules released by CTL activate the apoptotic pathways via the Fas/FasL interaction and destroy the infected cell. Cytotoxicity of NK cells and CTLs is often GrzB/perforin dependent. In the plasma membrane of targeted infected or tumor cells are perforin pores that permit the entry of serine-protease granzymes, such as GrzB that will cleave the caspase precursors and trigger apoptosis. This mechanism plays an important role in autoimmunity, immune responses to bacterial and viral infections, and tumor surveillance. Cytolysis of activated CTL can also be mediated via tumor necrosis factor family (TNFR) Fas receptor mechanisms (TNFRSF6, Apo-1, CD95) and Fas ligand (FasL) expressed on the target cell. The Fas-associated death domain allows activation of the pro-caspases 8 and 10, which will further activate the effector caspases 3, 6, and 7, that will lead to the cleavage of death substrates such as lamin A, lamin B1, lamin B2, PARP (poly-ADP ribose polymerase), and DNAPK (DNA-activated protein kinase) [5]. A deficiency of functional Fas–FasL interactions results in lymphoproliferation and autoimmunity. When $CD8^+$ T cells and NK cells recognize target cells, the contents of the lytic granules (perforin, granzymes, and granulysin) are secreted by degranulation. As a result of degradation by these lytic molecules, CD107 is exposed on the cell surface [6]. CD107a is a mobilization assay that allows for the detection of CTL with a novel MHC-Ib restriction that specifically recognize infected cells. This assay is a useful tool for detection of $CD8^+$ T cells that recognize a wide variety of intracellular pathogens. CD107a is also known as lysosome-associated membrane protein 1 (LAMP-1), a glycoprotein present in the cellular immune membrane of cytotoxic granules [6–10].

Measuring T cell immune functions is important for host defense, allergy, autoimmunity, transplant rejection, and tumor immunity. In this chapter we detail these cellular based assays and the methods used to characterize and quantify both phenotype and function of CTL [9–11].

2 Flow Cytometry

Flow cytometry assay is a laser-based, biophysical technology employed in cell counting, sorting, biomarker detection, and protein engineering, by suspending cells in a stream of fluid and passing them by an electronic detection apparatus. This allows simultaneous multi parametric analysis of the physical and/or chemical properties of a cell. This is an assay routinely used in the diagnosis of health disorders, especially blood cancers, but has many other applications in basic research, clinical practice, and clinical trials. A common variation is to physically sort particles based on their properties, so as to purify populations of interest. In history the first flow cytometry device used was the Coulter principle, and was disclosed in the US Patent issued in 1953, to Wallace H. Coulter. The first fluorescence-based flow cytometry device (ICP 11) was developed in 1968 by Wolfgang Göhde from the University of Münster and first commercialized in 1968–1969 by German developer and manufacturer Partec through Phywe AG in Göttingen. After that, instruments were developed, such as Cytofluorograph (1971) from Bio/Physics Systems Inc. (later: Ortho Diagnostics), the PAS 8000 (1973) from Partec, the first FACS instrument from Becton Dickinson (1974), the ICP 22 (1975) from Partec/Phywe, and the Epic from Coulter (1977–1978). The original name of the flow cytometry technology was "pulse cytophotometry" (from German: "Impulszytophotometrie") and in 1988, at the Conference of the American Engineering Foundation in Pensacola, Florida, the name was changed to "flow cytometry."

A flow cytometer has five main components: (1) a flow cell—liquid stream (sheath fluid), which carries and aligns the cells so that they pass single file through the light beam for sensing; (2) a measuring system—commonly used are measurement of impedance (or conductivity) and optical systems; (3) lamps (mercury, xenon); high power water-cooled lasers (argon, krypton, dye laser); low-power air-cooled lasers (argon (488 nm), red-HeNe (633 nm), green-HeNe, HeCd (UV)); diode lasers (blue, green, red, violet) resulting in light signals; (4) a detector and analogue-to-digital conversion (ADC) system—which generates FSC and SSC as well as fluorescence signals from light into electrical signals that can be processed by a computer; and (5) an amplification system—linear or logarithmic and a computer for analysis of the signals.

The principle of the flow cytometry is simple—a beam of light, LASER, of a single wavelength is directed onto a hydrodynamically focused stream of fluid. There are detectors aimed where the stream passes through the light beam: one in line with the light beam (forward scatter or FSC) and several perpendicular to it (side scatter or SSC) and one or more fluorescent detectors. The measurements that are made are FSC-proportional to cell size, SSC-proportional to cell granularity and fluorescence-as binding of fluorescent-labeled antibodies, Ca^{2+}-sensitive dyes within cells, fluorescent proteins expressed by cells, binding of DNA dyes. Each particle from 0.2 to 150 μm passing through the beam light, and fluorescent chemicals found in the particle or attached to the particle may be excited into emitting light at a longer wavelength than the light source. This combination of SSC and FSC light are properties picked up by the detectors, and, by analyzing fluctuations in brightness at each detector (one for each fluorescent emission peak), it is then possible to derive various types of information about the physical and chemical structure of each individual particle.

Flow cytometry assays study cells as they move in fluid suspension, allowing multiple measurements to be made per cell and FACS™ is the fluorescence-activated cell sorting. For this assay it is critical to run appropriate controls—such as instrument setup controls (e.g., CompBeads), CompBeads as single-color controls; gating controls and biological controls (e.g., unstimulated samples, healthy donors) and these will allow you to obtain consistent setup, compensation and to make appropriate biological comparisons and conclusions. Because the emission of different fluorescent dyes have spectral overlap, signals at the detectors have to be compensated electronically as well as computationally [8]. CompBeads provide a convenient way to create single-color compensation

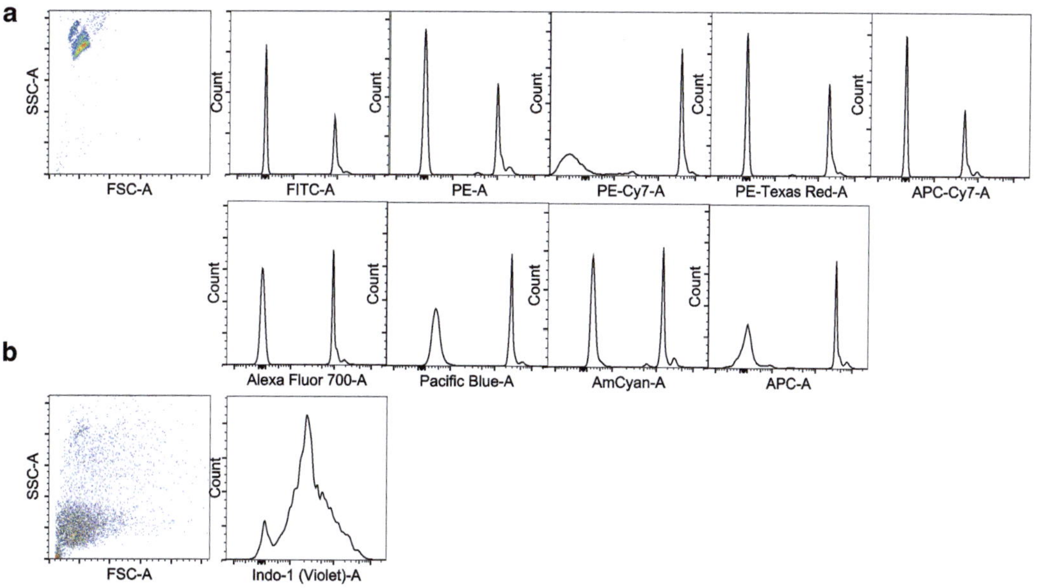

Fig. 1 CompBeads—a convenient way to create single-color automatic compensation control for ten-color multi-parametric measurement. (**a**) Representative FSC/SSC dot plot of the CompBeads and histograms of the CompBeads, each single color used in a multi-parametric measurement. (**b**) Representative FSC/SSC dot plot of PBMC and histogram of the live cells used for automatic compensation using a fixable dye as live/dead cell color control. For each sample, for compensation, 5,000 total events were acquired on a 4 LASERS flow cytometer (LSRFortesa; BD Biosciences Systems, San Jose, CA) equipped for the detection of 18 fluorescent parameters. Ab capture beads (BD Biosciences) were used as individual compensation tubes for each fluorophore in the experiment, and data analysis was performed using FlowJo version V10.0.1 (TreeStar, Ashland, OR)

controls. We often to use the same fluorochromes as in the experimental samples to create a bright and uniform positive fluorescent peak (Fig. 1). Another advantage of using CompBeads is conserving cells, since no cells are used and are optimal including experiments that use larger cell types using BD CompBead Plus, or for use in experiments in which tandem dye conjugates (PE-Cy™7, APC-Cy7) are stained (Fig. 1a) [11, 12].

BD™ CompBeads Set Anti-Mouse Igκ are polystyrene microparticles used to optimize compensation settings for multicolor flow cytometric assays using mouse cells. They contain two populations of microparticles, the BD™ CompBeads Anti-Mouse Igκ particles, which bind any mouse κ light chain-bearing immunoglobulin, and the BD™ CompBeads Negative Control (FBS), which has no binding capacity. When mixed together with a fluorochrome-conjugated mouse antibody, the BD™ CompBeads provide distinct positive and negative (background fluorescence) stained populations which can be used to set automatic compensation using instrument setup software. Compensation adjustments should be made using the same fluorochrome-labeled antibody used in the experiment for spectral overlap for any combination of fluorochrome-labeled Abs [12]. In Fig. 1 you can see the characteristic size, by dot plot analysis of beads (Fig. 1a), as well the bright single-color signal in histogram analysis (Fig. 1b) using CompBeads for each fluorochrome to perform automatic compensation (Fig. 1a, b).

2.1 CompBeads Assay Procedure

- Vortex BD™ CompBeads thoroughly before use.
- Label a separate 12 × 75 mm sample tube (BD Falcon™, Cat. #. 352008) for each fluorochrome-conjugated mouse Ig,κ Ab to be used in experiment.
- Add 100 μl of FACS buffer (PBS, 0.5–1 % BSA or 5–10 % FBS, 0.1 % NaN_3 sodium azide) or Stain BD buffer (BD Pharmingen Stain (FBS), Cat. # 554656, or BD Pharmingen Stain (BSA), Cat. # 554657) to each tube.
- Add one full drop (60 μl) of the BD™ CompBeads Negative Control (FBS*) and one drop of the BD™ CompBeads Anti-Mouse Igκ beads to each tube and vortex.
- Add 20 μl of each pre-diluted antibody stock (diluted to a concentration optimal for staining 10^6 cells) and vortex.
- Incubate for 15–30 min at room temperature. Protect from exposure to direct light (by covering the tube racks with aluminum foil).
- Set the flow cytometer instrument's PMT voltage settings using the target tissue for the experiment.
- Following the incubation step add 2 ml staining buffer to each tube and pellet by centrifugation at 200 × *g* for 10 min.

The important steps for flow cytometry assay are the following:

1. Configure your instrument.
2. Characterize your instrument.
3. Design your panel.
4. Optimize settings for your panel.
5. Run appropriate controls.
6. QC your data [8–10].

It is very important to titer antibodies with directly conjugated fluorochromes using a small staining volume (100 μl), number of cells (not critical up to ~5 × 10^6), staining time (15–30 min), temperature (e.g., 30 min RT for tetramer staining or 20 min 4 °C for surface staining), and type of sample (whole blood, PBMC, etc.). Acquisition of the data is mediated by a computer physically connected to the flow cytometer, and the software which handles the digital interface with the cytometer. The software is capable of adjusting parameters (i.e., voltage, compensation) for the sample being tested, and also assists in displaying initial sample information while acquiring sample data to insure that parameters are set correctly. Modern instruments usually have multiple lasers and fluorescence detectors. Increasing the number of lasers and detectors allows for multiple antibody labeling, and can more precisely identify a target population by their phenotypic markers.

Applications for flow cytometry are in a wide number of fields, including molecular biology, pathology, immunology, plant biology, and marine biology. There is a broad application of flow assay in medicine (especially in infectious diseases transplantation, hematology, tumor immunology and chemotherapy, prenatal diagnosis). In marine biology, the autofluorescent properties of photosynthetic plankton can be exploited by flow cytometry in order to characterize abundance and community structure. In protein engineering, flow cytometry is used in conjunction with yeast display and bacterial display to identify cell surface-displayed protein variants with desired properties. There is a long list of measurable parameters using flow cytometry and are constantly expanding:

- Cell surface antigens (cluster of differentiation (CD) markers)
- Intracellular antigens (various cytokines, secondary mediators, etc.)
- Nuclear antigens; enzymatic activity
- pH, intracellular ionized calcium, total DNA content (cell cycle analysis, cell kinetics, proliferation, ploidy, aneuploidy, endoreduplication, etc.)
- Total RNA content; DNA copy number variation (by flow-FISH or BACs-on-Beads technology)
- Protein modifications, phosphoproteins
- Transgenic products in vivo, particularly the green fluorescent protein or related fluorescent proteins; magnesium, membrane potential
- Membrane fluidity; apoptosis (quantification, measurement of DNA degradation, mitochondrial membrane potential, permeability changes, caspase activity)
- Protein expression and localization; cell viability
- Chromosome analysis and sorting (library construction, chromosome paint); used for confirming the diagnosis of chronic lymphocytic leukemia
- Volume and morphological complexity of cells
- Cell pigments such as chlorophyll or phycoerythrin
- Monitoring electropermeabilization of cells

- Oxidative burst; characterizing multidrug resistance (MDR) in cancer cells
- Glutathione; various combinations (DNA/surface antigens, etc.); cell adherence (for instance pathogen-host cell adherence)

3 General Gating Strategy of CTL

The data generated by flow cytometer can be plotted in a single dimension, to produce a histogram, or in two-dimensional dot plots or even in three dimensions. The regions on these plots can be sequentially separated, based on fluorescence intensity, by creating a series of subset extractions, termed "gates." Specific gating protocols exist for diagnostic and clinical purposes especially in relation to hematology. The plots are often made on logarithmic scales except the first characterization of population of interest in linear scale FSC/SSC depending on cell size that you analyzed (Fig. 2). Data accumulated using the flow cytometer can be analyzed using software, e.g., Flowjo, FACSDiva, CytoPaint (aka Paint-A-Gate), VenturiOne, CellQuest Pro, or Cytospec or FCS Express or both freeware WinMDI and Flowing Software. Exclusions of the doublets are necessarily after gating on cell population, for a better and clean analysis.

Live/Dead control. It is often important in experiment to use a dye that allows you to exclude the dead cells (Fig. 2). We highly recommend the LIVE/DEAD® Fixable Blue Dead Cell Stain Kit, for UV excitation if your machine is equipped with UV laser and can be

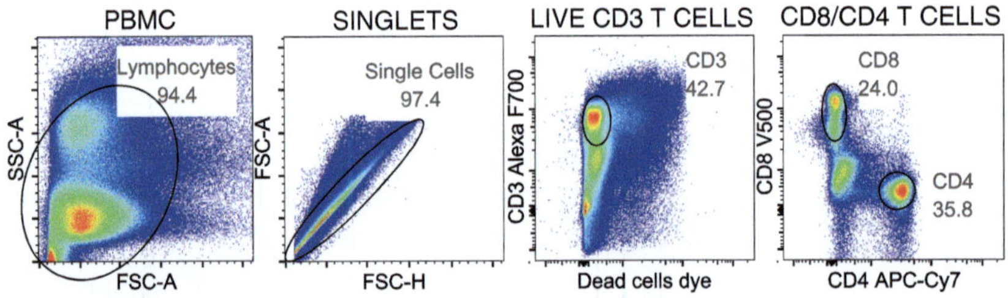

Fig. 2 Gating strategy used for 12-color multi-parametric measurement. Representative flow cytometric plots of gating strategy used to analyze the numbers of PBMC CD8+ or CD4+ T cells. Gating was done on PBMC cells with doublets and dead cell exclusion and on live/CD3+ T cells, we analyzed the subpopulation of T cells; *boxed numbers* indicate the frequencies of CD4+ or CD8+ T cell subpopulations. *Plots* are representative of 23 PBMC analyzed from individuals during chronic CMV infection. Samples were acquired on a 4 LASERS flow cytometer (LSRFortesa; BD Biosciences Systems, San Jose, CA) and data analysis was performed using FlowJo version V10.0.1 (TreeStar, Ashland, OR)

used in fixed cells too (Invitrogen Cat. # L-23105) [13]. The LIVE/DEAD® Fixable Dead Cell Stain Kit has amine-reactive fluorescent dye that allows you to evaluate mammalian cell viability by flow cytometry. In death, cells, ruptures in their membranes and the dye reacts with free amines either in the cell interior or on surface, yielding intense fluorescent staining. In viable cells, the dye's reactivity is restricted to the cell-surface amines, resulting in less intense fluorescence. The difference in intensity between the live and dead cell populations is typically greater than 50-fold, and this fluorescence intensity discrimination is completely preserved following formaldehyde fixation. Advantage of using this reactive dyes in the LIVE/DEAD® Fixable Dead Cell Stain Kits is that it is compatible with multiparameter staining experiments, because it has the blue-fluorescent reactive dye (L23105) with excitation and emission maxima of ~350–450 nm. If your flow cytometer does not have a UV laser you can also use LIVE/DEAD® Fixable Dead Cell Stain Kits that contain violet-fluorescent reactive dye (L34955), green-fluorescent reactive dye (L23101), and red-fluorescent reactive dye (L23102) (Fig. 2). It is important in your experiment to exclude dead cells and analyze live cells (Fig. 2) [13].

Gating strategy is an important step in data analysis. You can focus on the subset of your cells of interest, by gating the total cell population, excluding doublets and dead cells and finally gating on the subpopulation of your cells of interest (Fig. 2). Basically PBMCs purified based on gradient density using Ficoll were stimulated with/without the Ag of interest for 6 h, 37 °C, 5 % CO_2, in the presence of brefeldin A for the final 4 h. After that incubation cells were washed with FACS buffer (PBS, 0.5–1 % BSA or 5–10 % FBS, 0.1 % NaN_3 sodium azide) and stained for 20 min in the dark at 4 °C with surface Abs against various cell markers (CD3 Alexa Fluor 700, CD4 APC Cy7, and CD8 AmCyan or V400 all from BioLegend and BD Biosciences) [14]. After staining the cells were washed with FACS buffer and centrifuged at 1,500 rpm (e.g., 300×*g* at 4 °C). The pellet was stained with LIVE/DEAD® Fixable Dead Cell dye and incubated for an additional 20 min at RT in the dark. After this step cells were washed with FACS buffer, centrifuged at 1,500 rpm (e.g., 300×*g* at 4 °C), and fixed by resuspending cells in buffered paraformaldehyde (e.g., Cytofix Buffer; Cat. No. 554655) for 30 min at 4 °C, and finally washed, resuspended in FACS buffer, and stored at 4 °C (protected from light). For each sample, 1,000,000 total events were acquired on the flow cytometer (LSRFortesa; BD Biosciences Systems San Jose, CA) equipped for the detection of 18 fluorescent parameters. Ab capture beads (BD Biosciences) were used as individual compensation tubes for each fluorophore in the experiment, and data analysis was performed using FlowJo version V10.0.1 (TreeStar, Ashland, OR). To define positive and negative populations, we employed fluorescence minus one controls for each fluorophore used in this study, when initially developing staining protocols. In addition, we further optimized gating by examining known negative cell populations for background level expression [14] (Fig. 2).

4 Phenotype of CTL

4.1 Flow Cytometry Assay for Cell Surface Staining Protocol of Human PBMCs and Suspension Cell Lines (BD Biosciences Protocol) [15, 16]

- PBMCs or cell lines can be resuspended with FACS buffer (PBS, 0.5–1 % BSA or 5–10 % FBS, 0.1 % NaN_3 sodium azide) (do not add sodium azide to buffers if you are concerned with recovering cell function, e.g., if cells are to be collected for functional assays; it inhibits metabolic activity).
- Wash the cells twice in ice-cold FACS buffer and pellet the cells by centrifugation at 1,500 rpm (e.g., 300×*g* at 4 °C). Resuspend the cell pellet with cold FACS buffer to a final concentration of $1–5 \times 10^6$ cells/ml. It is always useful to check the viability of the cells which should be around 95 % but not less than 90 %.
- Distribute 100 μl aliquots of the cell suspension (10^6 cells) to either tubes 12×75 mm Polypropylene Round-Bottom Test (BD Falcon tubes cat # 352052). However, they can be stained in any container for which you have an appropriate centrifuge, e.g., polystyrene V-bottom 12×75 mm test tubes, Eppendorf tubes, and 96-well round-bottomed microtiter plates. The staining is recommended with ice-cold reagents/solutions moAb at 4 °C, since low temperature and presence of sodium azide prevent the modulation and internalization of surface antigens which can produce a loss of fluorescence intensity.
- *The blocking antibody,* step 3, *is optional but should be included if cells express high levels of Fc receptors which will contribute to nonspecific binding and background fluorescence.*

  Add 100 μl of Fc block to each sample (Fc block diluted in FACS buffer at 1:50 ratio). Incubate on ice for 20 min.
- *Centrifuge at 1,500 rpm* (e.g., *300×g at 4 °C) for 5 min at 4 °C. Discard supernatant.*
- Add 0.1–10 μg/ml of the primary labeled antibody.

  Dilutions, if necessary, should be made in FACS buffer. Determination of optimal antibody concentration may be necessary. For test size antibody products, add the recommended test size volume. Staining time may be increased (>45 min) depending on the avidity of the fluorescent antibody.
- Incubate for 20 min on ice, protected from light. Attention! For tetramer staining incubate for at least 30 min at room temperature or 37 °C.

This step will require optimization.

- Wash the cells two times with either 200 μl (for microwell plates) or 1 ml (for tubes) volumes of cold FACS buffer.
- Centrifuge cells at 1,500 rpm (300×*g*) for 5 min. carefully aspirate (for microwell plates or tubes) or invert and blot away (for tubes) supernatants from cell pellets.
- Resuspend them in 200 μl to 1 ml of ice-cold FACS buffer.
- Keep the cells in the dark on ice or at 4 °C in a fridge until your scheduled time for analysis.
- *If you use primary unlabeled antibody after completing* step 5 *do the following: Dilute the fluorochrome-labeled secondary antibody in FACS buffer at the optimal dilution (according to the manufacturer's instructions), resuspend cells in this solution, and incubate for at least 20–30 min at room temperature or 4 °C in the dark. Wash the cells three times by centrifugation at 500×g for 5 min and resuspend them in 200 μl to 1 ml of ice-cold FACS buffer. Keep the cells in the dark on ice or at 4 °C in a refrigerator until your scheduled time for analysis.*
- For extended storage (16 h) as well as for greater flexibility in planning time on the cytometer, resuspend cells in buffered paraformaldehyde (e.g., Cytofix Buffer; Cat. No. 554655) for 30 min at 4 °C. Researchers may need to verify if this fixation will affect antibody binding and fluorescence intensity.
- Washed samples, resuspended in FACS buffer, and then stored at 4 °C (protected from light use tin foil when on bench).
- Analyze the stained cell samples by flow cytometry.
- For PBMC preparation, use the manufacturer's directions for Ficoll products, and purification based on gradient density.
- For most applications, BSA as a blocking agent is sufficient, but investigators may use FBS if more stringent blocking is required.
- For the whole blood add appropriate volume of an erythrocyte lysing buffer (e.g., BD PharmLyse or BD FACS Lysing Solution). Follow the manufacturer's directions for incubation and washing.

5 Detection of Viral Specific CTL

5.1 Tetramer/Pentamer Staining

In immunology, MHC tetramers are used to quantify the numbers of antigen-specific T cells (especially $CD8^+$ T cells). MHC tetramers are class I or class II molecules that have been biotinylated or directly conjugated. These molecules are folded with the peptide of interest (like viral peptide described on the same HLA type of MHC) and β2M and tetramerized/pentamerized by a fluorescently labeled streptavidin. Tetramer can bind to three TCRs at once, allowing specific binding in spite of the low (10^{-6} mol) affinity of the typical class I-peptide-TCR interaction. MHC class II tetramers can also be made although these are more difficult to work with practically, because of a higher length of the peptide folded, so they can sometimes bind non-specifically. The tetramer will specifically label T cells that express T cell receptors that are specific for a given peptide-MHC complex. Antigen-specific responses can be measured as $CD8^+$, $tetramer^+$ T cells as a fraction of all $CD8^+$ lymphocytes. Also, there may be a need to correlate the $CD8^+$ antigen-specific $tetramer^+$ with functional response (cytokine release, transcription factor, cytotoxicity molecule released-GrzB, perforin, CD95, CD107) as well as with exhaustion anergic markers (PD1).

Tetramers can only identify T cells with single peptide/MHC specificities, while cytokine assays can determine the sum total of T cell responses to a particular protein or pathogen. In conclusion defining frequencies of the specific T cells is one of the primary goals of ex vivo T cell diagnostic, using this single cell assay that permits to count the numbers of antigen-specific T cells in cell material such as blood and can provide accurate frequency information which translates into the magnitude of antigen-specific T cell immunity.

For example (Fig. 3), in experiments using CMV-specific tetramers we can track only those CTLs that are CMV-specific and evaluate additional surface markers [17]. The following fluorochrome-labeled Abs for surface staining were used: APC-Cy7-conjugated anti-CD4, V-500-conjugated anti-CD8 (or AmCyan-conjugated anti-CD8), Alexa Fluor 700-conjugated anti-CD3, PerCP-conjugated anti-CD45RA, and appropriately conjugated isotype controls. The following PE-conjugated CMV-specific tetramers were purchased from Beckman Coulter: A1-VTEHDTLLY, A2-NLVPMVATV, B7-TPRVTGGGAM, B8-ELRRKMMYM, and B35-IPSINVHHY. Cell fluorescence was analyzed using a 4 LASERS flow cytometer (LSRFortesa; BD Biosciences Systems San Jose, CA). Data analysis was performed using FlowJo version V10.0.1 (TreeStar, Ashland, OR) (Fig. 3). During primary infection and viremia the majority of CMV $tetramer^+CD8^+$ T cells in the blood from those particular patients' LTRs no. 22 and no. 31 were $CD45RA^-$ and transition to $CD45RA^+$ during latent infection in the absence of viremia. In sharp contrast, CMV $tetramer^+CD8^+$ T cells in the lung allograft are $CD45RA^-$ ($CD45RO^+$; data not shown) during acute primary infection, with the majority of these cells maintaining this phenotype into latent infection. In total, we simultaneously analyzed five LTRs for PBMC sample tetramer responses during acute and chronic infection (1–3 months following resolution of viremia/active infection) for

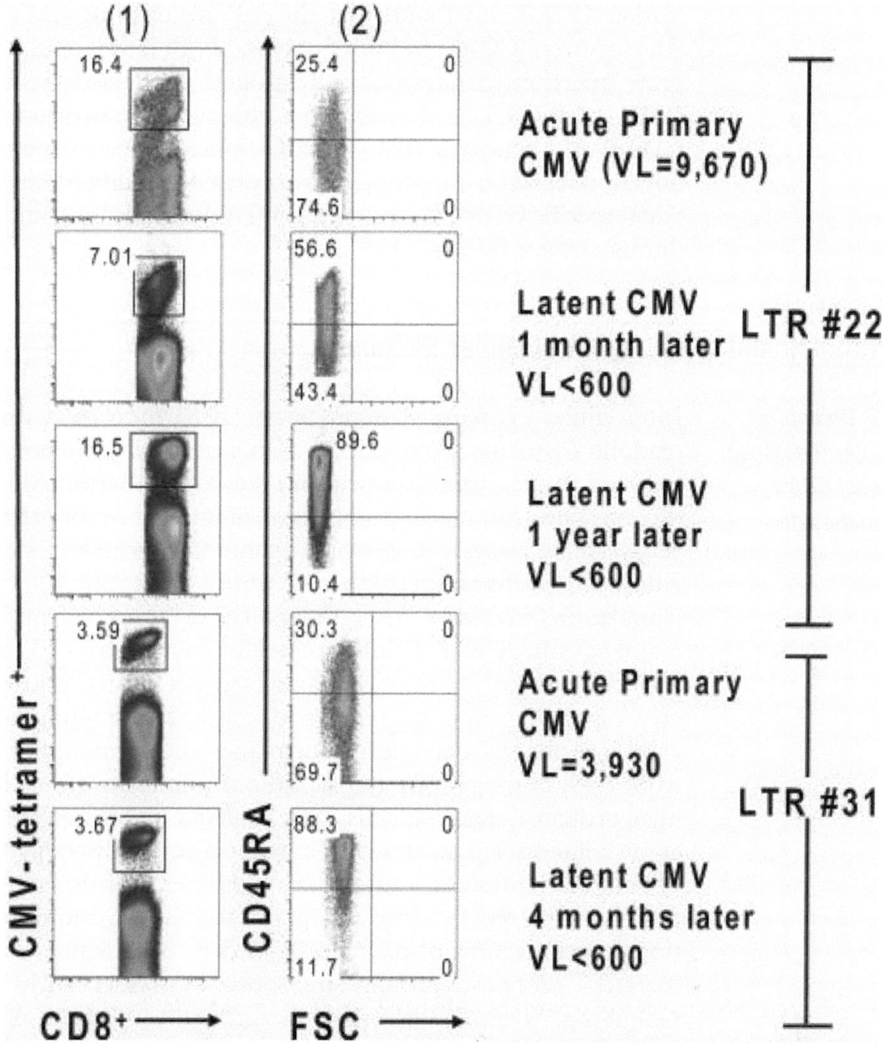

Fig. 3 Tetramer CMV-specific CD8+ T cells transition from a CD45RA− phenotype in the PBMC during viremia/acute infection to CD45RA+ during latent. Representative plots of CD8+CMV tetramer+ T cells in PBMC from LTRs#22 (both HLA-A2 and HLA-B7 pp65 tetramers) and LTR#31 (HLA-A2 pp65 tetramer) at the indicated time points during the transition from acute primary CMV infection into chronic infection. Gating is on CD3+CD8+tetramer+ T cells. *VL* Viral load. Samples were acquired on a 4 LASERS flow cytometer (LSRFortesa; BD Biosciences Systems San Jose, CA) and data analysis was performed using FlowJo version V10.0.1 (TreeStar, Ashland, OR)

CD45RA+ surface expression and found a significant mean increase in the percentage of CD8+CD45RA+tetramer+ cells in PBMC from 23.06 ± 4.24 % (SEM) to 72.5 ± 7.59 % ($p = 0.043$ by Wilcoxon signed-rank test) in acute vs. chronic infection, respectively [6]. Similar results were obtained when we analyzed CD8+IFN-γ+ effectors for CD45RA expression, as seen in Fig. 3. We should also mention that, as an additional control, we also assessed the memory marker CCR7 and found that the vast majority of CMV-specific effectors were CCR7⁻ in both the blood both during and following acute infection (data not shown). Together, these data show that CMV-specific $CD8^+$ T cells from the blood transition from a $CD45RA^-$ phenotype to a $CD45RA^+$ phenotype as viremia/acute infection resolves, indicating distinct phenotypic differences between CMV-specific $CD8^+$ effector memory T cells in the lung and PBMC during chronic infection [17].

6 Multifunctional of CTL by Intracellular Staining

6.1 ICS: Detecting Intracellular Cytokines in Activated $CD8^+$/ $CD4^+$ Lymphocytes

Intracellular cytokine staining assays (ICS) measure a functional readout (cytokine production) as opposed to tetramers, which measure antigen specificity without regard to function. Since some disease states can evoke populations of anergic (nonfunctional) T cells. Those assays can provide quantitative readouts since they enumerate antigen-specific cells without lengthy in vitro re-stimulation, necessary for proliferation or apoptosis or both. A major advantage of intracellular cytokine staining over ELISPOT is the ability to analyze multiple parameters per cell. ICS flow cytometry, especially when combined with cell surface staining, is a powerful tool for the detection of cytokines and transcription factors from both homogenous and mixed cell populations. For intracellular protein detection, cells must be fixed and permeabilized to allow a fluorescent antibody to enter and detect the target protein of interest. Different antigens have different sensitivities to and requirements for fixation and permeabilization, requiring additional optimization of protocols. To detect cytokines, which are secreted proteins, protein transport inhibitors such as BD GolgiStop™ (monensin) or BD GolgiPlug™ (brefeldin A) inhibitors are used to trap proteins inside the cell. Detection of degranulation by CD107 require monensin added to the system before cell stimulation versus cytokine detection or transfection factor expression that requires brefeldin A in the system for the last 4 or 6 h for stimulation of cells.

Activation of the cells: In the presence of brefeldin A, which inhibits intracellular transport of proteins, cytokines produced during activation will be retained inside the cell. The unstimulated control sample should also contain BFA. All activation procedures outlined are performed in 12 × 75-mm capped polystyrene test tubes (Falcon Catalog No. 2058). Incubate for 4 h at 37 °C, 7 % CO_2, with tube caps loosened to allow the entry of CO_2-containing air. (While a CO_2 incubator is preferred to ensure proper control of pH, the incubation can also be carried out in a water bath with each tube tightly capped.)

Activation of the cells requires some reagents such as the following:

- *Phorbol 12-Myristate 13 Acetate (PMA)* (Sigma Catalog No. P-8139): This can be used as positive control because activate all the T cell (unspecific) as maximum detection of intracellular cytokines. PMA needs to be reconstituted in DMSO at 0.1 mg/ml and stored in small aliquots (20 µl) at −20 °C. PMA is used by diluting the stock 1:100 in sterile PBS for each experiment at final concentration of 10 ng/ml of cell suspension.
- *Ionomycin* (Sigma Catalog No. I-0634) is another reagent needed to be used together with PMA as a positive control in experiments. This is reconstituted in EtOH at 0.5 mg/ml, stored same at -20 °C, and used by diluting the stock 1:10 in sterile PBS for experiment, at a final concentration of 1 µg/ml of cell suspension.
- *Staphylococcal enterotoxin B (SEB)* (Sigma Catalog No. S-4881) is a superantigen that stimulates polyclonal T cells of distinct vb families, so it is used as a positive control. SEB can be reconstituting in sterile PBS at 0.5 mg/ml. It can be stored at 4 °C or for longer time at -20 °C and is used in experiments at final concentration of 1 µg/ml of cell suspension.
- *Brefeldin-A (BFA)* (Sigma Catalog No. B-7651) is a protein transport inhibitor commonly used to enhance intracellular cytokine staining signals by blocking transport processes during cell activation. Especially useful for the intracellular staining of cytokines, BFA leads to the accumulation of most cytokines at the Golgi complex/endoplasmic reticulum [18, 19]. Typically, protein transport inhibitors are included during in vitro cell activation cultures for 4–24 h prior to harvest BFA is reconstitute in DMSO at 5 mg/ml. It can be stored in small aliquots (20 µl) at -20 °C. It is used by diluting the stock 1:10 in sterile PBS for each assay, at 10 µg/ml of cell suspension for the last 4–5 h of activation. Extensive incubation with BFA can reduce cell viability.
- *CD3/CD28* also can be used to activate T cells: Activate undiluted blood with immobilized CD3 in the presence of BFA. Incubate for 4–6 h at 37 °C. Use CD28 (BD Biosciences Catalog No. 340975) at 10 µg/ml to enhance activation responses to various stimuli, including SEB, CD3, and CD2/CD2R.
- *Peptides* can be used to activate specific T cells against different viruses, human CMV [14, 20], EBV [6, 21], BK [22, 23], RSV, HIV, and Flu. For example, PepMix HCMVA (pp65) or IE1 can be used for ex vivo stimulation of T cells (JPT Peptide Technologies, Berlin, Germany). According to JPT Peptide Technologies dissolve peptides in a minimum amount of pure

DMSO (approx. 40 μl) and dilute with PBS buffer to the final concentration—1 μg/ml (final concentration of DMSO must be below 1 % (v/v) to avoid toxicity in the biological system). The dissolved mix can be stored at −20 °C. It is recommended to make one single aliquot per test, and to make aliquots that can be conveniently handled (i.e., 4 μl rather than 0.4 μl), by avoiding repeated thawing/freezing cycles of stored aliquots. Use 1 μg/ml final concentration of each peptide per test for stimulating PBMC. For whole blood higher concentrations are generally required. Add 400 μl of cell suspension (containing 0.5×106–1×10^6 cells) to each tube. Place tubes in a rack and place the rack in a standard incubator (37 °C, H_2O-saturated 5 % CO_2 atmosphere) at a 5° slant (the tubes are almost laying horizontally). After 2 h, add 500 μl of supplemented media containing 10 μg of brefeldin A to each tube for a total of 6 h of stimulation [14, 20, 24].

CELLS used for ICS:

- *Whole blood*—collected into sodium heparin VACUTAINER tubes (BD VACUTAINER Catalog No. 367673). For best results, assay blood within 8 h of collection since a minor loss of activity can be expected beyond 8 h; typically, the percent of cytokine-positive cells is reduced by approximately 5 %. If blood cannot be used within 8 h, store VACUTAINER tubes horizontally at room temperature.
- *PBMCs in tissue culture medium*—can also be separated via Ficoll-Paque density-gradient centrifugation. Use standard techniques and resuspend at 2×10^6 cells/ml in RPMI-1640 with 10 % heat-inactivated fetal bovine serum (FBS) for activation.
- *Cell lines and T-lymphocyte clones*—For activation, 2×10^6 cells/ml in the fresh culture medium are typically used to grow the cells. Heat inactivate FBS or human serum to denature complement.
- *Frozen whole blood and PBMCs*—Lyse and fix activated whole blood or PBMCs using 1× FACS lysing solution; incubate for 10 min at room temperature and directly place the tubes in a freezer at −80 °C. After thawing, aliquot cells into staining tubes. Wash cells by adding 2–3 ml wash buffer and centrifuge for 5 min at $500 \times g$; then permeabilize with 1× FACS permeabilizing buffer.

Protocol for detecting intracellular cytokines using flow cytometry (ICS)

- Cells used for ICS can be obtained from whole blood (after lysis) or cells purified as PBMC (using density-gradient separation) or cells cultured can be used as fresh cells immediately after purification or cryopreserved in liquid nitrogen. Cells frozen could be thawed and washed twice in RPMI 1640 before stimulation.

- Cells are stimulated (at 2–3 × 10^6 cells/ml in 24-well plates, or V cone tubes in a 5 % CO_2 incubator for a total of 6 h in the presence for the last 4 h of 10 μg of brefeldin A (to enhance intracellular cytokine staining signals by blocking transport processes during cell activation) or for cytotoxicity detection of degranulation, CD107 as a cytolytic marker, will require 5 h with monensin to maximize CD107 detection. Also this technique needs to be done in the presence of anti-CD107a, before antigen stimulation.
- After stimulation cells are stained for surface markers (such as CD3, CD4, CD8, CD19, CD56) using the surface staining protocol.
- After surface staining, wash cells once 1× with 1 ml FACS buffer, and spin at 500 × *g* for 5 min at 4 °C.
- Label cells on ice with Live/Dead Fixable UV Dead Cell Stain (Invitrogen).
- Wash cells once 1× with 1 ml FACS buffer, spin at 1,400 rpm for 5 min at 4 °C, and resuspend cell pellets with 100 μl BD Cytofix/Cytoperm (BD Pharmingen, Cat # 51-2090KZ). You can keep them for up to 24–48 h, after fixing wash 1× with 1 ml FACS buffer, spin at 1,400 rpm for 5 min at 4 °C, and resuspend cell pellets with 100 μl FACS buffer however the intensity of staining may vary with time.
- Next day for ICS wash 1× with 1 ml 1× BD Perm/Wash and spin at 1,400 rpm for 5 min at 4 °C.
- Prepare intracellular stain mix and add 50 μL of mix per appro priate tube. For isotype tubes you must add isotype and buffer individually (for example Anti-IFNγ PE Cy7 (BD Pharmingen, clone XMG1.2) → 1:50 in 1× BD Perm/Wash buffer. Isotype → rat IgG_1 PE Cy7).
- Incubate on ice for 30 min in the dark.
- Wash 1× with 1 ml 1× BD Perm/Wash. Spin at 1,400 rpm for 5 min at 4 °C.
- Resuspend in 200 μl FACS buffer.
- Samples may be collected immediately or the next day.
- Store sealed with paraffin at 4 °C in the dark until samples are collected.
- *Attention!*—If you need to detect molecular transcription factors such as FoxP3 or Tbet we recommend to use special buffers from BD that have special transcription buffer that can be used for fixing and permeabilizing the cells.

- For each sample, 600,000–1,000,000 total events were acquired on a 4 LASERS flow cytometer Ab capture beads (BD Biosciences) are used as individual compensation tubes for each fluorophore in the experiment, and data analysis was performed using FlowJo software version V10-0.1 (TreeStar, Ashland, OR). Lymphocytes were identified by typical forward (FCS) versus side scatter (SSC), and cell doublets were excluded using forward scatter area-SSC A versus height SSC H. After gating on viable CD3$^+$, and subsequent on CD4$^+$, and CD8$^+$ subset cells, data were plotted for various cytokine combinations. Statistical markers were based on the staining of unactivated media control samples or SEB stimulation as positive control.

You can detect multifunctional frequencies of virus-specific CTL subsets looking at compartments such as lung and blood [25]. Greater frequencies of multifunctional CMV-specific CD4$^+$, but not CD8$^+$, T cells are present in the bronchoalveolar space over PBMC during chronic CMV infection. Because durable viral control likely requires the development and maintenance of CMV-specific memory T cells capable of producing other factors beyond IFN-γ, we evaluated the capacity for CD4$^+$ and CD8$^+$ T cells to produce an expanded panel of cytokines and chemokines that included IFN-γ, TNF-α, IL-2, and the CCR5-binding chemokine MIP-1β in 8 D$^+$R$^-$ LTRs during chronic infection [25]. A poly functionality of a cell can be determined and quantified using a software analysis SPICE (online available by courtesy of Dr. Roederer) [26]. As shown in a representative LTR, T cell effector memory responses for the entire panel were detected in CMV-specific CD4$^+$ (Fig. 4a) and CD8$^+$ (Fig. 4b) T cells during chronic CMV infection, with IL-2 being the cytokine least frequently detected. Because the functional quality of antigen-specific memory responses has been shown to be an important determinant of protection in various human and mouse models of infection, we next analyzed whether compartmental differences existed in the CMV-specific multifunctional cytokine$^+$/chemokine$^+$ populations producing IFN-γ, TNF-α, MIP-1β, and IL-2 from CD4$^+$ and CD8$^+$ T cells during chronic CMV infection using Boolean analysis. As shown in Fig. 4 both pp65-specific CD4$^+$ and CD8$^+$ T cells were found to include single (1+), double (2+), and triple (3+) cytokine/chemokine-producing populations in both tissue compartments, with CMV-specific CD4$^+$ T cells having a modestly wider array (8 vs. 5) compared to CD8$^+$ T cells (Fig 4c, d). Only CMV-specific CD4$^+$ T cells in the lung allograft were found to have a quadruple (4+) cytokine/chemokine-producing capacity attributable to the production of IL-2 among multiple CD4$^+$ T cell subsets, whereas detection of

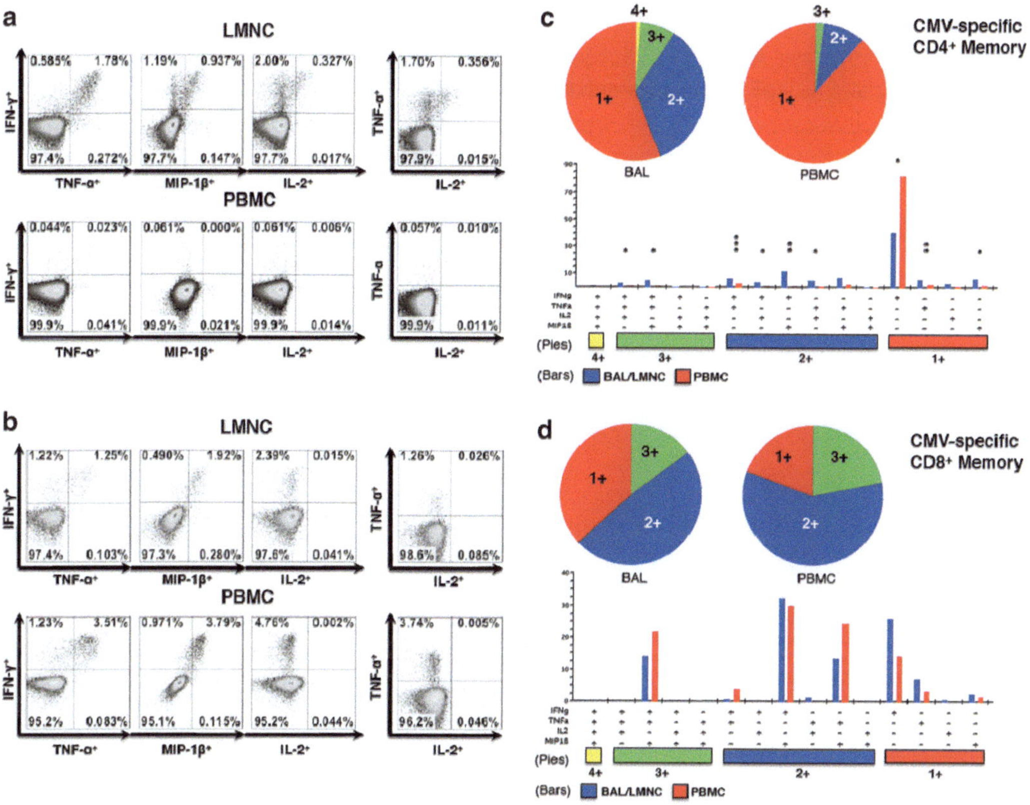

Fig. 4 Diverse multifunctional CMV-specific CD4$^+$ T cell effector memory populations are significantly increased in the lung during chronic infection but not among CD8$^+$ T cells. Representative multifunctional flow cytometric plots of (**a**) CD4$^+$ and (**b**) CD8$^+$ T cell LMNC and PBMC following re-stimulation with CMV antigen in two LTRs showing the frequency of IFN-γ by TNF-α, MIP-1β, and IL-2 as well as TNF-α by IL-2 during chronic infection. Individual *pie charts* show the percentage of pp65-specific CD4$^+$ (C) and CD8$^+$ (D) T cells that produce 1, 2, 3, or 4 functional responses. CMV-specific CD4$^+$ multifunctional responses to pp65-pooled peptides were significantly more frequent in the lung allograft than peripheral blood ($p<0.05$) (**c**), while CD8$^+$ multifunctional responses were equally distributed between the two compartments (**d**). Using Boolean analysis, the percentage of total for individual multifunctional subset responses for LMNC (*blue bars*) and PBMC (*red bars*) are shown in the *bar graph* for each of the 15 multifunctional subsets. Significant differences when comparing frequencies (mean ± SEM, not shown) of LMNC and PBMC pp65-specific single and multifunctional responses are indicated by a *$p<0.05$, **$p<0.01$, and ***$p<0.001$. *Figures* represent results from 8 LTRs. All *p*-values were determined by the Kruskal–Wallis one-way ANOVA or Wilcoxon signed-rank test

CD8$^+$IL-2$^+$ T cells was a rare event (<0.05 % observed frequency). Overall, when comparing the frequencies of multifunctional T cell memory responses between the LMNC and PBMC compartments, CMV-pp65-specific CD4$^+$ memory T cells showed significant preferential distribution to the lung in six different

Table I

Different T cells subtypes. All the T cell subset characteristics such as surface markers and specific transcription factors as well as the differentiation and effector cytokines

Type of cell	Tc	Th1	Th2	Th9	Th17	Tfh	Treg
Surface markers	CD8	CD4 CXCR3	CD4 CCR4 Crth2	CD4	CD4 CCR6	CD4 CXCR5	CD4 CD25
Differentiation cytokine	IFNγ IL-12 IL-27	IFNγ IL-2 IL-12 IL-18 IL-27	IL-4 IL-2 IL-33	Il-4 TGFβ	TGFβ IL-6 IL-1 IL-21 IL-23 IL-17A	IL-12 IL-6	TGFβ IL-12
Effector cytokines	IFNγ TNFα Ltα	IFNγ Ltα TNFα	IL-4 IL-5 IL-13	IL-9 IL-10	IL-17F IL-21 IL-22 TNFα CCL20	IL-21	TGFβ IL-10
Transcription factors	Tbet/ Eomes	Tbet STAT1 STAT6	GATA3 STAT5 STAT6	GATA3 Smads STAT6	RORγt RORα STAT3	Bcl6 MAF	FoxP3 Smad3 STAT5

multifunctional combinations as shown in Fig. 4c. In contrast, CMV-specific CD8+ T cells were found to have a similar distribution of T cell effector memory, when comparing 1+, 2+, or 3+ multifunctional cytokine/chemokine production between compartments, as shown in Fig. 4d. Together, these data demonstrate increased multifunctional capacities of CMV-specific CD4+, but not CD8+, memory T cells in the bronchoalveolar space compared to the blood during chronic infection [25, 26].

6.2 ICS for Transcription Factors

Another useful application of flow cytometry for CTL function detection is the molecular factors after ex vivo CMV-specific stimulation. As in Table I these molecular factors tetramer the type of immune response, such as Tbet or Eomes for type 1 or Gata3 for type 2 of immune response. In Fig. 5 you can see how the type 1 immune response using Tbet can be determined. For example in these experiments the following ten-color panel was used for UV LIVE/DEAD, CD3 Alexa Fluor 700, CD8 V500, CD4 APC-Cy7, CD107 PacBlue, Tbet PE, GranB PE Texas-Red TNFα FITC, IFNγ PE Cy7 (all BD Biosciences or BioLegend).

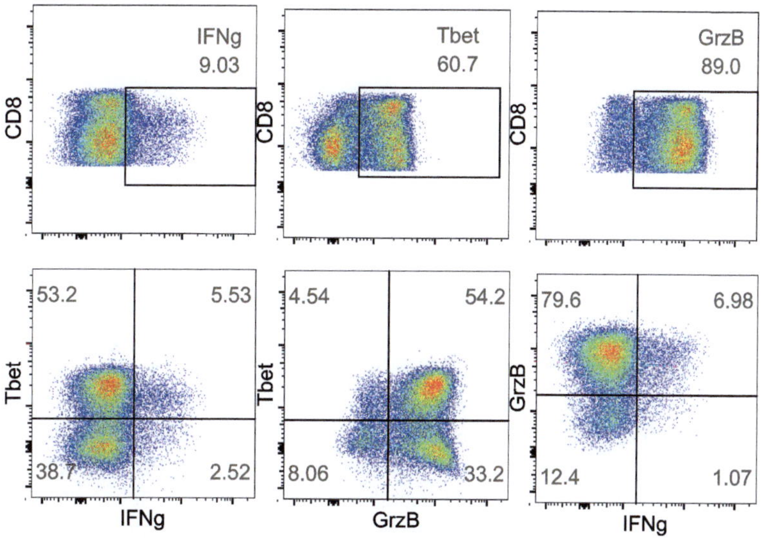

Fig. 5 Transcription factors and cytokine detection on CTL during CMV infection. Massive induction of molecular factor Tbet, IFNγ, and GrzB as a type 1 immune response signature in the peripheral CD8+ T cell pool, primary CMV infection. Here a representative experiment of a total of 23 patients after activation with CMV pp65-specific peptide. PBMC purified from the CMV donor were thawed and stimulated with CMV-specific peptide such as pp65 (or IE1 data not shown), for 6 h in the presence of brefeldin A (for the last 4 h). For each sample 1,000,000 total events were acquired on a 4 LASERS flow cytometer (LSRFortesa; BD Biosciences Systems, San Jose, CA) equipped for the detection of 18 fluorescent parameters. Ab capture beads (BD Biosciences) were used as individual compensation tubes for each fluorophore in the experiment, and data analysis was performed using FlowJo version V10.0.1 (TreeStar, Ashland, OR)

7 Proliferation of CTL

Proliferation assay using a green dye CFSE ([5- (and 6-) carboxyfluorescein diacetate succinimyl ester)].

Use of the intracellular fluorescent dye CFSE provides a powerful tool to monitor lymphocyte proliferation and cell migration, and to quantify cell division, because of the sequential decrease in fluorescent labeling in daughter cells. The lymphocytes stained with CFSE have been used to analyze the relationship between cell division and differentiation of cell function, or cell proliferation versus apoptosis, both in vivo and in vitro, and have allowed analysis of the site of response to antigens in vivo [27, 28]. CFSE molecules diffuse into cells and they are hydrolyzed by intracellular nonspecific esterases and bind to cellular components to become fluorescent products. Dead cells and cells without intact membranes

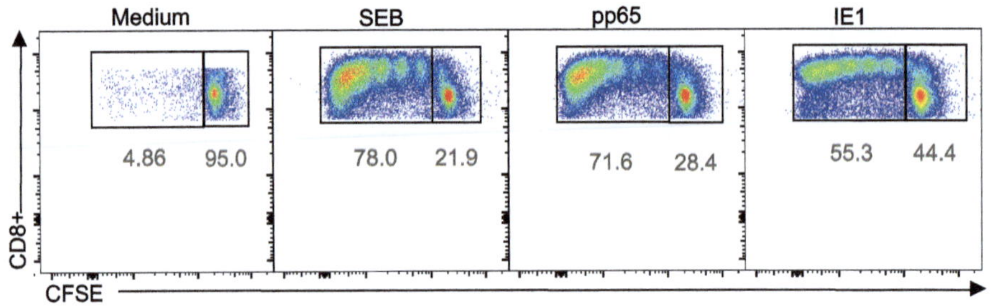

Fig. 6 Proliferation ability of CMV-specific CD8+ T cells using CFSE dilution assay. CD8+ cell proliferation in response of CMV-specific stimulation (pp65 or IE1) or not (medium as a control) or SEB as a control. Representative *plots* are showed from a total of 23 CMV-infected patients, and stimulated for 6 days in the presence of CFSE dye. After day 6 cells were given rest and re-stimulated for an additional 6 h with CMV-specific pp65 peptide or not or SEB as a control in the presence of brefeldin A. For each sample 1,000,000 total events were acquired on a 4 LASERS flow cytometer (LSRFortesa; BD Biosciences Systems, San Jose, CA) equipped for the detection of 18 fluorescent parameters. Ab capture beads (BD Biosciences) were used as individual compensation tubes for each fluorophore in the experiment, and data analysis was performed

do not label with these dyes and are not fluorescent. BD Bioscience has a new product, BD Horizon™ Violet Proliferation Dye 450 (VPD450), that is functionally similar to CFSE since it contains both an esterase-cleavable group VPD450 which can be used where either green fluorescent proteins or FITC-labeled antibodies are used. The VPD450 dye is excited by the violet laser compared to CFSE and its fluorescein analogs which utilize the same lasers and detectors as GFP, FITC, and Alexa Fluor® 488 (Fig. 6). It is straight forward to determine the frequency of proliferating cell subsets in conjunction with their poly-functionality and type of immune response.

7.1 CFSE Labeling Procedure [29, 30]:

- Prepare a single-cell suspension.
- Resuspend the single-cell suspension at 10–100 × 10^6/ml of PBS (pre-warmed to room temperature).
- Add an equal volume of 2× working solution of CFSE to final concentration of 5 μM,
- Prepare a 2× working solution by adding 2 μl of a 5 mM stock in 1.0 ml PBS.
- Immediately mix and incubate in the dark for 10 min at 37 °C.
- To quench the staining add 4.4 ml of ice-cold complete RPMI1640 media (10 % FCS).
- Pellet the cells by centrifugation.
- Wash once with fresh complete media.
- CFSE-labeled cells can be used for in vitro assay for 5–6 days.

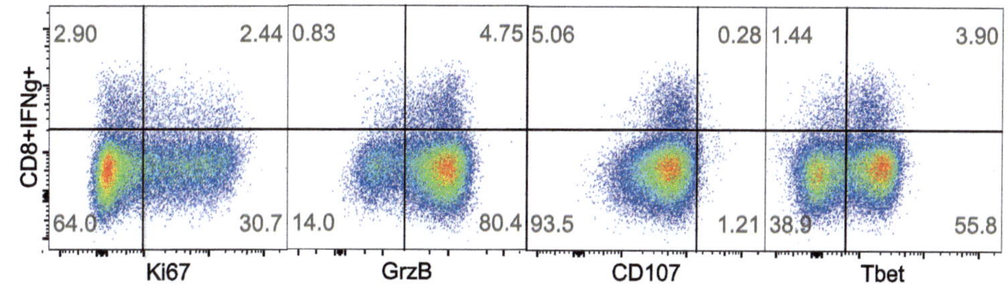

Fig. 7 CMV-specific IFNγ$^+$CD8$^+$ T cells directly correlate with cytotoxic phenotype (GrzB and CD107) during acute CMV infection. CD8$^+$ T cell response in acute CMV infection directly correlate between IFNγ secretion and GrzB and CD107 degranulation in response after activation with CMV-pp65-specific peptide. Also another marker for proliferating capacity of the cells is Ki67. PBMC were thawed and stimulated with CMV-specific peptide such as pp65 for 6 h in the presence of brefeldin A and monensin and CD107 Pacific Blue. For each sample 1,000,000 total events were acquired on a 4 LASERS flow cytometer (LSRFortesa; BD Biosciences Systems, San Jose, CA) equipped for the detection of 18 fluorescent parameters. Ab capture beads (BD Biosciences) were used as individual compensation tubes for each fluorophore in the experiment, and data analysis was performed using FlowJo version V10.0.1 (TreeStar, Ashland, OR)

7.2 KI 67

Another great marker that correlates with cell proliferation in the cell cycle analysis is the parameter Ki 67. Ki-67 protein (also known as MKI67). It is a cellular marker for proliferation (Fig. 7) and is strictly associated with cell proliferation. During interphase, the Ki-67 antigen can be exclusively detected within the cell nucleus, whereas in mitosis most of the protein is relocated to the surface of the chromosomes. Ki-67 protein is present during all active phases of the cell cycle (G_1, S, G_2, and mitosis), but is absent from resting cells (G_0). Overexpression is frequently seen in a variety of malignant tissues and is associated with worse survival of individuals with bladder, brain, breast, kidney, lung, ovary, prostate, or thyroid cancer. In addition, Ki-67 reactivity is included among other parameters in the World Health Organization's recommended grading system for neuroendocrine tumors of the pancreas and gastrointestinal tract. Ki-67 overexpression is associated with worse survival of individuals with a neuroendocrine tumor.

8 Cytotoxic Capacity of CTL

Detection of granules-Grz B, and annexin V, protocol, and example.

CD107a—In this method, the cells are cultured in the presence of CD107a monoclonal antibody before the 6-h antigen stimulation, which enables sensitive detection of CD107a as measuring degranulation of T cells by cell-surface expression of IFNγ [29, 30]. Cells stimulate in the presence of 5 μg/ml each of brefeldin A and monensin. Monensin helps maximize the CD107 readout, whereas brefeldin A helps maximize the IFNγ readout. Dissolve monensin (Sigma #5273) at 5 mg/ml in methanol, and then dilute 1:10 in PBS on the day of use, followed by 1:100 dilutions into the culture medium. Add antibody to CD107a in fluorochrome that gives the brightest signal (such as Pacific Blue or PE-Cy5). Add the antibody, at 10 ml per 200 ml of cell stimulation culture, at the beginning of the activation period, and activate for 5–6 h. Continue with processing for surface, and after fixing and permeabilization, continue with ICS for cytokine or transcription factor as desired. As an example (Fig. 7) we can detect at different time points in the same patient the CMV acute/chronic infection response by simultaneous detection of gamma-producing CMV-specific T cell ($CD8^+IFN\gamma^+$) with lytic degranulation of CMV-specific $CD8^+CD107a^+$ T cells after in vitro stimulation with pp65/or IE1 peptide-specific CMV (Fig. 7). Also we can measure the lytic degranulation by GrzB detection in $pp65^+$ CMV-specific $CD8^+$ T cells and correlate with the $CD8^+Tbet^+$ T cells.

Apoptosis—There are two ways that a cell can die: by necrosis and by apoptosis.
Necrosis— Occurs when a cell is damaged by an external force (e.g. ischemia). The death causes inflammation that can cause further distress or injury within the body [21, 27, 28, 31, 32].

Apoptosis, or *programmed cell death*, is a naturally occurring process in the body, a genetically determined cell self-destruction that is marked by the fragmentation of nuclear DNA. This normal physiological process eliminates DNA-damaged, superfluous, or unwanted cells (as immune cells targeted against the self in the development of self-tolerance), and when stopped (by genetic mutation) may result in uncontrolled cell growth and tumor formation [28, 31]. During apoptosis, a cell triggers a process that will allow it to "commit suicide." In this process, the cell undergoes a reduction in size as its cellular components break down and condense. This process is mediated by proteolytic enzymes called caspases. Those enzymes are present in all cells as procaspases, as inactive precursors. By cleavage by other caspases they are usually activated, as a proteolytic caspase cascade. This activation signal is initiated by death signals, which cause intracellular adaptor molecules to aggregate and activate procaspases. Caspase activation is regulated by members of the Bcl-2 and IAP protein families.

In apoptotic cells, the phospholipid membrane of phosphatidylserine is translocated from the inner to outer leaflet of the plasma membrane [27, 28, 31]. Exposing phosphatidylserine to the external cellular environment can be detected by Annexin V that is a $Ca2^+$-dependent phospholipid-binding protein (35–36 kDa). Annexin V has high affinity and binds PS to cells that expose PS. Annexin V may be conjugated to fluorochromes including BD Horizon™ V450 from BD Biosciences or Pacific Blue from

BioLegend and is used as a sensitive probe for flow cytometric analysis of apoptotic cells at an earlier stage based on nuclear changes and DNA fragmentation [27, 28]. This staining precedes the loss of membrane integrity which accompanies the latest stages of cell death resulting from apoptotic or from necrotic processes. Annexin V V450 or Pacific Blue is typically used in conjunction with a vital dye such as propidium iodide (PI) or 7-amino-actinomycin (7-AAD) to allow them to identify early apoptotic cells (PI^-, PacBlue Annexin V^+). Viable cells with intact membranes exclude PI (PI^-, PacBlue Annexin V^-), whereas the membranes of dead are permeable to PI (PI^+, PacBlue Annexin V^-) or damaged cells or late apoptotic cells (PI^+, PacBlue Annexin V^+). The movement of cells through these three stages suggests apoptosis [27, 28].

There are also several kits available that contain recombinant annexin V conjugated to one of the fluorophores (FITC, Alexa Fluor® 488 dye) to provide the maximum sensitivity. The kit includes a ready-to-use solution of the red-fluorescent PI nucleic acid-binding dye. PI is impermeable to live cells but stains late apoptotic and dead cells with red fluorescence, binding tightly to the nucleic acids in the cell. After staining a cell population with Annexin V and PI apoptotic cells show green fluorescence, dead cells show red and green fluorescence, and live cells show little or no fluorescence. After cells are stained with Ab specific for extracellular markers they can be stained in a particular buffer for apoptosis (containing Ca^{2+}) with Annexin V conjugated with a fluorochrome.

8.1 Annexin V Staining Protocol [21, 32]

- Cells that were labeled with Ab for surface staining, and with LIVE/DEAD® Fixable Dead Cell dye for UV laser, are not fixed and washed twice with cold FACS buffer by centrifugation at 1,500 rpm ($300 \times g$) for 5 min at 4 °C.
- Then carefully resuspend the cells in Annexin V-binding buffer (cat # 422201) at a concentration of 1×10^6 cells/ml.
- Transfer 100 μl of cell suspension in 5 ml test tube.
- Add 5 μl of Pacific Blue™ Annexin V.
- Gently vortex the cells and incubate for 15 min at RT (25 °C) in the dark.
- Add 400 μl of Annexin V-binding buffer (cat # 422201) to each tube.
- Analyze by flow cytometry.

9 Conclusions

Intracellular cytokine detection by flow cytometry has emerged as the premier technique for studying cytokine production at the single-cell level. It detects the production and accumulation of cytokines within the endoplasmic reticulum after cell stimulation, allowing direct T cell subsets determination. Also T cell polarization and plasticity can be detected using a combination of flow cytometry protocols for immunophenotyping using cell surface markers or MHC tetra/pentamers to identify antigen-specific response, making it a flexible and versatile method [33–37]. This capability, combined with the high throughput inherent in the instrumentation, gives intracellular cytokine staining an enormous advantage over existing single-cell techniques such as ELISPOT, limiting dilution, and T cell cloning.

Understanding the complexity of CTL function along with expression of key transcription factors, further defines these cells [35, 38, 39]. All of these aspects lead to a better understanding of T cell immunology, achieved by single-cell analysis using flow cytometry [37–41].

References

1. Williams MA, Bevan MJ (2007) Effector and memory CTL differentiation. Annu Rev Immunol 25:171–192, doi: 0.1146/annurev.immunol.25.022106.141548
2. Kurtulus S, Tripathi P, Hildeman DA (2012) Protecting and rescuing the effectors: roles of differentiation and survival in the control of memory T cell development. Front Immunol 3:404. doi:10.3389/fimmu. 2012. 00404, Epub 2013 Jan 23
3. Kahan BD (2003) Individuality: the barrier to optimal immunosuppression. Nat Rev Immunol 3:831–838. doi:10.1038/nri1204
4. Kapsenberg ML (2003) Dendritic-cell control of pathogen-driven T-cell polarization. Nat Rev Immunol 3:984–993
5. McElroy DS, Badstibner AM, D'Orazio SEF (2007) Use of the CD107 mobilization assay reveals that cytotoxic T lymphocytes with novel MHC-Ib restriction are activated during Listeria monocytogenes infection. J Immunol Methods 328(1–2):45–52
6. Betts MR, Brenchley JM, Price DA, De Rosa SC, Douek DC, Roederer M, Koup RA (2003) Sensitive and viable identification of antigen-specific CD8+ T cells by a flow cytometric assay for degranulation. J Immunol Methods 281(1–2):65–78
7. Popescu I, Macedo C, Abu-Elmagd K, Shapiro R, Hua Y, Thomson AW, Morelli AE, Storkus WJ, Metes D (2007) EBV-specific CD8+ T cell reactivation in transplant patients results in expansion of CD8+ type-1 regulatory T cells. Am J Transplant 7(5):1215–1223, Epub 2007 Feb 27
8. Sarkar S, Kalia V, Haining WN, Konieczny BT, Subramaniam S, Ahmed R (2008) Functional and genomic profiling of effector CD8 T cell subsets with distinct memory fates. J Exp Med 205(3):625–640.doi:10.1084/jem.20071641, Epub 2008 Mar 3
9. Maecker HT, Frey T, Nomura L, Trotter J (2004) Selecting fluorochrome conjugates for maximum sensitivity. Cytometry A 62:169
10. Maecker HT, Trotter J (2006) Flow cytometry controls, instrument setup, and the determination of positivity. Cytometry A 69:1037
11. Roederer M (2008) How many events is enough? Are you positive? Cytometry A 73: 384–385
12. Crowther EJ, Stall A, Bishop JE, Sasaki D (2002) A setup system for compensation: BD CompBeads plus BD FACSDiva software Presented at ISAC XXI, San Diego, *CA, 4–9 May* Poster No. 57644
13. BD™CompBead and BD™CompBead Plus compensation particles, BD Biiosciences website: http://www.bdbiosciences.com/external_files/pm/doc/mkt_lit/salesSheets/live/web_enabled/23-13303-01.pdf
14. Molecular Probes Invitrogen web site: http://products.invitrogen.com/ivgn/product/L23105
15. Pipeling MR, Popescu ID, Orens JB, Pilewski JM, McDyer JF (2013) Dynamic changes in dominant antigen responses following primary CMV infection in lung transplant recipients. J Heart Lung Transplant 32(4):S298
16. BD Biosciences web site tutorial protocol: http://www.bdbiosciences.com/resources/flowcytometry/index.jsp
17. Pipeling MR, West EE, Osborne CM, Whitlock AB, Dropulic LK, Willett MH, Forman M, Valsamakis A, Orens JB, Moller DR, Lechtzin

N, Migueles SA, Connors M, McDyer JF (2008) Differential CMV-specific CD8+ effector T cell responses in the lung allograft predominate over the blood during human primary infection. J Immunol 181(1):546–556

18. Gordy C et al (2011) Regulation of steady-state neutrophil homeostasis by macrophages. Blood 117:618
19. Jia W et al (2011) Autophagy regulates endoplasmic reticulum homeostasis and calcium mobilization in T lymphocytes. J Immunol 186:5313
20. Parish CR (1999) Cancer immunotherapy: the past, the present and the future. Immunol Cell Biol 77(6):499–508
21. BioLegend website for Annexin V Pacific Blue protocol: http://www.biolegend.com/pacific-blue-annexin-v-5476.html
22. Hoegh-Petersen M, Roa L, Liu Y, Zhou F, Ugarte-Torres A, Louie P, Fonseca K, Khan F, Russell JA, Storek J (2012) Low cytomegalovirus-specific T-cell counts at reactivation are associated with progression to high-level viremia or disease in seropositive recipients of hematopoietic cell grafts from seropositive but not seronegative donors. Cytotherapy 14(2):194–204. doi:10.3109/14653249.2011.634402, Epub 2011 Dec 7
23. Wiesmayr S, Webber SA, Macedo C, Popescu I, Smith L, Luce J, Metes D (2012) Decreased NKp46 and NKG2D and elevated PD-1 are associated with altered NK-cell function in pediatric transplant patients with PTLD. Eur J Immunol 42(2):541–550. doi:10.1002/eji.201141832. Epub 2011 Dec 16
24. Macedo C, Orkis EA, Popescu I, Elinoff BD, Zeevi A, Shapiro R, Lakkis FG, Metes D (2009) Contribution of naïve and memory T-cell populations to the human alloimmune response. Am J Transplant 9(9):2057–2066. doi:10.1111/j.1600-6143.2009.02742.x, Epub 2009 Jul 16
25. Akulian JA, Pipeling MR, John ER, Orens JB, Lechtzin N, McDyer JF (2013) High-quality CMV-specific CD4+ memory is enriched in the lung allograft and is associated with mucosal viral control. Am J Transplant 13:146–156
26. Roederer M (2011) SPICE: exploration and analysis of post-cytometric complex multivariate datasets. Cytometry A 79(2011-01-01):167–174
27. Parish CR, et al. (2009) Use of the intracellular fluorescent dye CFSE to monitor lymphocyte migration and proliferation. Curr Protoc Immunol Unit 4.9
28. Miller MJ et al (2002) Two-photon imaging of lymphocyte motility and antigen response in intact lymph node. Science 296:1869
29. Jung T, Schauer U, Heusser C, Neumann C, Rieger C (1993) Detection of intracellular cytokines by flow cytometry. J Immunol Methods 159(1–2):197–207
30. Foster B, Prussin C (2012) Current protocols in immunology. Wiley, New York, NY), Unit 6.24; (NIAID, NIH Bethesda MD)
31. Alberts B, Johnson A, Lewis J et al (2002) Molecular biology of the cell, 4th edn. Garland Science, New York
32. BD website for Annexin V V500 methods: http://www.bdbiosciences.com/external_files/pm/doc/tds/human/live/web_enabled/561501.pdf
33. Maeckerlab Weblog. http://maeckerlab.typepad.com/maeckerlab_weblog/2006/05/detecting_cd107.html
34. Ramaswami B, Popescu I, Macedo C, Luo C, Shapiro R, Metes D, Chalasani G, Randhawa PS (2011) The Polyomavirus BK large T-antigen-derived peptide elicits an HLA-DR promiscuous and polyfunctional $CD4^+$ T-cell response. Clin Vaccine Immunol 18(5):815–824. doi:10.1128/CVI.00487-10, Epub 2011 Mar 2
35. Ramaswami B, Popescu I, Macedo C, Metes D, Bueno M, Zeevi A, Shapiro R, Viscidi R, Randhawa PS (2009) HLA-A01-, -A03-, and -A024-binding nanomeric epitopes in polyomavirus BK large T antigen. Hum Immunol 70(9):722–728. doi:10.1016/j.humimm.2009.05.003, Epub 2009 May 14
36. Zhu J, Yamane H, Paul WE (2010) Differentiation of effector CD4 T cell populations. Annu Rev Immunol 28:445–489
37. Zhou L, Chong MM, Littman DR (2009) Plasticity of CD4+ T cell lineage differentiation. Immunity 30:646–655
38. Chatenoud L, Bach JF (2006) Adaptive human regulatory T cells: myth or reality? J Clin Invest 116:2325–2327
39. Mitchell P, Afzali B, Lombardi G, Lechler RI (2009) The T helper 17-regulatory T cell axis in transplant rejection and tolerance. Curr Opin Organ Transplant 14:326–331
40. Chang SH, Dong C (2009) IL-17 F: regulation, signaling and function in inflammation. Cytokine 46:7–11
41. Pearce EL, Mullen AC, Martins GA, Krawczyk CM, Hutchins AS, Zediak VP, Banica M, DiCioccio CB, Gross DA, Mao CA, Shen H, Cereb N, Yang SY, Lindsten T, Rossant J, Hunter CA, Reiner SL (2003) Control of effector CD8+ T cell function by the transcription factor Eomesodermin. Science 302(5647):1041–1043

Chapter 4

Intracellular Signaling of CTLs

Sharon Natasha Cox

Abstract

Extracellular signals are transmitted to intracellular targets thanks to a complex network of interacting proteins that regulate a large number of cellular processes. The signaling mechanisms that occur in CTLs are initiated by T cell receptors (TCRs) that recognize antigens presented in the groove of class I histocompatibility (MHC) molecules of target cells. The strength of this interaction and the consequent activation of intracellular mechanisms determine the fate of the developing T cells. The intracellular mediators of activation can be easily detected using a classical methodology such as western blot. Here we describe this technique bearing particular attention to these mediators using SNAP i.d., a newly developed protein detection system.

Key words CTL intracellular signaling, Protein phosphorylation, SDS-polyacrylamide gel electrophoresis, SNAP i.d. immunoblotting

1 Introduction

Signal transduction from the extracellular space to cytoplasmic molecules is initiated by T cell receptors (TCRs) that recognize antigens presented on class I histocompatibility (MHC) complex of target cells. The TCR ligands are binary proteins containing an MHC moiety and a peptide antigen, termed peptide-MHC or pMHC. The strength of TCR-pMHC interactions determines the fate of the developing T cells [1]; weak interactions exert a positive selection (clonal expansion) and maturation, while strong interactions result in negative selection and T cell death. These processes implicate the differential activation of regulatory molecules in the cytoplasm or in the nucleus and initiation of proliferation or cell death. CTLs are derived from activated naive $CD8^+$ cells, proliferate after activation, and can expand their number a thousand times at the peak of a primary immune response. Destruction of pathogenic cells by CTL is obtained prior to cell contact with the target cell and Ag recognition, thus initiating the release of cytolytic granules into the immunological synapse. The major pathways

Elena Ranieri (ed.), *Cytotoxic T-Cells: Methods and Protocols*, Methods in Molecular Biology, vol. 1186,
DOI 10.1007/978-1-4939-1158-5_4,

activated in CTLs by the TCR-pMHC interaction are on one hand the $Ca2^{+}$-dependent perforin/granzyme-mediated apoptosis, and on the other $Ca2^{+}$-independent Fas ligand/Fas-mediated apoptosis. The interaction induces the production of several second messengers that convey the signal to the cytoplasm from the cell surface. The signal transduction that leads to degranulation takes place in a relatively short time scale and does not require new gene expression. After TCR activation various intracellular events and signaling proteins are activated such as phosphatidylinositol 3-kinase (PI3K) [2], mitogen-activated protein kinase (MAPK), and protein kinase C (PKC) [3], and the protein activation can be evaluated easily by Western blotting. At first both Lck and Fyn, the predominant *src* family kinase, are activated upon TCR activation and are central to the initiation of TCR signaling pathways; their activated form, in turn, activates ZAP-70 [4]. These proteins can be detected by immunoblotting with specific p56lck (Lck) and p59fyn antibodies important in evaluating T cell activation differentiation, tolerance, and anergy [5]. A transmembrane adaptor called linker for activated T cells (LAT) is activated through ZAP-70 and plays an essential role in bridging the TCR engagement to downstream signaling events such as calcium mobilization and Ras-Erk activation. LAT, on one hand, binds directly to GADS and phospholipase C-1 (PLC-γ1) and serves as a docking protein for the complex Shc-Grb2-SOS as well as indirectly associates with SLP-76, Vav, and other proximal TCR-signaling components [6]. PLC-γ1 generates inositol triphosphate (IP3) and diacylglycerol (DAG) as second messengers to trigger Ca^{++} mobilization and protein kinase θ (PKCθ) activation, respectively. Phosphoinositol 3-kinase (PI3K) activation is also important for CTL signaling leading to perforin/granzyme-mediated apoptosis, but not Fas ligand-mediated killing [7]. Furthermore, PI3K activation is not required for the process of degranulation per se, but its activation is fundamental for ERK activation [2].

Once we have obtained purified CTLs using positive or negative selection techniques, as described in the previous chapter, these cells can be harvested and protein extracts can be obtained using detergents. After quantization of the proteins these will be resolved on sodium dodecyl sulfate (SDS) polyacrylamide gels and then transferred electrophoretically to adsorbent membranes such as polyvinylidene difluoride (PVDF). A faster method for protein immunodetection will be described here using the instrument SNAP i.d. At this point we will be able to detect even small concentrations of proteins in a quicker time and in a very versatile way.

1.1 Preparation of Protein Extracts from CTLs with RIPA Buffer

This phase of the protocol consents the resuspension of the cells in a RIPA (radio-immunoprecipitation assay) buffer that contain detergents. These alter the integrity of cell membranes, thereby facilitating lysis of cells and extraction of soluble proteins. As soon as lysis occurs, proteolysis, dephosphorylation, and denaturation begin.

Phosphorylation of a protein is a reversible protein posttranslational modification. Protein kinases catalyze the transfer of the negatively charged γ-phosphate group from ATP to a hydroxyl side chain of serine, threonine, or tyrosine residues of the protein, changing the protein's conformation and activity; this activated status can be easily detected by specific antibodies with Western blot. The reverse reaction, phosphate removal from the protein, or dephosphorylation is performed by protein phosphatases and should be avoided to evaluate correctly the activation status of the protein; this can be prevented supplementing the buffer with fresh phosphatase inhibitors. Furthermore, protease inhibitors should also be added to avoid proteolysis and these events can be slowed down tremendously if samples are kept on ice or at 4 °C at all times. The RIPA buffer described in this protocol is without sodium deoxycholate and SDS because some protein kinases and other enzymes may be sensitive to these components of the standard RIPA buffer, resulting in decreased activity. We can also add 1 % of *n*-dodecyl β-D-maltoside to the RIPA buffer that is known to solubilize better detergent-insoluble membrane fractions since this detergent has dual-hydrophobic/hydrophilic properties that facilitate lipid displacement and provide a lipid-like environment for membrane proteins [8].

1.2 Determination of Protein Concentration

Samples prepared with RIPA buffer can be easily quantified with the Bradford protein assay. The quantification is needed in order to load the same amount of protein on the same SDS-PAGE. An accurate protein concentration of each sample can be obtained when determined analytically with this method so that identical amounts of proteins from the different samples can be compared, and thus the relative amount of specific proteins in each sample can be compared accurately. If samples are compared based on cell number, differences of up to 20 % in the amount of protein may result. Such differences may cause even larger ones in the following steps when phosphorylation is assessed immunologically. The Bradford protein assay uses Coomassie blue G-250 reagent. Without protein, the solution is acidic and is red–brown; when the protein binds, the pKa of the dye shifts causing the dye to become blue. The dye is then measured at 595 nm with a spectrophotometer. Generally, more protein in a sample the higher the absorbance. The linear concentration range is 0.125–1 mg/ml of protein, using BSA (bovine serum albumin) as the standard protein. Protein concentrations are estimated by reference to absorbance obtained from a series of standard protein dilutions, which are assayed alongside the unknown samples (Table 1).

1.3 SDS-Polyacrylamide Gel Electrophoresis (SDS-PAGE) and Western Blotting (Protein Blotting)

SDS-polyacrylamide gel electrophoresis (SDS-PAGE) and Western blotting (protein blotting) is a well-known technique to detect and characterize proteins. Sodium dodecyl sulfate (SDS) is a detergent that can dissolve hydrophobic molecules and solubilize proteins reducing them to their primary structure and at the same time the sulfate group confers proteins a negative charge making them

Table 1
Preparation of a six-point standard curve

Eppendorf tube	1	2	3	4	5	6
BSA concentration (mg/ml)	0	0.1	0.3	0.5	0.8	1
BSA (μl)	0	10	30	50	80	100
H_2O (μl)	50	90	70	50	20	0

migrate towards the positive pole when placed in an electric field. The polyacrylamide gel, on the other hand, consists of acrylamide and bisacrylamide that can be added at different ratios; in particular, we use the 29:1 ratio.

Two gels are actually used; the top gel, called the stacking gel, is slightly acidic (pH 6.8) and has a low acrylamide concentration that makes a porous gel that is needed to pack up the proteins and make sharp defined bands. The lower gel, called the separating or the resolving gel, is more basic (pH 8.8), and has a higher polyacrylamide content. The acrylamide concentration of this gel generally ranges from 7.5 to 20 %. Lower percentage gels are better for resolving very-high-molecular-weight molecules, while higher percentages are needed to resolve smaller proteins. Proteins resolved on SDS gels are then transferred electrophoretically to adsorbent membranes such as nitrocellulose or PVDF membranes.

1.4 Immunodetection Protocol Using SNAP i.d

The SNAP i.d. Protein Detection System is a new method for immunodetection that applies a vacuum to actively drive reagents through the membrane. This methodology is much quicker and gives equal or better signal-to-noise ratios compared to the standard conventional Western blotting where diffusion is the primary means of reagent transport. The difference is that the blocking step takes only 20″ and the primary and secondary antibody incubation steps are reduced to only 10 min.

We use the same amount of primary and secondary antibodies used in standard immunodetection, but in, respectively, 1/3–1/5 the volume of antibody at a three- to fivefold higher concentration (Table 2).

Generally, for primary and secondary antibodies we multiply, respectively, by three and five the concentration suggested by the antibody specification sheet.

This method seems to be very versatile since we can perform up to six different incubation steps contemporarily using the triple wells. In fact if we separate the protein marker properly we have the possibility to cut the PVDF membrane in three pieces in order to detect proteins at different molecular weights contemporarily. For example, we are able to detect anti-PLCγ1 at 155 KDa, anti-Akt at 60 kDa, and anti-ERK1/2 at 42–44 kDa if we cut the membrane as shown in Fig. 1.

Table 2
Antibody optimization guidelines

	Standard immunodetection	SNAP i.d. system	Standard immunodetection	SNAP i.d. system
	Primary antibody	**Primary antibody**	**Secondary antibody**	**Secondary antibody**
Ab stock concentration	1 mg/ml	1 mg/ml	1 mg/ml	1 mg/ml
Volume of Ab used	10 ml	3 ml	50 ml	10 ml
Final Ab dilution	1:10,000 (0.1 μg/ml)	1:3,333 (0.33 μg/ml)	1:50,000 (0.02 μg/ml)	1:10,000 (0.1 μg/ml)
Mass of antibody used	0.1 μg/ml × 10 ml = 1 μg	0.33 μg/ml × 3 ml = 1 μg	0.02 μg/ml × 50 ml = 1 μg	0.1 μg/ml × 10 ml = 1 μg

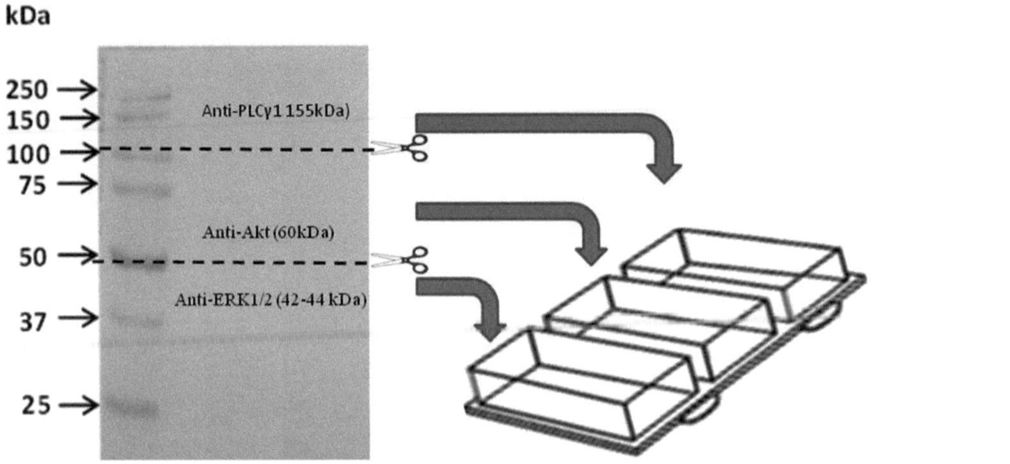

Fig. 1 Western blot showing Precision Plus Protein Dual Color Marker from BIORAD resolved using 10 % in-house SDS-PAGE. The PVDF membrane can be cut into three pieces as shown to detect three different proteins at three different molecular weights contemporarily. For example, we are able to detect anti-PLCγ1 at 155 KDa, anti-Akt at 60 kDa, and anti-ERK1/2 at 42–44 kDa contemporarily using the triple-well blot holder of the SNAP i.d.

2 Materials

All solutions must be prepared with ultrapure water (obtained purifying deionized water at a sensitivity of 18.2 MΩ at 25 °C) and analytical grade reagents. Prepare and store all reagents at room temperature (unless indicated otherwise). All waste disposal regulations must be followed when disposing waste materials.

2.1 Preparation of Protein Extracts from CTLs with RIPA Buffer

1. RIPA buffer (must be kept at 4 °C):
2. Tris–HCl pH 7.4, 20 mM.
3. NaCl 150 mM.
4. Ethylenediaminetetraacetic acid (EDTA# E9884) 5 mM.
5. Sodium orthovanadate 1 mM (Na_3VO_4, Sigma-Aldrich #S6508).
6. NP-40 1.5 % (Tergitol, Sigma-Aldrich).
7. Before using the RIPA buffer add protease inhibitors; for every ml add aprotinin, leupeptin, and pepstatin by adding 1 μl of each at an initial concentration of 10 mg/ml and phosphatase inhibitor cocktail (100×, Pierce #78420).
8. *n*-Dodecyl β-D-maltoside (Sigma-Aldrich, #D4641).
9. Refrigerated centrifuge.
10. Precooled 1.5 ml Eppendorf tubes.

2.2 Determination of Protein Concentration

1. Bio-Rad Protein Assay Kit II (450 ml dye reagent concentrate, bovine serum albumin (BSA) standard, BIORAD #500-0002).
2. Disposable cuvettes (BIORAD #223-9955).
3. Spectrophotometer set at 595.

2.3 SDS-Polyacrylamide Gel Electrophoresis (SDS-PAGE) and Western Blotting (Protein Blotting)

1. Mini PROTEAN® 3 System (BIORAD).
2. 30 % Acrylamide/Bis Solution (#161-0157, BIORAD).
3. Lower (separating) buffer: 1.5 M Tris–HCl, 0.4 % SDS, pH 8.8.
4. Upper (stacking) buffer: 0.5 M Tris–HCl, 0.4 % SDS, pH 6.8.
5. 20 % Ammonium persulfate (APS, GIBCO #15703, freshly prepared in water).
6. 10 % Sodium dodecyl sulfate (SDS, prepared in water).
7. Tetramethylethylenediamine (TEMED, BIORAD #161-0801).
8. 5/10 ml Syringe.
9. Sample buffer (4× concentrated): 200 mM Tris–HCl pH 6.8, 40 % glycerol, 10 % SDS, 0.2 %.
10. Bromophenol blue.
11. Running buffer 10×: 25 mM Tris base (Sigma-Aldrich, #T1503), 192 mM glycine (Sigma-Aldrich, #G8898), 0.1 % SDS, pH 8.3.
12. Protein marker: Precision Plus Protein™ Dual Color Standards (BIORAD #161-0374).
13. Rotary shaker.
14. Mini Trans-Blot® Cell (BIORAD).
15. Transfer buffer 10×: 30.0 g Tris base (Sigma-Aldrich, #T1503), 144 g Glycine (Sigma-Aldrich, #G8898).
16. Transfer apparatus.
17. PVDF membrane (Millipore, #IPVH00010).
18. 3 MM Whatman paper.

2.4 Preparation, Blot Assembly, and Immunodetection Protocol Using SNAP i.d.

1. Vacuum source: Pump or other uniform vacuum sources that generate a minimum pressure of 410 millibar (12 in. Hg) and 34 l/min.
2. Vacuum flask (capacity 1 l or more) with stopper.
3. Vacuum tubing to connect vacuum flask to vacuum source.
4. Spacer.
5. Forceps.
6. Blot holders: Single Blot Holder (Millipore #WBAVDBH01), Double Blot Holder (Millipore #WBAVDBH02), Triple Blot Holder (Millipore #WBAVDBH03).
7. Blot roller.
8. Washing buffer: PBS, 0.1 % Tween-20 (Sigma-Aldrich, #P1379).
9. Blocking buffer: PBS, 0.1 % Tween-20, 1 % bovine serum albumin (BSA, Sigma-Aldrich, #A8022).

10. Primary antibody solution diluted in antibody diluents: T-PBS, 0.1 % Tween-20, 0.5 % BSA.
11. Secondary antibody solution diluted in antibody diluents: T-PBS, 0.1 % Tween-20, 0.5 % BSA.

3 Methods

3.1 Preparation of Protein Extracts from CTLs with RIPA Buffer

1. Purified CTLs should be washed in PBS and spun down at 300 × *g* for 5′ at 4 °C (*see* **Note 1**).
2. The supernatant must be carefully and completely removed by gently inverting the falcon on blotting paper.
3. Flick the tube to break up the cell pellet.
4. Add 1 μl of each of the protease inhibitors (aprotinin, leupeptin, and pepstatin) and 10 μl phosphatase inhibitors when investigating phosphorylation events for every ml of RIPA buffer (*see* **Note 2**).
5. Add 100 μl of RIPA buffer on the resuspended cells.
6. Vortex periodically for 60″ at least three times.
7. Transfer to precooled appropriately labeled Eppendorf tubes, and leave on ice for 30′.
8. Spin the samples at 1,500 × *g* for 10 min at 4 °C, to pellet nuclei.
9. Transfer supernatant to new, labeled, precooled Eppendorf tubes and determine protein concentrations (*see* **Note 3**).

3.2 Determination of Protein Concentration

1. Dilute the BIORAD assay dye 1:5 with, mix well, and filter through the Whatman filter paper to remove particulates (*see* **Note 4**).
2. Prepare enough BIORAD assay dye for the standard curve and the unknown protein samples and the blank. Assay the protein standards and protein solutions in duplicate.
3. Reconstitute the lyophilized BSA with deionized water to a final concentration of 1 mg/ml and store frozen in 1 ml aliquots for quick use.
4. Prepare a range of protein standards diluting the BSA stock solution (1 mg/ml) with water as indicated in Table 1.
5. Samples should also be diluted if the concentration of the sample is not found in the linear range of the assay (*see* **Note 5**).
6. Add 1 ml of the diluted BIORAD assay dye directly in the cuvette.
7. Using a fresh tip for each sample, pipet 20 μl of each standard into the appropriate cuvette (20 μl of RIPA for "blank"). Then pipet 20 μl of each protein solution into the appropriate cuvette.

8. Cover each cuvette with parafilm and invert each three times to mix.
9. Let stand for 5 min.
10. Place the cuvette in the reader and determine the optical density of the samples at 595 nM.
11. Plot the optical densities of the protein standards against the concentration and calculate by linear regression ($y = ax + b$) the slope (a) and constant (b). Calculate the protein concentrations of the samples by the formula protein conc. (mg/ml) = (a × sample OD − b) × dilution factor.

3.3 SDS-Polyacrylamide Gel Electrophoresis (SDS-PAGE) and Western Blotting (Protein Blotting)

1. Glass plates and spacers should be cleaned with ethanol and completely dried before being assembled.
2. Prepare 10 % polyacrylamide separating gel (10 ml): Mix 3.33 ml of acrylamide mixture, and 3.8 ml water in a disposable falcon, and then add 2.5 ml of lower (separating) buffer, 100 μl SDS.
3. Mix well and add 200 μl APS. Mix and add 20 μl TEMED.
4. Mix the solution and cast the gel. Allow space for stacking the gel and gently overlay with isopropanol (*see* **Note 6**).
5. Allow gel to polymerize (about 10–15 min), rinse out the isopropanol with a squirt bottle containing ultrapure water, and dry with a small strip of 3 MM Whatman paper.
6. Prepare 5 ml of 3 % polyacrylamide stacking gel: 660 μl Acrylamide stock solution, 1.26 ml of upper buffer, 3.0 ml of water, and 50 μl SDS.
7. Mix and add 25 μl APS. Mix well and add 20 μl TEMED.
8. Mix the solution and cast the gel.
9. Insert the 10-well gel comb from one angle to the other, making sure not to create bubbles and allow polymerization (10–15 min).
10. Vertically lift the comb gently, and wash each well with a 5/10 ml syringe (*see* **Note 7**).
11. Prepare samples: Mix 30 μg protein extract with 1:3 of 4× concentrated sample buffer. Boil the samples for 5 min, immediately place on ice for 5 min, and spin down the samples in order to recover the entire condensate.
12. Assemble gel in apparatus, add running buffer to the upper chamber, and watch for leaks.
13. Add buffer to the lower chamber.
14. Load samples; we generally load protein standards in the first and last wells (*see* **Note 8**).
15. Run gel: Connect the wire leads to the power supply. Turn the power supply on and run the gel at 150 V (constant voltage) for about 75 min.

16. End run when the bromophenol-blue dye reaches the bottom, and turn off the power supply.
17. Cut two pieces of 3 MM Whatman papers and the PVDF membrane. The size should be the same as the glass plates used to cast the gels.
18. Activate the PVDF membrane: Immerge the membrane for 1′ in methanol, then 5′ in water, and for at least 5′ in transfer buffer (*see* **Note 9**).
19. Once the dye has reached the end of the gel, take the gel care fully out from between the glass plates.
20. Cut off the stacking gel.
21. Gel and all components of the transfer sandwich should be equilibrated in new transfer buffer for 30′.
22. Assemble the transfer sandwich: Put a wet scotch-bright pad on the black side of the transfer sandwich and add a 3 mm paper on top of it. Put the SDS-gel on the 3 mm paper, put the wet PVDF membrane on the gel, and discard bubbles. Put the other 3 mm paper on the PVDF membrane. Add another wet scotch-bright pad on top of the transfer sandwich, and close the transfer sandwich. Take care not to trap air bubbles between the gel and the other components.
23. Place the transfer sandwich into the transfer apparatus filled with 500 ml of 1× transfer buffer.
24. Close the transfer apparatus, insert it into a container filled with ice, and connect it to the power supply (*200 mA constant current, 60 min*).
25. At the end of the protein transfer, remove the PVDF membrane from the transfer sandwich. Cut a small wedge from the top left side of the marker lane for orientation purposes and to know exactly on which side of the membrane the proteins are spotted.
26. Wash the membrane three times for 5′ with T-PBS on a rotary shaker and proceed to the next step. If desired the process can stop here and the membrane can be dried out and placed in Whatman paper in the fridge at 4 °C until needed.

3.4 Preparation, Blot Assembly, and Immunodetection Protocol Using SNAP i.d.

1. Since immunodetection in the SNAP i.d.® system is performed in a short period of time, blocking, primary and secondary antibody dilutions should be prepared before starting the procedure (Table 3).
2. If the PVDF membrane has been dried out, re-wet the blot with 100 % methanol 1′, and then wash with distilled water for 5′ prior to assembly.
3. Open the blot holder lid taking care not to damage the inner white surface.

Table 3
Blocking, antibody, and wash volumes required

	Single well (7.9 × 8.8 cm)	Double well (4.6 × 8.8 cm)	Triple well (3.2 × 8.8 cm)
Blocking solution volume	30 ml/well	15 ml/well	10 ml/well
Antibody volume	3 ml/well	1.5 ml/well	1 ml/well
Wash buffer* volume	30 ml/well	15 ml/well	10 ml/well

*Tris- or phosphate-buffered saline solutions, supplemented with 0.1% Tween® 20 surfactant

4. Wet the inner white face of the blot holder with a squirt bottle containing ddH_2O, and remove excess liquid using the blot roller (*see* **Note 10**).
5. Position carefully the pre-wet blot membrane in the center of the blot holder with the forceps, ***protein side down***, and remove excess liquid and air bubbles with the blot roller (*see* **Note 11**).
6. Place the spacer on top of the blot making sure to cover all edges and use the blot roller to ensure that all the bubbles are eliminated and that the blot spacer with blot membrane is in complete contact.
7. Close the blot holder firmly at the base of the tab area in order to securely close the lid.
8. Place the blot holder in the system chamber with the well side up and with proteins facing upwards. You must align the blot holder tabs with the notches of the chamber and then close the system lid.
9. Add the appropriate volume of blocking solution (Table 2). In the case of a single well add 30 ml blocking solution; no incubation step is needed and immediately turn on the vacuum using the vacuum control knob.
10. After the wells have completely dried out (10–20 s) turn the vacuum off; at this point it is possible to add the antibody collection tray beneath the blot holder if you desire to recover the primary antibody solution.
11. Apply 3 ml (for single well) of primary antibody evenly and across the surface of the blot holder with a disposable stripette. The vacuum must be off (Table 4).
12. Incubate for 10 min at room temperature. Solution will be absorbed into the blot holder and surface may appear dry. Do not apply vacuum during the 10′ incubation.
13. Turn the vacuum on and wait for 10–20 s to make sure that antibody solution has completely emptied from the blot holder. At this point recover the antibody collection tray if it has been used.

Table 4
Primary antibody dilutions of main proteins involved in intracellular signaling of CTLs in standard immunodetection vs. SNAP i.d. immunodetection

Primary antibody name	Produced by	Cat. no.	Host[b]	Predicted MW (kDa)	Standard Ab dilution	SNAP i.d. Ab dilution
Anti-Akt1/PKBα	Millipore	05-796	Rb	60	1:1,200–1:2,000	1:400
Anti-Fyn	Abcam	AB1881	M	59	1:1,000	1:300
Anti-lck	Abcam	AB3623	Rb	57	1:1,000	1:300
Anti-LAT	Millipore/Upstate	06-807	Rb	36/38	1:1,000	1:300
Anti-p-LAT(y191)	Millipore/Upstate	07-278	Rb	36/38	1:500	1:150
Anti-Zap70 (y315+y319)	Abcam	AB12869	Rb	74.3	1:1,000	1:300
Anti-GADS/grap2	Millipore/Upstate	06-983	Rb	40	1:2,000	1:600
Anti-GRB2	Millipore/Upstate	05-372	M	23–25	1:500	1:150
Anti-SOS	Millipore/Upstate	07-337	Rb	175	1:2,000	1:600
Anti-PLCγ1	Cell Signaling	2822	Rb	155	1:1,000	1:300
Anti-pPLCγ1	Cell Signaling	2821	Rb	155	1:1,000	1:300
Anti-PKCθ	Cell Signaling	12206	Rb	78	1:1,000	1:300
Anti-p-PKCθ (Thr538)	Cell Signaling	9377	Rb	79	1:1,000	1:300
Anti-SLP76/LCP2	Cell Signaling	4958	Rb	76	1:1,000	1:300
Anti-vav1	Millipore/Upstate	07-192	Rb	98	1:500	1:166
Anti-ERK1/2	Cell Signaling	4695	Rb	44/42	1:1,000	1:300
Anti-pERK1/2 (Thr202/Tyr204)	Cell Signaling	4370	Rb	44/42	1 :2,000	1:600
Anti-c-jun	Abcam	AB32137	Rb	36	1:1,000–1:10,000	1:300–1:3,000
Anti-Akt	Cell Signaling	9272	Rb	60	1:1,000	1:300
Anti-p-Akt (Thr308)	Cell Signaling	7271	Rb	60	1:1,000	1:300
Anti-phospho-Akt (Ser473)	Millipore	05-1003	M	60	1:2,000	1:600
Anti-β actin	Sigma	A1978	M	42	1:4,000–1 2,000	1:1,300–1:600

[b] Host species in which the antibody was produced; M= Mouse, Rb = Rabbit

Table 5
Examples of secondary antibody dilution in standard immunodetection vs. SNAP i.d. immunodetection (Millipore)

Secondary antibody[a]	Host[b]	Cat. no.	Standard Ab dilution	SNAP i.d. Ab dilution
Anti-mouse IgG	Gt	AP124P	1:50,000	1:10,000
Anti-rabbit IgG	Gt	AP132P	1:200,000	1:30,000
Anti-sheep IgG	Rb	AP147P	1:50,000	1:20,000
Anti-goat IgG	Rb	AP106P	1:80,000	1:10,000

[a] Horseradish peroxidase conjugate
[b] Host species in which the antibody was produced; Gt = Goat, Rb = Rabbit

14. With vacuum running continuously, add 30 ml of wash buffer. Repeat the washing step two more times (total of three washes). When the frame is completely empty, *turn vacuum off.*
15. Apply 3 ml of secondary antibody evenly across the blot holder surface. Incubate for 10 min at room temperature with vacuum off (Table 5). Again, solution will be absorbed into the blot holder and surface may appear dry.
16. Incubate for 10 min at room temperature. Solution will be absorbed into the blot holder and surface may appear dry. Do not apply vacuum during the 10′ incubation.
17. Turn the vacuum on and wait for 10–20 s to make sure that antibody solution has completely emptied from the blot holder. At this point recover the antibody collection tray if it has been used.
18. With vacuum running continuously, add 30 ml of wash buffer. Repeat the washing step two more times (total of three washes). When the frame is completely empty, *turn vacuum off.*
19. Remove blot holder from the system, place it on the bench with the well side down, open the lid with forceps, and remove and discard the spacer. Remove blot and incubate with the appropriate HRP detection reagent.

4 Notes

1. The culture medium must be washed away completely because some components (fetal calf serum, etc.) may interfere with protein detection.
2. Add 1 % of dodecyl β-D-maltoside if you intend to evaluate proteins that are present in the inner leaflet of the plasma

membrane and in lipid raffs, because this detergent efficiently solubilizes lipid rafts.

3. The protein concentration of each sample should be determined so that identical amounts of proteins from the different samples can be loaded onto SDS-polyacrylamide gels.
4. Remove the Bradford reagent from 4 °C storage and let it warm to ambient temperature.
5. For example, if the unknown sample is expected to have a concentration of 5 mg/ml and the linear range of your assay is 0.1–1 mg/ml, then the unknown sample needs to be diluted tenfold so that it is in the middle of the linear range.
6. This overlay with isopropanol helps to level the gel solution and limits the contact with atmospheric oxygen (which inhibits acrylamide polymerization).
7. If the gel is to be used the next day, do not remove the comb and place the gel on three-layer tissue paper soaked with running buffer and wrapped completely with aluminum foil.
8. Once the proteins are electrotransferred we cut the PVDF membrane at a certain kDa more precisely from one end to the other based on the migration of Precision Plus Protein™ Dual Color Standards positioned in the first and last wells.
9. The activation should be done on a rotary shaker in order to be sure to activate the membrane uniformly.
10. If using double- or triple-well blot holder, the unused wells should also be wet.
11. The wedge on the top left side of the marker lane can be used for orientation purposes.

Acknowledgments

This work was supported by grants from the MiUR (PON-REC ONEV 134/2011; FIRB RBAP11B2SX) and Regione Puglia (BISIMANE project, H31D08000030007).

References

1. Beal AM, Anikeeva N, Varma R, Cameron TO, Vasiliver-Shamis G, Norris PJ, Dustin ML, Sykulev Y (2009) Kinetics of early T cell receptor signaling regulate the pathway of lytic granule delivery to the secretory domain. Immunity 31:632–642
2. Robertson LK, Mireau LR, Ostergaard HL (2005) A role for phosphatidylinositol 3-kinase in TCR-stimulated ERK activation leading to paxillin phosphorylation and CTL degranulation. J Immunol 175:8138–8145
3. Pardo J, Buferne M, Martínez-Lorenzo MJ, Naval J, Schmitt-Verhulst AM, Boyer C, Anel A (2003) Differential implication of protein kinase C isoforms in cytotoxic T lymphocyte degranulation and TCR-induced Fas ligand expression. Int Immunol 15:1441–1450
4. Salmond RJ, Filby A, Qureshi I, Caserta S, Zamoyska R (2009) T-cell receptor proximal signaling via the Src-family kinases, Lck and Fyn, influences T-cell activation, differentiation, and tolerance. Immunol Rev 228:9–22

5. Welke J, Zavazava N (2002) P59(fyn) is upregulated in anergic CD8+ T cells. Hum Immunol 63:834–843
6. Jordan MS, Singer AL, Koretzky GA (2003) Adaptors as central mediators of signal transduction in immune cells. Nat Immunol 4:110–116
7. Fuller CL, Ravichandran KS, Braciale VL (1999) Phosphatidylinositol 3-kinase-dependent and -independent cytolytic effector functions. J Immunol 162:6337–6340
8. Falahati R, Leitenberg D et al (2007) Changes in the role of the CD45 protein tyrosine phosphatase in regulating Lck tyrosine phosphorylation during thymic development. J Immunol 178:2056–2064

Chapter 5

Monitoring Antigen-Specific T Cell Responses Using Real-Time PCR

Devin B. Lowe, Jennifer L. Taylor, and Walter J. Storkus

Abstract

Flow cytometry-, ELISA-, and ELISpot-based in vitro assays have played important roles in assessing the frequencies and functional competence of antigen-specific T cells in the setting of infectious disease and cancer. Such methods have helped in the development of antigen-specific vaccines for human disease prevention/treatment and have also served as a foundation for the monitoring of patients' immune responsiveness based on antigen-induced T cell expression of effector molecules (such as cytokines, chemokines, or proteins associated with cytolysis) as a consequence of therapeutic intervention.

The following method outlines a protocol employing quantitative real-time PCR (qRT-PCR) with SYBR® green technology to examine antigen-specific CD8⁺ T cell responses based on their rapid up-regulation of IFN-γ mRNA transcription following in vitro stimulation with peptide (antigen)-loaded, autologous peripheral blood mononuclear cells (PBMCs). The advantages of the current qRT-PCR approach over protein-based detection methods include the sensitivity to distinguish resident CD8⁺ T cell responses against multiple antigens without the need to artificially pre-expand T cell numbers ex vivo, as is commonly required for the latter in vitro assay systems. Following qRT-PCR setup and run, the level of human IFN-γ transcript is normalized to CD8 transcript expression level, with data reported as the relative fold change in this index versus a patient-matched PBMC sample stimulated with a negative control peptide (e.g., HIV NEF).

Key words Quantitative real-time PCR, CD8⁺ T cell, Peptide-restricted response, Cancer

1 Introduction

Over the past several decades, a number of immunologic techniques have been used to document and quantitate antigen-specific responses among CD8⁺ T cells harvested from patients with cancer [1]. These include in vitro sensitization (IVS) procedures in which T cells are first preincubated with antigens for typically 5–7 days, prior to the measurement of their "specific" production/secretion of effector cytokines (e.g., interleukin (IL)-2, interferon (IFN)-γ, tumor necrosis factor (TNF)-α, among others) by means of enzyme-linked immunosorbent assay [ELISA]) and/or the cytolysis of antigen-expressing target cells, which both provide

Elena Ranieri (ed.), *Cytotoxic T-Cells: Methods and Protocols*, Methods in Molecular Biology, vol. 1186,
DOI 10.1007/978-1-4939-1158-5_5, © Springer Science+Business Media New York 2014

indices of T cell functionality. The enzyme-linked immunosorbent spot (ELISPOT) assay remains a separate but related technique in distinguishing protein expression at the individual T cell level and, thus, it provides information regarding T cell functionality, but also a quantitative index of antigen-specific T cell frequencies in the bulk population. Additionally, flow cytometric methods, incorporating fluorescently labeled MHC class I-peptide multimers (e.g., tetramer and dextramer technologies), allow for the determination of the frequency of T cells reactive against a given MHC class I-presented peptide complex. When combined with procedures that stain for intracellular expression of T cell effector molecules (e.g., cytokines, chemokines, lytic molecules such as perforin and granzyme B, or lytic granule release based on translocation of the CD107 marker to the T cell surface) a quantitative readout of antigen-specific T cell functionality may also be established [2–4].

Unfortunately, for detection of T cell responses that are rare events against a range of low-to-moderate immunogenic antigens, substantial cell (PBMC) yields, and prior IVS may limit the range of specificities that may be investigated and/or necessitate in vitro expansions that may deviate the nature and frequency of analogous responses in vivo [5]. In the following method, we describe a quantitative real-time PCR (qRT-PCR)-based approach to assess peptide-specific, type 1 $CD8^+$ T cell responses based on the quantitation of acute differences in IFN-γ mRNA expression levels in the absence or the presence of antigen-specific stimulation. The strength of this method lies in its ability to rapidly (within 2 h) quantitate a range of antigen-specific T cell responses in a given patient, without prior in vitro manipulations, using a small sample size in comparison to the aforementioned immunologic techniques. Our experience with this method, to date, has involved the analysis of low-frequency $CD8^+$ T cell responses against peptide epitopes derived from antigens differentially expressed by blood vessel cells within the tumor microenvironment in HLA-$A2^+$ patients with renal cell carcinoma (RCC). We envision this technique to be useful in the longitudinal assessment of type 1 T cell response in cancer patients undergoing any form of immunomodulatory therapy, including specific vaccination approaches [5–7]. However, one can also readily envision the application of this qRT-PCR technique of monitoring T cell responsiveness in the settings of infectious disease, autoimmunity, and organ transplantation [8–11].

2 Materials

1. Ficoll-Hypaque density gradient solution (GE Healthcare).
2. Phosphate-buffered saline (PBS).
3. Complete culture medium (CM) (IMDM [Life Technologies] supplemented with 10 % heat-inactivated normal human serum

[Sigma], 10 mmol/l L-glutamine, 100 U/ml penicillin, 100 μg/ml streptomycin, and nonessential amino acids [all from Life Technologies]).

4. RNeasy plus micro Kit (Qiagen).
5. High Capacity RNA-to-cDNA Kit (Life Technologies).
6. SYBR® Green Master Mix (Life Technologies).
7. Human CD8 forward and reverse primers.
8. Human IFN-γ forward and reverse primers.
9. PCR thermocycler.
10. qRT-PCR system.

3 Methods

3.1 Human Peripheral Blood Mononuclear Cell (PBMC) Isolation and Culture Setup

The collection and handling of human blood should be performed in accordance to institutional rules and guidelines. Assume that all blood products contain infectious material.

1. Human whole blood should be transferred from heparinized tubes to a T75 culture flask (do not exceed 50 ml). Blood should be diluted at a 1:2 ratio with PBS, mixed thoroughly, and 30 ml aliquoted into a 50 ml conical tube (*see* **Note 1**).
2. Gently add 12 ml Ficoll-Hypaque to the bottom of the tube so that the diluted blood overlays the density gradient solution.
3. Centrifuge tubes at 800 × *g* for 20 min at room temperature.
4. Carefully aspirate the interphase layer containing the leukocytes without disturbing the erythrocyte pellet at the bottom of the tube and transfer to a new 50 ml conical tube (*see* **Note 2**).
5. Add PBS up to 50 ml, mix sufficiently, and centrifuge at 500 × *g* for 10 min at 4 °C.
6. Decant the supernatant, resuspend the leukocyte cell pellet in 5 ml PBS, and repeat **steps 5** and **6** for a total of two wash steps.
7. Resuspend the PBMCs in CM and adjust to 2.7×10^6 cells/ml.
8. Place 150 μl into each well of a 96-well U-bottom plate depending on the number of desired replicates and peptides to be analyzed (*see* **Note 3**).

3.2 PBMC Peptide Stimulation

Peptides are solubilized in DMSO at a concentration of 10 mg/ml and placed at −20 °C for long-term storage. Temporary peptide storage (<1 month) is recommended at 4 °C.

1. Pipette 50 μl of CM containing a desired peptide (at a final concentration of 10 μg/ml per well) into each well containing PBMCs. Gently tap the sides of the plate to evenly distribute the well components (*see* **Notes 4** and **5**).

2. Incubate the plate at 37 °C with 5 % CO_2 for an optimal period of time, which is generally between 2 and 4 h (*see* **Note 6**).
3. Centrifuge the plate at 300 × *g* for 5 min at 4 °C.
4. Carefully aspirate the CM from wells while leaving the cell pellet intact.

3.3 RNA Isolation and cDNA Generation of Peptide-Stimulated PBMCs

1. Proceed with isolating genomic DNA-free RNA from each designated well as indicated by the RNeasy plus micro kit. The final column pass will result in 12 μl eluate (purified RNA in H_2O). For short-term storage, maintain the purified RNA on ice (*see* **Note 7**).
2. Generate cDNA for each sample using the High Capacity RNA-to-cDNA Kit as recommended by the manufacturer. Briefly, add the 2× RT buffer, 20× enzyme mix, RNA sample, and nuclease-free H_2O to 20 μl total volume per tube. Any unused RNA should be immediately stored at −80 °C (*see* **Note 8**).
3. Incubate the tube in a PCR thermocycler at 37 °C for 60 min followed by a stop reaction cycle at 95 °C for 5 min. The tube can be temporarily placed at 4 °C until use in a downstream qRT-PCR reaction. However, the generated cDNA should be held at −20 °C for long-term storage.

3.4 qRT-PCR Performance and Analysis

qRT-PCR primers used for SYBR® green technology must conform to several guidelines in order to guarantee specific and quality amplification. Primer length is recommended to be between 18 and 24 nucleotides and specifically amplify a target that is 50–150 bp long. Melting temperatures for primer pairs should be compatible (Tm of 58–60 °C) and contain approximately 50 % GC content. Additionally, primer pairs must be designed to avoid hybridization (i.e., primer-dimer amplification) and either anneal to exons with an internal intron region or span an exon/exon boundary. Primers are also usually dissolved in water at a working stock concentration of 20 μM, and qRT-PCR trial runs incorporating primers between 0.05 and 0.9 μM will typically yield optimum primer pair concentrations for qRT-PCR assay conditions.

1. Mix the SYBR® Green Master Mix, IFN-γ or CD8 forward/reverse primers, H_2O, and cDNA together in the appropriate tube on a cold block following the specific guidelines of a qRT-PCR system as diagramed in Fig. 1. Assays should also include a no-template control (NTC) and no-reverse-transcriptase control in order to rule out contamination (*see* **Notes 9–12**).
2. The following cycling parameters for PCR amplification are utilized on the StepOnePlus™ Real-Time PCR System (Life Technologies) (with melting curve analysis immediately

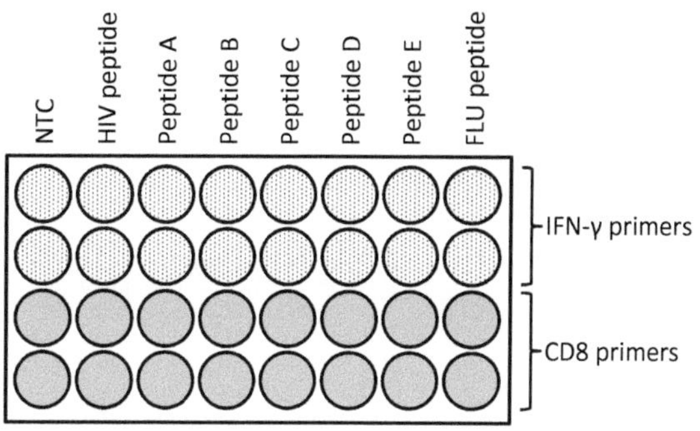

Fig. 1 Example of a qRT-PCR reaction plate setup. After generating high-quality cDNA from peptide-stimulated cells, the qRT-PCR components (outlined in Subheading 3.3) must be added individually to the appropriate qRT-PCR tubes on a cold block. The diagrammed plate includes NTC wells for both IFN-γ and CD8 primers (minus cDNA) in order to affirm the absence of gene-specific amplification. Although IFN-γ primer products will provide index of peptide-specific gene activation in responder T cells, the data must first be normalized to CD8 mRNA expression levels in order to register peptide responsiveness to the presence of $CD8^+$ T cells and to correct for interwell/interassay variability. A negative control peptide (HIV NEF) is used to establish the baseline (negative) IFN-γ response so that relative IFN-γ fold change differences can be calculated for peptides A–E following the comparative CT (ΔΔCt) method. This representative plate also includes positive control wells in which PBMCs were initially exposed to a virus-derived peptide, such as FLU M1, against which a majority of individuals exhibit type 1 immunologic memory

following in order to confirm the absence of nonspecific amplification):

- 20 s at 95 °C.
- 3 s at 95 °C followed by 30 s at 60 °C for 35 cycles.

3. Using specific software from the qRT-PCR system, assign a baseline range that demonstrates little to no fluorescent activity up to the cycle before amplification becomes evident (usually cycles 3–15). Additionally, modify the threshold level to capture Ct (threshold cycle) values in the linear portion of the amplification curve (*see* Fig. 2).
4. Following a successful qRT-PCR run, calculate IFN-γ gene expression values using an appropriate quantitation method (i.e., absolute or relative quantitation). We employ the comparative CT (ΔΔCt) method for relative quantitation and report IFN-γ expression (corrected to CD8 mRNA) as the relative fold change (increase or decrease) versus an HIV peptide-stimulated control sample as demonstrated in Fig. 3 (*see* **Notes 13–15**).

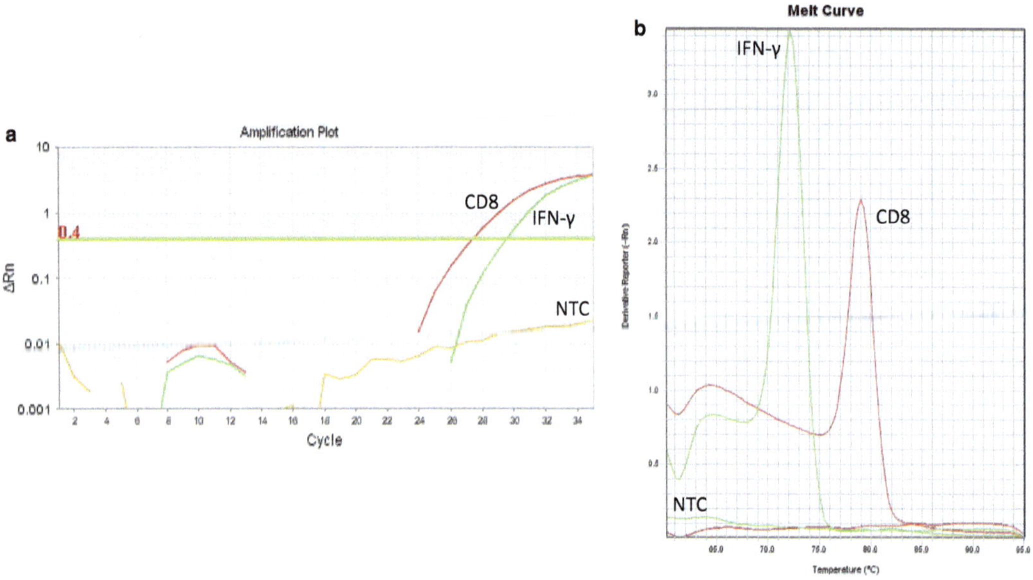

Fig. 2 Representative qRT-PCR amplification and melting curve plots for the human IFN-γ- and CD8-specific amplicons. (**a**) CD8 and IFN-γ were amplified from cDNA of a normal HLA-A2⁺ human donor through qRT-PCR using the StepOnePlus™ Real-Time PCR System (Life Technologies). Ct values were obtained following baseline subtraction (cycles 3–15) and threshold assignment within the linear portion of the amplification curves. (**b**) Melting curve analysis revealed gene-specific products at 79 °C and 72 °C for the CD8 and IFN-γ primers, respectively. NTC wells containing either CD8 or IFN-γ primers (along with all other reaction components as indicated in Subheading 3.4, **step 1**) did not demonstrate observable double-stranded DNA products as determined by amplification and melting curve plots

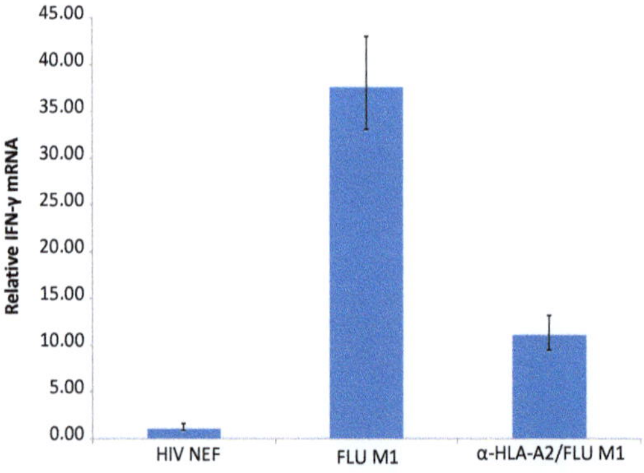

Fig. 3 qRT-PCR can detect relative fold change differences in IFN-γ expression following HLA class I-restricted peptide stimulation. PBMCs from a normal HLA-A2⁺ donor were stimulated with 10 μg/ml of either HIV NEF (AFHHVAREL) or FLU M1 (GILGFVFTL) peptide for 2 h at 37 °C. In a parallel reaction, HLA class I molecules on PBMCs were first blocked using the anti-HLA-A2 antibody BB7.2 for 1 h prior to FLU M1 peptide stimulation. Cells were immediately lysed following a 2-h incubation period, with total RNA purified, and corresponding cDNA generated as detailed in Subheading 3.3. Following the procedure outlined in Subheading 3.4, qRT-PCR was performed in duplicate using primers specific to IFN-γ and CD8. IFN-γ Ct values were normalized to CD8 mRNA for all assay conditions, and final data are reported as the relative IFN-γ fold change compared to PBMCs stimulated with HIV NEF peptide using the comparative CT (ΔΔCt) method

4 Notes

1. Although freshly harvested PBMCs are recommended, particularly for expected rare-event CD8+ T cell responses, we have successfully analyzed CD8+ T cell reactions from PBMCs cryopreserved (in 90 % fetal bovine serum/10 % DMSO) in liquid nitrogen. Frozen PBMCs are first thawed and maintained (at 4×10^5 cells) in 96-well U-bottom plates in 150 μl CM overnight prior to being stimulated with peptides as in Subheading 3.2, **step 1**.
2. If erythrocyte contamination is evident in the harvested interphase layer following density gradient centrifugation, perform a red blood cell lysis step using ACK lysing buffer.
3. Duplicates are typically run for each peptide analyzed to conserve SYBR® green reagent and to limit PBMC material use in order to expand the range of peptide-specific responses that may be investigated. Assuming consistent pipetting technique, qRT-PCR Ct values should be well below a standard deviation of 0.5.
4. Since the goal of this method is to assess intrinsic CD8+ T cell responses in HLA-A2+ individuals, peptides should be 8–10 amino acids long and bind the HLA-A2 peptide domain. With appropriate modification, this method may be used for the analysis of antigen-specific CD4+ or CD8+ T cell responses in many species [12]. Our laboratory has successfully used a peptide prediction tool (http://www-bimas.cit.nih.gov/molbio/hla_bind/) to determine the potential immunogenic peptide sequences derived from proteins of interest based on HLA-binding affinity scores.
5. Situations may arise where resident antigen-presenting cells (APCs) in the plated PBMCs are either abnormally low or deficient in their ability to directly present exogenous peptide to CD8+ T cells (e.g., immunocompromised individual). In these cases, an artificial APC may be used to generate an adequate type 1 immunologic response [13, 14]. The HLA-A2+ TAP-deficient cell T2 (ATCC # CRL-1992) can be loaded with peptide for 3–4 h, added to individual wells containing PBMCs at a 5:1 E:T ratio (i.e., 8×10^4 T2 cells per well), and centrifuged at $250 \times g$ for 2 min as a modification to Subheading 3.2, **step 1**.
6. In preliminary studies, we observed that HLA-A2+ patient CD8+ T cells against the influenza (FLU) M1 peptide (e.g., GILGFVFTL) were generally rather high after 2 h of T cell stimulation in culture (*see* Fig. 3). This incubation time conforms to independent data supporting maximal IFN-γ transcript

expression in responder T cells within a 2–4-h period, with IFN-γ mRNA levels dropping precipitously after this time point [5].

7. The RNeasy plus micro Kit calls for adding RLT buffer to disrupt and lyse cells. Owing to the volume constraints of wells in the 96-well U-bottom plate, cell pellets are resuspended in 200 μl RLT buffer and transferred to a sterilized 1.5 ml microcentrifuge tube containing 200 μl RLT buffer. Samples are then further homogenized by vortexing for 1 min.
8. We generally use 3 μl of RNA sample per cDNA conversion reaction. However, optimum RNA volumes are user dependent and should be determined empirically.
9. Although this qRT-PCR method employs SYBR® green to quantify PCR amplification, the use of an alternate fluorogenic strategy (i.e., TaqMan) may also be readily adopted, assuming that the appropriate primer/probe sets are designed/utilized [5, 13].
10. The qRT-PCR system usually recommends certain master mixes and consumables for optimum performance. We use the StepOnePlus™ Real-Time PCR System (Life Technologies) and incorporate the "Fast" setting for all qRT-PCR runs. As such, our laboratory incorporates the Fast SYBR® Green Master Mix along with MicroAmp® Fast tubes (all from Life Technologies) for Subheading 3.4, **step 1**.
11. In our experience, 2 μl of cDNA per qRT-PCR reaction is sufficient to amplify CD8 and IFN-γ mRNA within a run of 35 cycles (Fig. 2). However, the user should determine an optimum cDNA volume, particularly for low-copy genes.
12. Specific human primer sequences are as follows:

    CD8 (used at 0.05 μM for each primer pair).

    Forward—ACTTGTGGGGTCCTTCTCCT.

    Reverse—GTCTCCCGATTTGACCACAG.

    IFN-γ (used at 0.9 μM for each primer pair).

    Forward—TGGAAAGAGGAGAGTGACAGAA.

    Reverse—TCTTTTGGATGCTCTGGTCAT.

    Melting curve analysis following qRT-PCR reveals specific Tm values of approximately 79 °C and 72 °C for CD8 and IFN-γ, respectively (Fig. 2).
13. Absolute quantitation incorporates serial dilutions of a standard curve (of known quantity) in order to assign copy numbers to a gene of interest. Relative quantitation determines the fold change difference of a gene of interest in experimental samples relative to an untreated (i.e., normal) sample. To correct for qRT-PCR variability among samples, gene amplification values are typically normalized to a gene target that remains

unchanged among experimental and normal groups (e.g., housekeeping gene expression).

14. Our laboratory incorporates the comparative CT ($\Delta\Delta$Ct) method for relative quantitation. The caveat to this approach is that the amplification efficiencies for both the gene of interest (e.g., IFN-γ) and normalizer gene (e.g., CD8) are identical. The general formula for calculating $\Delta\Delta$Ct is

$$2^{\Delta\Delta Ct} = 2^{(Ct,IFN-\gamma-Ct,CD8)control-(Ct,IFN-\gamma-Ct,CD8)treatment}$$

where Ct,IFN-γ is the threshold cycle of IFN-γ, and Ct,CD8 is the threshold cycle of the normalizer gene product CD8. Control refers to a "normal" patient specimen whereas treatment designates a sample from the same patient undergoing a therapy in study. For a more detailed explanation on obtaining relative fold change differences, see the review by Schmittgen and Livak [15].

15. CD8 is designated as the normalizer gene in order to correct for sample variations of IFN-γ expression. Since HLA-A2-restricted peptides are used for stimulation purposes, $CD8^+$ T cells are expected to represent the primary effector cell population synthesizing IFN-γ mRNA. We have not observed substantial differences in CD8 mRNA levels pre/posttreatment in human PBMCs, indicating that CD8 transcript levels remain relatively constant among our patient cohorts. However, since $CD8^+$ T cell frequencies in individuals change over time for a variety of reasons (e.g., pathogen insult, immunodeficiency), normalizing to CD8 mRNA maintains the sensitivity of the qRT-PCR assay as opposed to inappropriately normalizing to the expression of a housekeeping gene (e.g., β-actin) that remains stable over time regardless of a patient's general health status.

Acknowledgments

This work was supported by NIH R01 grant CA140375 (W.J.S.) and a Postdoctoral Fellowship (PF-11-151-01-LIB) from the American Cancer Society (D.B.L.). The authors declare no conflicts of interest.

References

1. Lemonnier FA (2013) Evaluating $CD8^+$ T cell responses in vitro. Methods Mol Biol 960:261–277
2. Betts MR, Brenchley JM, Price DA, De Rosa SC, Douek DC, Roederer M, Koup RA (2003) Sensitive and viable identification of antigen-specific CD8+ T cells by a flow cytometric assay for degranulation. J Immunol Methods 281(1–2):65–78
3. Rao A, Taylor JL, Chi-Sabins N, Kawabe M, Gooding WE, Storkus WJ (2012) Combination therapy with HSP90 inhibitor 17-DMAG

reconditions the tumor microenvironment to improve recruitment of therapeutic T cells. Cancer Res 72(13):3196–3206

4. Berrien-Elliott MM, Jackson SR, Meyer JM, Rouskey CJ, Nguyen TL, Yagita H, Greenberg PD, DiPaolo RJ, Teague RM (2013) Durable adoptive immunotherapy for leukemia produced by manipulation of multiple regulatory pathways of CD8+ T-cell tolerance. Cancer Res 73(2):605–616
5. Kammula US, Marincola FM, Rosenberg SA (2000) Real-time quantitative polymerase chain reaction assessment of immune reactivity in melanoma patients after tumor peptide vaccination. J Natl Cancer Inst 92(16):1336–1344
6. Wheeler CJ, Black KL, Liu G, Mazer M, Zhang XX, Pepkowitz S, Goldfinger D, Ng H, Irvin D, Yu JS (2008) Vaccination elicits correlated immune and clinical responses in glioblastoma multiforme patients. Cancer Res 68(14): 5955–5964
7. Xu Y, Theobald V, Sung C, DePalma K, Atwater L, Seiger K, Perricone MA, Richards SM (2008) Validation of a HLA-A2 tetramer flow cytometric method, IFNgamma real time RT-PCR, and IFNgamma ELISPOT for detection of immunologic response to gp100 and-MelanA/MART-1 in melanoma patients. J Transl Med 6:61
8. Provenzano M, Mocellin S, Bonginelli P, Nagorsen D, Kwon SW, Stroncek D (2003) Ex vivo screening for immunodominant viral epitopes by quantitative real time polymerase chain reaction (qRT-PCR). J Transl Med 1(1):12
9. Trojan A, Urosevic M, Hummerjohann J, Giger R, Schanz U, Stahel RA (2003) Immune reactivity against a novel HLA-A3-restricted influenza virus peptide identified by predictive algorithms and interferon-gamma quantitative PCR. J Immunother 26(1):41–46
10. Trojan A, Giger R, Rist N, Speck RF (2004) Impaired CD8+ T-cell reactivity against viral antigens in cancer patients with solid tumors. Infection 32(5):287–292
11. Schultz-Thater E, Frey DM, Margelli D, Raafat N, Feder-Mengus C, Spagnoli GC, Zajac P (2008) Whole blood assessment of antigen specific cellular immune response by real time quantitative PCR: a versatile monitoring and discovery tool. J Transl Med 6:58
12. Hempel DM, Smith KA, Claussen KA, Perricone MA (2002) Analysis of cellular immune responses in the peripheral blood of mice using real-time RT-PCR. J Immunol Methods 259(1–2):129–138
13. Rentzsch C, Kayser S, Stumm S, Watermann I, Walter S, Stevanoviç S, Wallwiener D, Gückel B (2003) Evaluation of pre-existent immunity in patients with primary breast cancer: molecular and cellular assays to quantify antigen-specific T lymphocytes in peripheral blood mononuclear cells. Clin Cancer Res 9(12): 4376–4386
14. Wang A, Chandran S, Shah SA, Chiu Y, Paria BC, Aghamolla T, Alvarez-Downing MM, Lee CC, Singh S, Li T, Dudley ME, Restifo NP, Rosenberg SA, Kammula US (2012) The stoichiometric production of IL-2 and IFN-γ mRNA defines memory T cells that can self-renew after adoptive transfer in humans. Sci Transl Med 4(149):149ra120
15. Schmittgen TD, Livak KJ (2008) Analyzing real-time PCR data by the comparative C(T) method. Nat Protoc 3(6):1101–1108

Chapter 6

CTL ELISPOT Assay

Elena Ranieri, Iulia Popescu, and Margherita Gigante

Abstract

Enzyme-linked immune absorbent spot (Elispot) is a quantitative method for measuring relevant parameters of T cell activation. The sensitivity of Elispot allows the detection of low-frequency antigen-specific T cells that secrete cytokines and effector molecules, such as granzyme B and perforin. Cytotoxic T cell (CTL) studies have taken advantage with this high-throughput technology by providing insights into quantity and immune kinetics. Accuracy, sensitivity, reproducibility, and robustness of Elispot resulted in a wide range of applications in research as well as in diagnostic field. Actually, CTL monitoring by Elispot is a gold standard for the evaluation of antigen-specific T cell immunity in clinical trials and vaccine candidates where the ability to detect rare antigen-specific T cells is of relevance for immune diagnostic. The most utilized Elispot assay is the interferon-gamma (IFN-γ) test, a marker for $CD8^+$ CTL activation, but Elispot can also be used to distinguish different subsets of activated T cells by using other cytokines such as T-helper (Th) 1-type cells (characterized by the production of IFN-γ, IL-2, IL-6, IL-12, IL-21, and TNF-α), Th2 (producing cytokines like IL-4, IL-5, IL-10, and IL-13), and Th17 (IL-17) cells.

The reliability of Elispot-generated data, by the evaluation of T cell frequency recognizing individual antigen/peptide, is the core of this method currently applied widely to investigate specific immune responses in cancer, infections, allergies, and autoimmune diseases. The Elispot assay is competing with other methods measuring single-cell cytokine production, e.g., intracellular cytokine by FACS or Miltenyi cytokine secretion assay. Other types of lymphocyte frequency and function assays include limiting dilution assay (LDA), cytotoxic T cell assay (CTL), and tetramer staining. Compared with respect to sensitivity the Elispot assay is outranking other methods to define frequency of antigen-specific lymphocytes. The method described herein would like to offer helpful and clear protocols for researchers that apply Elispot. IFN-γ and perforin Elispot assays are described.

Key words Elispot, T cell, Cytokines, Cancer

1 Introduction

Czerkinsky in 1983 was the first who described—Elispot—a new method to enumerate frequency of B hybridoma cells secreting an antigen-specific immunoglobulin. In 1988 again, Czerkinsky was the first to develop an ELISA spot assay measuring the frequency of T lymphocytes secreting a specific lymphokine. Later in 1988 was described a dual-color Elispot for the first time to use computer imaging for analyzing and counting spots as well the first

Elena Ranieri (ed.), *Cytotoxic T-Cells: Methods and Protocols*, Methods in Molecular Biology, vol. 1186,
DOI 10.1007/978-1-4939-1158-5_6, © Springer Science+Business Media New York 2014

membrane bottomed plate to perform Elispot assays. The future development of this assay is represented by Fluorescent multicolor Elispot and high-throughput immune toxicological studies in drug development.

1.1 Principle

Elispot method is based on the sandwich enzyme-linked immunosorbent assay (ELISA) technique by using high-affinity antibodies directed against different epitopes of the same molecule in order to assess cell activation. It was introduced in 1983 by Sedgwick and Holt [1]. Monoclonal or polyclonal antibody for specific cytokines is usually coated onto a PVDF (polyvinylidene difluoride)-backed microtiter plate that dramatically increased the Elispot sensitivity, and less frequently on polystyrene microplate with cellulose nitrate membranes. Responding to stimulation of specific antigen or non-specific mitogen, T cells are placed directly on the bottom of 96-well Elispot plates and incubated into a humidified 37 °C CO_2 incubator for a specific period of time. During this incubation phase, T cells secret the cytokine that is quickly captured by the antibody immobilized on the membranes.

After removal of the cells by washing, a detection antibody is added to the wells. The antibody is directly conjugated with enzyme [horseradish peroxidase (HRP) polyclonal antibody specific for the chosen analyte, or alkaline-phosphatase (ALP) conjugated], or biotinylated. In the latter case, after removing the unbound antibody with repeated washes, a third step with enzyme-conjugated streptavidin is required. Unbound enzyme is subsequently removed by washing and substrate solution is added. BCIP/NBT (for ALP) or TMB (for HRP) is the most sensitive substrate but also Fast Red and AEC (for HRP) are used, taking into account that different substrates give different colors and may also yield different sensitivities.

Colored insoluble precipitate forms, according to the substrate utilized, and appears as spot at the sites of cytokine secretion, with each individual spot representing a single producing cell. The spots can be counted with an automated Elispot reader system or manually, using a stereomicroscope (Fig. 1).

1.2 Elispot Pros

Elispot assay is a very sensitive and robust method for performing individual tests as well as large-scale trials, taking into account that limited number of cells is necessary compared to other cellular assays [2]. Regarding the sensitivity, that depends on the cytokine analyzed, Elispot assay is between 20 and 200 times more sensitive than a conventional ELISA and the detection levels can be as low as one cell in 100,000/1,000,000. Such added sensitivity is decisive, since antigen-specific T cells typically occur in low frequencies in vivo.

On the other hand, although Elispot and RT-PCR analysis reveal similar sensitivity, Elispot has an added value by detecting

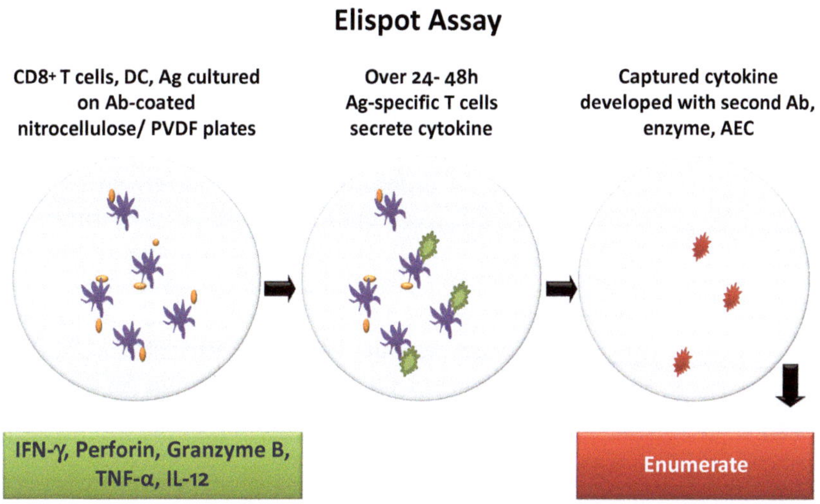

Fig. 1 ELISPOT assay principle. A monoclonal antibody for specific cytokine is pre-coated onto a polyvinylidene difluoride (PVDF)-backed microplate. CD8+ T cells are pipetted into the wells along with DCs and individual peptides and the microplate is placed into a humidified 37 °C CO_2 incubator for a period ranging from 24 to 48 h. During incubation, the immobilized antibody binds the cytokine secreted from the cells. After washing, a detection antibody specific for the chosen analyte is added to the wells. Following the washes, enzyme conjugated to streptavidin is added and a substrate is added. A colored precipitate forms, according to the substrate utilized, and appears as spot at the sites of cytokine secretion, with each individual spot representing a single producing cell

the protein and not the mRNA. For cytokine analyses this is of advantage since many cytokines are translationally regulated.

The comparison of the Elispot to other methods, such as the tetramer and pentamer analysis, takes to the conclusion that, overall, Elispot is a superior method of investigation because it overcomes the identification of the single epitopes and their MHC class I restriction [3]. In addition, the tetramer/pentamer approach does not provide the number of functional T cells and their effector function, a critical information for the immunological monitoring [4–6]. Actually, standardization, simplification, and validation of the technique are the major focus for the application of this test in the clinical settings. Predictably, it will require the automation of the steps of the Elispot protocol (i.e., precoated plates, automated cell counters, automated cell separators, cell sorters, and automated Elispot reader), as well as a reference laboratory with a highly trained personnel able to test hundreds of samples for reactivity to various antigens in a very short time [7, 8].

Another additional feature is that it is possible to test frozen stocks of human lymphocytes without loss of function. Pre- and posttreatment samples can be tested side by side and the results can be reproduced. Further, T cells can be retested for gaining supplementary information in follow-up assays because they survive Elispot assays unaffected [8].

1.3 Positive Controls and Antigen Formats

Here are reported some of the antigenic formats utilized for the Elispot assay and stimuli/positive controls relevant for testing the proper functionality of the assay system and the viability of the cells used. Usually a polyclonal T cell activator can serve as a positive control, such as anti-CD3 antibody or the CEF peptide pool. This pool contains 32 different peptides that cover 15 different HLA class I-restricted T cell epitopes (defined as common $CD8^+$ T cell epitopes), derived from human cytomegalovirus, Epstein-Barr virus, and influenza virus. The CEFT pools instead cover the applications based on HLA class II-restricted T cell responses. Other commonly used stimuli comprise phytohemagglutinin (PHA), lipopolysaccharide (LPS), and concanavalin A (Con A).

Antigen Formats:

- Freeze and thaw lysate.
- Class I and class II peptides.
- Recombinant proteins.
- RNA.
- Recombinant virus vectors.

Stimuli/positive controls:

Phytohemagglutinin (PHA)	2–5 μg/ml	IFNγ
Pokeweed mitogen extract (PWM)	0.1 μg/ml	IFNγ
Concanavalin A (ConA)	2 μg/ml	IFNγ
Anti-CD3	100 ng/ml	IFNγ
Staphylococcus enterotoxin B (SEB)	10 μg/ml	IFNγ
Tetanus toxoid toxin (TT)	5 μg/ml	IFNγ
CEF peptide pool	2 μg/ml	IFNγ
Saccharomyces cerevisiae (SAC)	0.001 % v/v	IFNγ
Candida albicans	10 μg/ml	IFNγ
Lipopolysaccharide (LPS)	10 μg/ml	IFNγ
Ionomycin	500 ng/ml	Perforin
Phorbol myristate acetate (PMA)	1 ng/ml	Perforin

2 Materials

1. Cytokine-specific primary coating Ab (primary Ab).
2. Coating buffer (1× PBS/carbonate).
3. Biotinylated detection Ab (secondary Ab).

4. Complete culture medium.
5. 1× Phosphate-buffered saline (PBS) (washing buffer I).
6. 1× Phosphate-buffered saline (PBS) + 0.05 % Tween (washing buffer II).
7. Phosphate-buffered saline (PBS) + 1 % FCS or 5 % BSA (blocking solution).
8. 1× Hanks' balanced salt solution (HBSS) + 1 mM EDTA (anti-aggregate wash buffer).
9. Dilution buffer.
10. Avidin-horseradish peroxidase (AP) complex (Vectastain Elite Kit Vector).
11. Aminoethyl carbazole (AEC) solution.

3 Methods

3.1 Interferon γ Elispot Assay

COATING (First DAY)

All solutions and equipment coming into contact with cells must be sterile and aseptic procedures should be used accordingly. Please consider that performance of the assay can be affected by alterations of temperatures, incubation timing, number of washing steps, and specified reagent preparation volumes.

1. Dilute coating antibody in sterile 1× PBS according to Table 1 (*see* **Note 1**).
2. Vortex.
3. Add 100 μl of diluted antibody in the wells of Elispot microplate.
4. Seal the plate with parafilm or alternatively use the lid.

Table 1
List of antibodies mainly used for Elispot assays and technical specifications for their use

Cytokine	Coating antibody clone	Final concentration (μg/ml)	Coating incubation time (h)	Secondary antibody clone	Final concentration (μg/ml)
IFN-γ	mAb 1-D1K	10	16–20	mAb 7-B6-1	2
Perforin	mAb Pf-80/164	30	16–20	mAb Pf-344 biotin	1
Granzyme B	mAb HC-4	15	16–20	mAb HC-2 biotin	1
TNF-α	mAb TNF3/4	15	16–20	mAb TNF5 biotin	0.5
IL-12	mAb IL-12-I	15	16–20	mAb IL-12-II biotin	1.25

5. Store microtiter plate overnight at 4 °C or alternatively incubate the microplate at 37 °C for 2 h.

PLATE PREPARATION (Second DAY)

6. Discard the antibody with a bang, opening the plate quickly out of the hood.
7. Rinse the plate four times with 180 µl of sterile 1× PBS per well, 7 min for each wash (*see* **Note 2**).
8. Firmly shake out the excess liquid from plate and pat the bottom of plate with adsorbent tissue.
9. Block the membrane with 180 µl per well of RPMI supplemented with 10 % human serum AB^+ (heat inactivated at 56 °C for 30 min) in order to saturate the remaining binding sites (*see* **Note 3**).
10. Incubate for at least 1 h at 37 °C.
11. Discard with vigorous shake the blocking solution, by opening the plate outside the sterile hood.
12. Add 10–20 µl of cell culture complete medium in each well to avoid drying of the membrane.
13. Prepare antigen or mitogen (i.e., peptide, proteins) or other stimuli as positive control for desired T cell activation, dilute in complete culture medium, and add 100 µl/well. Unstimulated cells are used to detect background cytokine production (*see* **Notes 4** and **5**).
14. Plate cell suspensions serially diluted (i.e., ranging from 10^6 or 10^5 to 10^4 cells/well) according to the ongoing experiment, in a maximum volume of 100 µl (*see* **Note 6**).
15. Replace lid.
16. Incubate Elispot plate at 37 °C, 5 % CO_2, and 100 % humidity (*see* **Note 8**). Duration of the incubation time can differ (20–40 h) upon the type of cells used and nature of stimulus and cytokine kinetics as well. Please refer to Table 1 (*see* **Note 7**).

DEVELOPMENT (Third DAY)

From this point onwards, it is possible to use non-sterile conditions.

17. Discard with vigorous shake the medium from the plate.
18. Wash extensively the wells with 400 µl of PBS-Tween 20 0.05 % six times (*see* **Note 9**).
19. After the last wash, remove excess liquid from the plate and pat the bottom of the plate with dry absorbent paper to completely remove the drops of buffer from the wells.
20. Dilute the secondary biotinylated antibody in non-sterile 1× PBS-BSA 0.5 % according to Table 1 (*see* **Note 10**).

21. Add 100 μl to the wells of Elispot plate.
22. Incubate the plate for 2 h at 37 °C.
23. 10 min Prior to the end of the incubation, prepare the solution of avidin-horseradish peroxidase (AP) complex and keep it at room temperature for 30 min before using (*see* **Note 11**).
24. In the meanwhile discard antibody from the microplate and wash the wells with 400 μl of 1× PBS-Tween 20 0.05 % six times.
25. After the last wash, tap repeatedly the plate on absorbent paper to completely remove the drops of buffer from the wells.
26. Add 100 μl of AP complex per well and incubate for 1 h at room temperature in the dark.
27. At the end of the incubation wash the plates and at the same time prepare AEC solution under chemical hood (*see* **Note 12**).
28. Discard with vigorous shake the AP complex solution from the plate.
29. Wash three times with 400 μl of 1× PBS-Tween 20 0.05 %.
30. Wash three times with 400 μl of 1× PBS.
31. After the last wash, tap repeatedly the plate on absorbent paper to completely remove the drops of buffer from the wells.
32. Add 100 μl of AEC per well and incubate at room temperature for 4–5 min (*see* **Note 13**).
33. Stop the reaction by putting the plate under tap water.
34. Let the plate dry to better visualize the spots.
35. Count spots manually by using a dissecting microscope or automatically using an image analysis system.

3.2 Perforin Elispot Assay

COATING (First DAY)

1. Prewet PVDF plates with 50 μl/well of 70 % ethanol and incubate for 2 min at room temperature (*see* **Note 14**).
2. Decant solution from wells and rinse the plate three times with 200 μl of sterile water per well and two times with 200 μl per well 1× PBS.
3. Dilute 100 μl of coating antibody in 10 ml of 1× PBS. Mix and pipet 100 μl into each well, cover the plate with plastic lid, and incubate overnight at 4 °C.

PLATE PREPARATION (Second DAY)

4. Discard the solution from wells and wash once with 100 μl of 1× PBS.
5. Add 100 μl of 2 % skimmed dry milk in 1× PBS or RPMI 1640 with 10 % FCS into wells, cover, and incubate for 2 h at room temperature.

6. Decant the blocking solution with vigorous shake and tap the plate on absorbent paper.
7. Rinse plate once with 1× PBS.
8. Dispense into wells 100 μl of cell suspensions serially diluted and use positive controls to monitor the Elispot performance. Cells may have been previously in vitro stimulated with appropriate antigens (see the abovementioned list). Cover the plate with a plastic lid and incubate cells at 37 °C, 5 % CO_2, and 100 % humidity for an appropriate length of time (15–20 h) (*see* **Notes 5** and 7).

DEVELOPMENT (Third DAY)

From this point onwards, it is possible to use non-sterile conditions.

9. Shake excess liquid from the plate and pat the bottom of the plate with adsorbent paper.
10. Rinse wells three times with PBS-0.1 % Tween 20.
11. Dilute 10 μl of detection antibody into 10 ml of PBS-1 % BSA. Pipet 100 μl in wells, cover the plate, and incubate for 1 h 30 min at room temperature (*see* **Note 15**).
12. Decant solution from wells and wash three times with PBS-0.1 % Tween 20.
13. Add 100 μl of streptavidin-alkaline phosphatase dilution (1:5,000) in each well. Seal the plate with an adhesive cover and incubate for 1 h at room temperature.
14. Discard and wash three times with PBS-0.1 % Tween 20.
15. Remove the washing buffer by repeated tapping on absorbent paper.
16. Distribute 100 μl of BCIP/NBT buffer in wells (*see* **Note 16**).
17. Let the reaction go for about 10–20 min and then stop the reaction with distilled water by washing three times.
18. Let the plate dry to better visualize the spots (*see* **Note 17**).
19. Count the spots manually by using a dissecting microscope or automatically using an image analysis system (*see* **Note 18**).

4 Notes

1. Before use quick-spin vials to recover the entire volumes.
2. Plates can be washed manually with multichannel pipet or by automated ELISA plate washer with washing head length and flow rate adapted so that membranes and spots are not damaged.
3. Do not touch membrane of the plate with pipet tips to avoid damage and alterations of the reading.

4. Each experimental condition must be in triplicate for accurate data; first plate cytokine-secreting cells to detect (Fig. 2, panels c, d).
5. When analyzing antigen-specific T cell responses in Elispot, controls are of relevance. Besides the use of the negative control consisting of cells in medium without antigen or other stimuli, the positive control of the immunoassay, both for cell viability and functionality, should be a polyclonal T cell activator such as anti-CD3 or alternatively an antigen (usually PHA).
6. Although freshly harvested cells are recommended, it is possible to plate cryopreserved PBMCs or T cells (in 90 % FCS/10 % DMSO) in liquid nitrogen and recent publications showed no difference between frozen and fresh cells used. The cells must be frozen in 1–2 ml vials containing 10^7–10^8 cells/vial. When needed, thaw frozen PBMCs in a 37–40 °C water bath by shaking the cryovial. Take the vial from the water bath when there is still a very small piece of ice in the suspension. Wipe outside of vial with alcohol (for asepsis) and place in hood. The PBMCs or T cells should be transferred in a 15 ml conical tube containing 10 ml of warm (37 °C) cell culture medium adjusting the cell number to the concentration as requested for the assay (e.g., 2×10^6 PBMC/ml if 2×10^5 PBMCs are to be plated in 100 μl/well).
7. The incubation time is merely experimental because it will depend on the pre- and/or activation of the T cells.
8. During the incubation time do not agitate or move the plate and try to place the plate on a plane surface at 37 °C to avoid spot development just on one side of the well.
9. First wash of the microtiter plate should be fast; the following washes can be done by putting the plate on rotation for 3 min/each wash.
10. Work under sterile hood to keep the antibody sterile.
11. Avidin binds biotin with a non-immunological bond but the affinity is 1,000-fold compared to antigen-antibody bond which is an irreversible bond. After the incubation, add hydrogen peroxide and chromogenic substrate (AEC). Peroxidase hydrolyzes H_2O_2 and generated O_2 that oxidizes the substrate. Dark red spots are generated. Preparation of AP complex solution:

1× PBS	10 ml
Tween 20	10 μl
Vortex	
Reagent A	One drop
Reagent B	One drop

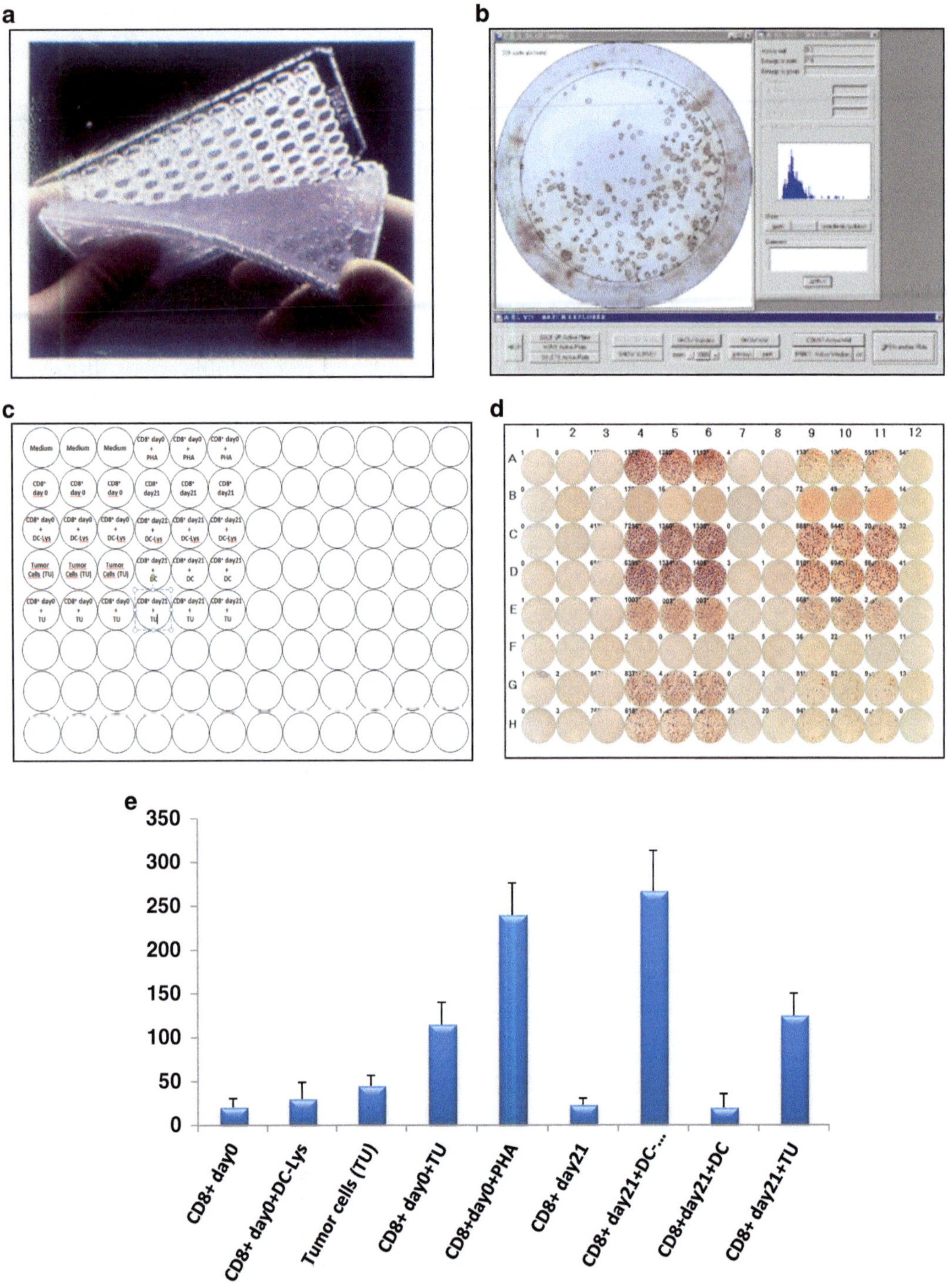

Fig. 2 Example of an ELISPOT assay plate setup. Determinations are performed in triplicate in multiscreen PVDF (polyvinylidene difluoride)-backed microplate plates (**a**) and spots are counted using an ELISPOT plate reader (**b**). In quadrant (**c**) is represented a representative Elispot experiment preformed in our lab to evaluate the capability of ex vivo-generated DCs to promote specific CTL responses in renal cell carcinoma (RCC) patients, by secretion of IFN-γ. CD8+ T cells were cultured along with autologous DC pulsed with renal tumor lysate (at a 10:1 T cell:DC ratio), in the presence of 1 ng/ml IL-12p70 and 1,000 UI/ml IL-6. Responder

12. Preparation of aminoethyl carbazole (AEC) solution:
    - AEC tablet (it must be taken with plastic tweezers or let it drop directly in the vial/cap; never use metal tweezers).
    - Dimethylformamide 2.5 ml:
    Dissolve the tablet in a 50 ml Falcon tube and then add acetate buffer 50 mM pH 5 (47.5 ml). Filter with 0.45 μm filter. The solution can be stored at +4 °C in the dark up to 1 month. Prior to use add 25 μl of H_2O_2 30 % and vortex.

    The acetate buffer (50 mM pH 5.0) should be prepared fresh for every experiment under the following conditions:

Acetic acid 0.2 N	4.6 ml
Sodium acetate 1 M	2.2 ml
ddH_2O	49.427 ml

13. Work rapidly, possibly with multichannel pipet.
14. If the ethanol treatment is not performed, the quality of spots is poor (with grayish and blurry spots); thus the pre-activation of the plates is mandatory.
15. It is recommended to use 0.22 μm filter for the diluted detection antibody solution just before use.
16. BCIP/NBT buffer is potentially carcinogenic and should be disposed appropriately. Caution: Handle this reagent carefully. Always wear gloves.
17. Read the spots only after the membrane is completely dried; they will be better visible and for the counting.
18. The spots may become sharper after one night at +4 °C. Background in the spots is sometimes an undesirable event. It is recognized by specific designed software for spot counts and can be automatically corrected. It is also recommended to store the plate at a dry place in the dark, to prevent spot bleaching.

Fig. 2 (continued) lymphocytes were re-stimulated for 3 weeks on a weekly schedule with mature DC in RPMI/10 % human serum AB supplemented with IL-2 and IL-7. On day 21, CD8+ cells were assessed for their effector cytokine profiles using h-IFNγ-ELISPOT assays. T cells were added to ELISPOT wells along with tumor lysate-loaded DC at a 10:1 T cell:DC ratio. The diagrammed plate includes wells for positive and negative controls. The positive control was represented by CD8+ T cells at day 21 stimulated with 5 μg/ml of PHA while negative controls were medium, CD8+ T cells at time 0, CD8+ T cells at day 21, CD8+ T cells at time 0 plus DC without lysate, and CD8+ T cells at day 21 plus DC without lysate. In quadrant (**d**) are represented the frequencies of responder T cells reactive against RCC and results represent the average (±S.D.) of triplicate wells of values

Acknowledgments

This work was supported by Progetto Strategico Regione Puglia grant (E.R., 2008), Ministero dell'Istruzione, dell'Università e della Ricerca (MiUR) FIRB, CAROMICS grant (E.R., 2011), and a Postdoctoral Fellowship by MiUR, PROGRAMMA OPERATIVO NAZIONALE (PON) RICERCA E COMPETITIVITÀ 2007–2013 PONa3_00395 "BIOSCIENCES AND HEALTH" (B&H) (M.G., 2013). The authors declare no conflicts of interest.

References

1. Sedgwick JD, Holt PG (1983) A solid-phase immunoenzymatic technique for the enumeration of specific antibody-secreting cells. J Immunol Methods 57:301–309
2. Zhang W, Caspell R, Karulin AY, Ahmad M, Haicheur N, Abdelsalam A, Johannesen K, Vignard V, Dudzik P, Georgakopoulou K, Mihaylova A, Silina K, Aptsiauri N, Adams V, Lehmann PV, McArdle S (2009) ELISPOT assays provide reproducible results among different laboratories for T-cell immune monitoring even in hands of ELISPOT-inexperienced investigators. J Immunotoxicol 6:227–234
3. Ramaswami B, Popescu I, Macedo C, Luo C, Shapiro R, Metes D, Chalasani G, Randhawa PS (2011) The polyomavirus BK large T-antigen-derived peptide elicits an HLA-DR promiscuous and polyfunctional CD4 T-cell response. Clin Vaccine Immunol 18:815
4. Tigno JT, Lehmann PV, Tary-Lehmann M (2009) Dissociated induction of cytotoxicity and DTH by CFA and CpG. J Immunother 32:389
5. Nowacki TM, Kuerten S, Zhang W, Boehm BO, Lehmann PV, Tary-Lehmann M (2007) Granzyme-B production, but not cytokine signatures distinguish recently activated CD8 memory cells from resting memory cells. Cell Immunol 247:36–48
6. Kuerten S, Kleen T, Assad RJ, Lehmann PV*, Tary-Lehmann M* (*contributed equally) (2007) Dissociated production of perforin, granzyme B and IFN-γ by HIV-specific CD8+ cells in HIV infection. AIDS Res Hum Retroviruses 24:62–71
7. Kuerten S, Rottlaender A, Rodi M, Velasco VB Jr, Schroeter M, Kaiser C, Addicks K, Tary-Lehmann M, Lehmann PV (2010) The clinical course of EAE is reflected by the dynamics of the neuroantigen-specific T cell compartment in the blood. Clin Immunol 137(3):422–432
8. Butterfield LH, Palucka AK, Britten CM, Dhodapkar MV, Hakansson L, Janetzki S, Kawakami Y, Kleen TO, Lee PP, Maccalli C, Maecker HT, Maino VC, Maio M, Malyguine A, Masucci G, Pawelec G, Potter DM, Rivoltini L, Salazar LG, Schenedel DJ, Slingluff CL, Song W, Stroncek DF, Tahara H, Thurin M, Trinchieri G, van Der Burg SH, Whiteside TL, Wigginton JM, Marincola F, Khleif S, Fox BA, Disis ML (2011) Recommendations from the iSBTc-SITC/FDA/NCI Workshop on Immunotherapy BioMarkers. Clin Cancer Res 17:3064–3076

Chapter 7

Methods of Purification of CTL-Derived Exosomes

Angela Montecalvo, Adriana T. Larregina, and Adrian E. Morelli

Abstract

Exosomes are membrane nanovesicles (approximately <120 nm in size) released by most, if not all, living cells and in particular by leukocytes. They originate within the endocytic compartment by invagination of the endosome membrane. Therefore, they have a different biogenesis and molecular composition than microvesicles (>0.2 μm) shed from the plasma membrane. Although the functions of exosomes in vivo are beginning to be elucidated, increasing evidence suggests that exosomes constitute a mechanism of cell-to-cell communication, transferring antigens, proteins, mRNAs, and noncoding RNAs among cells. Interestingly, effector T cells including cytotoxic T lymphocytes (CTLs) release death-inducing molecules of the TNF superfamily through exosomes contained in their cytotoxic granules. The present chapter provides basic protocols for purification of exosomes secreted by CTLs.

Key words Exosomes, T cells

1 Introduction

CD8 T cells are potent killer cells also known as cytotoxic T lymphocytes (CTLs). One of the main functions of CTLs during elicitation of the immune response is to kill infected, tumor or allogeneic cells via the perforin-dependent apoptotic pathway. Perforins and other mediators are released into the enclosed intracellular space formed by the immunological synapse between the effector CTL and its target cell [1]. While it is well accepted that the CTL lytic content is released as soluble mediators, CTLs also deliver death-inducing molecules through vesicles known as exosomes [2].

1.1 The CTL Synapse

T-Cell activation has always been an intriguing process from a biological perspective, as a result of the complex and restricted fashion in which T cells encounter their specific antigenic peptide that is loaded inside MHC molecules expressed on the antigen (Ag)-presenting cell (APC) surface. Due to this and the fact that the affinity of the T-cell receptor (TCR) for its cognate peptide/MHC

Elena Ranieri (ed.), *Cytotoxic T-Cells: Methods and Protocols*, Methods in Molecular Biology, vol. 1186,
DOI 10.1007/978-1-4939-1158-5_7, © Springer Science+Business Media New York 2014

complex is quite low, there are a number of other receptor–ligand interactions between the T cell and the APC that increase the overall sensitivity of the T cell and the efficiency of T-cell activation. Monks and colleagues [3] described the supramolecular activation cluster (SMAC) as a stereotypical structure at the interface between the T cell and the APC. Within the immunological synapse between CD8 T cells and APCs, the central (c)-SMAC concentrates proteins that participate in Ag-recognition, CTL-activation, signaling, and/or degranulation (i.e., CD4, CD28, TCR, and associated Lck and PKC-θ). Surrounding the c-SMAC, adhesion molecules required for CTL-to-target cell interaction (i.e., the integrin CD11a/CD18 and associated talin on the CTL) arrange in a ring-shaped domain termed peripheral (p)-SMAC [4]. Unlike the synapses between APCs and CD4 T cells, those between effector CTLs and their targets are short-lived since the target cells are killed within minutes [4]. Another important difference of the CTL synapse is that it harbors an extra secretory domain located next to the c-SMAC and within the p-SMAC ring [1, 4]. The secretory domain of the CTL synapse is the only site where the cytotoxic granules of the CTLs release their lytic content into the gaps formed between the CTL and target cell (Fig. 1). These intercellular gaps form part of a larger cleft-shaped space in the otherwise tight immunological synapse. Thus, the CTL synapse is critical for the release of cytotoxic granules in a polarized fashion against the target cell [1]. It also provides a constricted intercellular seal that prevents diffusion of cytotoxic mediators contained in the cytotoxic granules, therefore avoiding killing of bystander cells [1].

1.2 Cytotoxic Granules

The cytotoxic granules of CD8 T cells are single membrane vesicles of approximately 700 nm in diameter that contain the lytic proteins perforin, granzymes, and death-inducing molecules of the TNF superfamily [5–8]. Each cytotoxic granule has one or multiple dense cores and an electron-lucent area, which contains small intraluminal vesicles (ILVs) ranging between 40 and 70 nm in diameter [5] (Fig. 1). The dense cores are enriched in perforin, granulysin, and granzymes complexed with chondroitin sulfate-rich proteoglycans, whereas the enzyme cathepsin D is present in the electron lucent area between the ILVs [5, 9].

The peripheral membrane of the cytotoxic granule expresses the lysosomal proteins Lamp-1, Lamp-2, and CD63, while only a low percentage of the granules are positive for the endosomal marker mannose 6-phosphate receptor [5]. Fas-ligand (L) and other members of the TNF superfamily (i.e., TRAIL) are expressed on the limiting membrane of the granule and on the surface of the ILVs [7, 8]. Cytotoxic granules of CTLs are often referred to as secretory lysosomes because they are organelles with lysosomal features capable of releasing regulated exocytosis pre-synthesized lytic proteins stored in their lumen [10]. Cytotoxic granules are closely

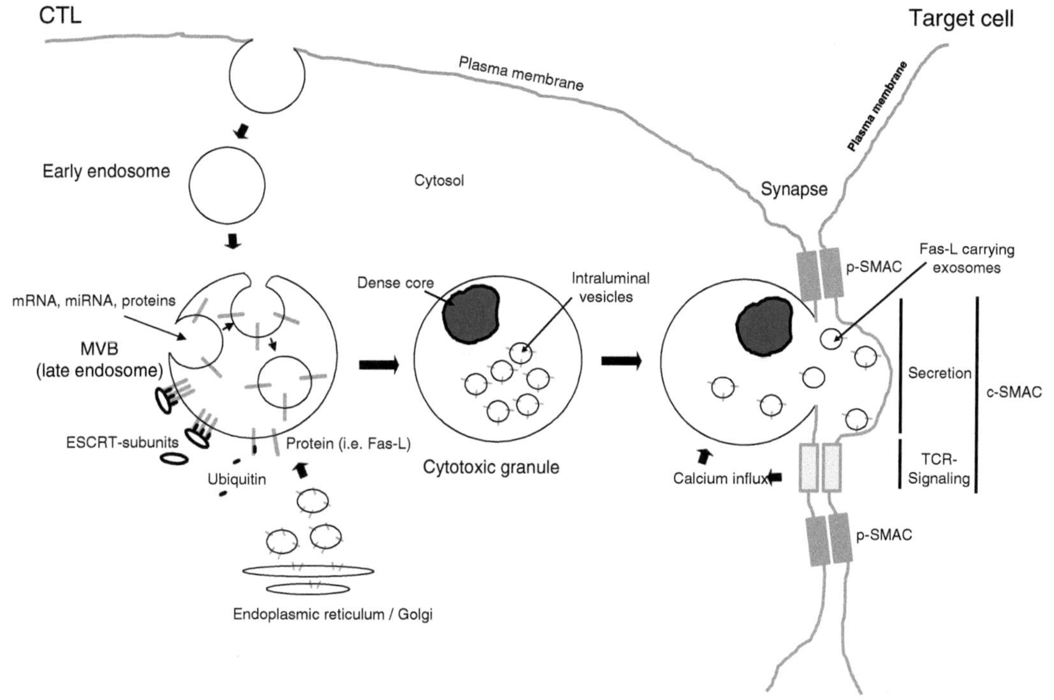

Fig. 1 Biology of exosomes in effector CTLs. Exosomes originate by reverse budding of the limiting membrane of early endosomes, which then become MVBs with ILVs inside. Proteins transported from the Golgi (in this case Fas-L) and bearing specific sorting signals are ubiquitylated on their cytosolic domains and sorted into the forming MVBs. The ESCRT machinery, composed of multiple subunits and accessory molecules, binds the ubiquitylated proteins, concentrates the proteins in micro-domains in the MVB limiting membrane, triggers the reverse budding of the peripheral membrane of MVBs, and cleaves the nascent vesicles into free ILVs within the lumen of MVBs. During this process, certain cytosolic proteins, mRNAs, and noncoding RNAs (including microRNAs) are transferred into the lumen of the nascent ILVs. Besides ILVs, cytotoxic granules contained one or a few dense cores. Upon recognition of the target cell and buildup of the CTL synapse, cytotoxic granules mobilize to the c-SMAC and release their Fas-L-bearing ILVs into the secretory domain of the c-SMAC, where the secreted ILVs are now termed exosomes. Release of exosomes within the confined space of the CTL synapse limits diffusion of the vesicles carrying death-inducing molecules, preventing killing of bystander cells

related to the multivesicular bodies (MVBs) described in most cell types. MVBs are endosomal/lysosomal compartments containing ILVs. When MVBs fuse their limiting membrane with the plasma membrane, they release their content of ILVs as exosomes into the extracellular space [11, 12] (Fig. 1).

1.3 Biology of Exosomes

Exosomes are membrane nanovesicles (approximately <120 nm in diameter) generated by reversed budding or evagination of the limiting membrane of endosomes. When the nascent vesicles are pinched off the endosome membrane, they accumulate as ILVs in the lumen of the endosome that then becomes a MVB (Fig. 1). Once ILVs are released into the extracellular space, the vesicles are termed exosomes [11, 12]. The MVBs may undertake either a secretory or degradative/lysosomal pathway [13, 14]. In the secretory route, MVBs fuse with the cell membrane releasing their content into the extracellular milieu. Cells can release exosomes constitutively or in a regulated fashion, the latter as a result of activation of surface receptors that increase the content of cytosolic calcium. Alternatively, MVBs fuse with lysosomes, where the MVB content is degraded. Unlike bigger vesicles or microvesicles (approximately >0.2 μm) released by shedding of the plasma membrane of living cells (i.e., ectosomes, microparticles) [15], or dying cells undergoing apoptosis (apoptotic cell blebs), exosomes originate in the endocytic compartment of living cells [11, 12]. Despite exosomes have been described originally in maturing reticulocytes [16], most if not all, types of cells release exosomes, in particular leukocytes (i.e., B cells, dendritic cells, mast cells, and T cells), platelets, epithelial cells, and tumor cells [17–22]. Moreover, exosomes are also detected in most bodily fluids [23–26]. Once released, exosomes may bind either to neighboring cells or to the extracellular matrix. Alternately, they can mobilize passively via blood or organic fluids. Circulating exosomes in blood are captured swiftly by phagocytes of the lung, spleen, and liver [27–29].

Because of their endocytic origin, the composition of exosomes differs from that of microvesicles shed from the plasma membrane. Proteins enriched in exosomes likely participate in ILV biogenesis (i.e., Tsg101, Hrs, Alix, annexins, Rab proteins), cytoskeleton organization (i.e., actin, tubulin), protein arrangement inside membrane micro-domains (i.e., the tetraspanin protein family including CD9, CD63, CD81), protection from lysis by complement factors (i.e., CD55, CD56), Ag-presentation or Ag-transport (i.e., MHC molecules, heat shock proteins), binding of exosomes to target cells or the extracellular matrix (i.e., milk fat globule-E8 [MFG-E8]/lactadherin, integrins), and signal transduction (i.e., kinases, G-proteins) [30]. Some of these proteins (i.e., tetraspanins, Tsg101, heat shock proteins) are used as exosomes markers. Other proteins are targeted or enriched in exosomes depending on the lineage or stage of maturation, differentiation, infection, or transformation of the parent cell.

Due to the mechanism of origin of the ILVs, the proteins expressed on the exosome membrane (i.e., tetraspanins, MHC molecules, integrins) maintain the same topology displayed on the cell surface with their extracellular domains facing outwards. In CTLs, the topology of those proteins expressed on the exosome membrane is particularly critical for membrane-bound cytolytic proteins of the TNF superfamily (i.e., Fas-L). In order to kill the target cell, the death-inducing domains of the cytolytic proteins transported by the exosomes must be oriented towards the exosome surface. The exosome membrane also contains externalized phosphatidylserine and lipid rafts rich in sphingolipids, ceramide, and cholesterol [31, 32]. Exosomes transport mRNAs, and noncoding RNAs including microRNAs in the vesicle lumen, which protects the "exosome shuttle RNAs" from enzymatic degradation [33–37].

1.4 Role of Exosomes in the Immune System

Although the function(s) of exosomes in vivo has not been elucidated, increasing evidence strongly suggests that they constitute a mechanism of cell-to-cell communication to transfer functional proteins (i.e., Ags, prions, morphogens), mRNAs, and noncoding regulatory RNAs among cells in normal and pathological conditions [38–42]. Dendritic cells transfer Ags and functional miRNAs to neighboring APCs through exosomes [28, 43, 44]. APC-derived exosomes can function as Ag-presenting vesicles for primed T cells [45, 46]. Follicular dendritic cells, within B-cell follicles, bind exosomes likely secreted by neighboring B cells [47]. This may represent a mechanism of Ag-presentation to B-lymphocytes to promote/maintain B-cell memory. T cells, upon TCR activation, release exosomes bearing the TCR/CD3/ζ complex and intracellular proteins of the TCR-transduction machinery, probably as a mechanism to downregulate TCR-signaling following T-cell stimulation [48]. Activated T cells secrete exosomes bearing death-inducing molecules of the TNF superfamily to trigger apoptosis of neighboring activated T cells during activation-induced cell death [7, 8]. Effector CTLs kill target cells by releasing exosomes expressing death-inducing molecules on their surface (see below).

Due to their immune-regulatory potential, exosomes released by immunogenic or immunosuppressive APCs have been employed for vaccination against tumors or pathogens [49, 50], and for negative immunization for prevention/therapy of autoimmune disorders, allergy, or transplant rejection [51–53] in murine models. Immunization with tumor-derived exosomes carrying tumor-Ags has been proved to stimulate antitumor CTL responses [22]. In situ, tumors release exosomes that restrain innate and adaptive immunity against the tumor as a mechanism of immune escape. Tumor-derived exosomes released in the tumor microenvironment promote differentiation of myeloid-derived suppressor cells, increase T-cell apoptosis, downregulate T-cell function, block cytotoxicity of NK cells and CTLs, and enhance the function and inhibit apoptosis of regulatory T cells [54–62].

1.5 Effector CTLs Release Exosomes Carrying Death-Inducing Molecules

Following recognition of the target cell and buildup of the CTL synapse, the cytotoxic granules fuse with the surface membrane of the CTL, releasing their dense core(s), soluble mediators, and exosomes into the gaps formed between the CTL and target cell [2] (Fig. 1). Exosomes released by T cells have been shown to bear on their surface death-inducing molecules of the TNF superfamily including Fas-L and TRAIL that trigger apoptosis of target cells [7, 8]. The cytoplasmic tail of Fas-L contains a proline-rich domain flanked by lysines responsible for sorting Fas-L from the trans-Golgi network to MVBs/secretory lysosomes without transiting the cell surface [63]. Tyrosine phosphorylation and mono-ubiquitylation of the lysine groups control sorting of Fas-L into MVBs [64]. When mono-ubiquitylated, cytosolic domains of trans-membrane proteins are recognized by the endosomal-sorting complex for transport (ESCRT), they are sorted first into the limiting membrane of MVBs, and next into the membrane of ILVs [65, 66] (Fig. 1).

The membrane-bound forms of death-inducing molecules of the TNF superfamily are notoriously the most effective cytolytic variants. By contrast, the soluble counterparts generated via cleavage by metallo-proteases on the cell surface result to be much less toxic and likely constitute a mechanism to downregulate their lytic activity. Secretion of these molecules via exosomes in a regulated fashion following TCR activation prevents surface expression and therefore nonspecific killing by T cells. Importantly, since TNF superfamily molecules are released on the exosome surface, they are able to form multimers to activate their corresponding death-inducing receptors that indeed function as trimers. Secretion of TNF superfamily molecules via exosomes also augments their local concentration, reduces their degradation by proteases, and facilitates their retention in the extracellular milieu through binding of the exosomes to the extracellular matrix. T cells also release exosomes bearing death-inducing molecules of the TNF superfamily as a mechanism to downregulate the T-cell response by activation-induced cell death [7, 8]. In certain circumstances, Fas-L-bearing exosomes released by activated CD8 T cells instead of promoting apoptosis of tumor cells, they facilitate tumor invasion by increasing tumor expression of the matrix metalloproteinase 9 through a Fas-signaling pathway [67]. Not only CTLs, but also NK cells and dendritic cells kill target cells via release of exosomes carrying Fas-L and perforin [68, 69].

Cells of immune-privileged sites like the placenta trophoblast [70] and malignant tumors [54, 55] secrete Fas-L-bearing exosomes as a mechanism of immune escape. In those cells with abundant MVBs, like cells of hematopoietic lineage, Fas-L is sorted preferentially to MVBs and ILVs, avoiding surface expression. Alternatively, in cells poor in MVBs, Fas-L is sorted by default into the cell membrane, as occurs in parenchymal cells of some immune-privilege sites [63].

Cytolytic nanovesicles similar to exosomes have been generated in vitro. Retroviral packaging cell lines expressing transgenic Fas-L release (infective and noninfective) retroviral particles carrying functional Fas-L on their surface [71]. When mixed with Fas-expressing target cells, these particles trigger apoptosis through Fas-L. Under these circumstances, the exosome-like viral particles are not confined within the enclosed space of the immunologic synapse since they are dispersed in the culture medium by Brownian motion. Thus, their cytotoxic potential can be enhanced by addition of (a) bridging antibodies that will on one end recognize ligands on the vesicle surface and on the other end will link the target cells via FcR, or (b) polybrene or poly-L-lysine, two polycationic molecules that facilitate binding between the negatively charged surfaces of the target cells and the Fas-L-bearing vesicles [72]. These cytolytic vesicles, bearing bioactive Fas-L, are commercially available as a lyophilized powder (Millipore Upstate, catalogue # 01-210) for in vitro studies of cytotoxicity.

In summary, exosomes carrying death-inducing molecules play a critical role in the regulation of the immune response during the steady-state and pathological conditions. Through the past two decades, improvements in techniques to obtain highly pure exosomes together with the better understanding of exosome biogenesis, their molecular composition and differences between exosomes and other types of cell-derived vesicles transformed the field of exosomes into a hot area of basic and applied research. This chapter describes techniques required to purify exosomes from effector CTLs.

2 Materials

Solutions, plasticware, and dissecting instruments must be sterile.

2.1 Human Samples and Animals

C57Bl/6 (B6) mice and BALB/c/cByJ mice, 8–12 week old. Human whole blood.

2.2 Material and Reagents

1. Phosphate-buffered saline (PBS 1×) without Ca and Mg.
2. Plasticware: pipettes, 15 and 50 ml conical tubes, tissue culture grade vented flaks (175 cm^2).
3. Biosafety cabinet, pipette aids, refrigerated benchtop centrifuge, freezer (−80 °C). Ultracentrifuge equipped with fixed angle or swinging-bucket rotors.
4. RPMI-1640 culture medium, with sodium bicarbonate, without L-glutamine, sterile-filtered, endotoxin tested. Supplement the medium with 10 % v/v heat-inactivated fetal calf serum (FCS), L-glutamine (2 mM), nonessential amino acid solution (1×), sodium pyruvate (0.11 mg/ml,) HEPES (10 mM), 2-mercapthoethanol (0.55 mM), and penicillin and streptomycin (100 U each).
5. Human recombinant IL-2 (PrepoTech). It exerts cross-reactivity on mouse T cells.
6. Mouse CD3+ T Cell Enrichment Columns (R&D Systems).
7. Dynabeads® Mouse Pan T (Thy1.2) (Dynal® at Invitrogen).

8. Lympholyte®-M (Cedarlane Laboratories).
9. Mouse CD8+ T Cell Enrichment Columns (R&D Systems).
10. Ficoll-Paque PREMIUM (GE Healthcare Life Sciences).
11. Phytohemagglutinin M (Sigma-Aldrich).
12. Human CD8+ T Cell Enrichment Columns (R&D Systems).
13. Protease inhibitor cocktail for use in tissue culture media, DMSO solution containing aprotinin, bestatin, E-64, leupeptin, and pepstatin A (Sigma-Aldrich).
14. Tubes for SW41 ultracentrifuge rotor: Ultra-Clear™ tubes 9/16 × 3½ in. (14 × 89 mm) (Beckman).
15. Deuterium oxide (heavy water, D_2O) (Cambridge Isotope Laboratories Inc).
16. Sucrose/D_2O solution. Dissolve 15 g of protease-free sucrose and 1.2 g Tris base in 25 ml of heavy water (D_2O). Adjust pH to 7.5–8 with 10 N HCl drops. Adjust final volume to 50 ml with D_2O. Filter the solution through a 0.2 μm syringe filter. Keep the solution in the fridge.
17. Gradient maker model #GM-20 (C.B.S. Scientific Co., Del Mar, CA, USA), or similar model.
18. Magnetic stir plate.
19. Peristaltic pump.
20. NanoDrop 2000c spectrophotometer (Thermo Scientific).
21. LM10 NanoSight's instrument equipped with a high-sensitivity EMCCD camera and the NTA 2.0 software (NanoSight).
22. Refractometer.

3 Methods

CTL-derived exosomes are purified from T-cell culture supernatants by ultracentrifugation. Because naïve T cells or resting CTLs do not have lytic activity, exosomes must be purified from culture supernatants of human or mouse CTL lines or clones, or from activated/effector CTLs. There are multiple methods to generate activated/effector CD8 T cells, which are outside the scope of this chapter. As an example of generation of allo-reactive CTLs in mice, T cells purified with mouse CD3+ T Cell Enrichment Columns from spleens of C57Bl/6 mice are stimulated with CD3-depleted (by negative selection with Dynabeads® Mouse Pan T), γ-irradiated (2,000 rads) splenic APCs from BALB/c mice (1 T cell:1 APC ratio) in complete medium supplemented with IL-2 (100 U/ml). After 5 days, viable CTLs are separated on a Lympholyte-M gradient, rinsed and cultured in complete culture medium (10^6 cells/ml) with IL-2 (100 U/ml). Seven days later, CTLs are re-stimulated with splenic BALB/c APCs, as aforementioned. The process can be repeated to increase the CTL yield [4]. Before use, CD8 T cells are purified with mouse CD8+ T Cell Enrichment Columns.

As an example of generation of activated/effector CTLs in humans, T-cell blasts are generated by stimulating peripheral blood mononuclear cells (PBMCs, isolated by Ficoll-Paque gradient) with PHA (10 μg/ml) in complete medium (2×10^6 cells/ml). After 1 day, PBMCs are washed and resuspended in complete medium supplemented with IL-2 (100 U/ml) and cultured for 6 days, with changes of medium with IL-2 every 2 days [8]. Before use, (day 7) CD8 CTLs are purified with human CD8+ T Cell Enrichment Columns.

3.1 Generation of Culture Supernatants Containing CD8 T Cell-Derived Exosomes

1. Purified CD8 T cells are washed in PBS and resuspended (2×10^7 cells/ml) in culture medium with 10 % *exosome-free* FCS (*see* **Note 1**) supplemented with PHA (50 μg/ml). Place the cells back in the incubator (37 °C, 5 % CO_2).
2. After 5 min, the cells are rinsed off the PHA with PBS and cultured in medium with 10 % *exosome-free* FCS (without PHA) supplemented with a protease inhibitor cocktail (*see* **Note 2**).
3. One hour later, centrifuge the T cells at 2,500×*g* (20 min, 4 °C) and collect the supernatant for exosome purification. Maintain the supernatant in a tube on ice. Keep the tube on ice between the following steps to minimize protein degradation (in particular cleavage of molecules of the TNF superfamily on the exosomes).

3.2 Concentration of Exosomes from Culture Supernatants of CD8 T Cells (See Note 3)

1. Remove microvesicles bigger than exosomes and cell debris by transferring the supernatant with a pipette (*see* **Note 4**) to the appropriate sterile tubes and centrifuge at 10,000×*g* (30 min, 4 °C). When using a fixed-angle rotor, after adjusting the tube caps, make a mark or orient tube caps as a reference for identification of the small pellet of debris on the tube wall.
2. Harvest the supernatant containing the exosomes with a pipette (*see* **Note 4**). Keep the supernatant in a tube on ice.
3. The cleared supernatant is transferred to a sterile Ultra-Clear™ (14×89 mm) Beckman tube, and centrifuged at 100,000×*g*, for 60 min, at 4 °C in a SW41 rotor, with the brake set at low (*see* **Note 5**). If necessary, fill up the rest of the tube with sterile PBS.
4. After centrifugation, discard gently the supernatant with a pipette, leaving the exosome pellet and the bottom 100–200 μl of liquid. Resuspend the pellet in 1 ml of PBS supplemented with the protease inhibitor cocktail. Keep the exosome preparation in a tube on ice.

3.3 Purification of Exosomes Released by CD8 T Cells (See Note 6)

To remove protein aggregates and debris, the T-cell exosomes must be further purified on a 30 % sucrose/D_2O gradient [73] or on a continuous sucrose gradient [17].

3.3.1 Purification of T-Cell Exosomes on a 30 % Sucrose/D_2O Gradient

1. The T-cell exosomes concentrated by ultracentrifugation (**step 4** in Subheading 3.2) are placed on top of 2 ml 30 % sucrose/D_2O cushion without disrupting the interface, in a sterile Ultra-Clear™ (14 × 89 mm) Beckman tube. Fill up the rest of the tube with sterile PBS. Centrifuged at 100,000 × *g* (60 min, 4 °C) in a SW41 rotor with the bake set at low.
2. The interphase with the exosomes (a whitish band barely visible on the upper area of the sucrose cushion) is harvested in a 15 ml tube. Adjust to 11 ml with sterile PBS supplemented with the protease inhibitors and (optional) fungizone and 0.1 % Na azide (to prevent contamination).
3. The sucrose is removed from the exosomes by placing the 15 ml tube in a horizontal or orbital shaker (slow motion) for a minimum of 30 min (at 10 °C, in the fridge or cold room).
4. After 30 min (or alternatively the next day), the exosomes are transferred to a sterile Ultra-Clear™ (14 × 89 mm) Beckman tube, and pelleted by centrifugation at 100,000 × *g* (60 min, 4 °C).
5. Remove the supernatant gently, leaving the exosome pellet untouched with approximately 100–200 μl of liquid in the tube. Resuspend the pellet with a micropipettor avoiding bubbles and transfer the liquid to a 1.5 ml RNase-free microcentrifuge tube (in case you need the exosomes for RNA extraction), and keep the tube on ice.
6. Determine the quantity of exosomes (based on their protein content) with a NanoDrop 2000c spectrophotometer. The exosomes size and concentration can be measured by nanoparticle tracking analysis with a NanoSight's instrument (NanoSight) [74]. The quality of the exosomes can be evaluated by electron microscopy, and/or by analysis of exosome markers (surface and intraluminal) by western blot analysis on exosome lysates, or by flow cytometric analysis of surface markers on immune-labeled exosomes attached to latex or iron beads [75].
7. For RNA extraction, add TRIzol® (final volume of 700 μl in the microcentrifuge tube), pipet up and down gently to dissolve the exosomes, and keep it at −80 °C until RNA extraction (*see* **Note 6**). For functional studies, keep the exosomes in PBS and use them preferable the same day, or keep them in the fridge o/n (*see* **Note 7**).

3.3.2 Purification of T-Cell Exosomes on a Continuous Sucrose Gradient

1. Exosomes float at a density between 1.15 and 1.19 g/ml. Per continuous sucrose gradient, prepare 5 ml of 2 M sucrose (by adding 1 ml of HEPES stock solution to 4 ml of HEPES/sucrose solution), and 5 ml of 0.25 M sucrose (by mixing 4.5 ml of HEPES stock solution to 0.5 ml of HEPES/sucrose solution).
2. In a sterile Ultra-Clear™ (14×89 mm) Beckman tube, add 1.5 ml of HEPES/sucrose solution (2.5 M).
3. Attach an outlet valve (luer type) followed by tubing to the gradient maker. Connect the tubing to a peristaltic pump to deliver slowly the sucrose gradient to the sterile Ultra-Clear™ (14×89 mm) Beckman tube. Place a magnetic spin-bar into the chamber closer to the gradient maker outlet. Close the valve of the gradient maker and the outlet valve. Place the gradient maker on a magnetic stir plate on a surface higher than the bench.
4. Add 5 ml of 2 M sucrose solution to the compartment next to the gradient maker outlet. Turn on the magnetic stir plate at low speed. Open the gradient maker valve (inside valve) to allow bubbles to escape. Allow approximately 1 ml of solution to backflow into the empty chamber and close the gradient maker valve. Remove with pipette and place the 2 M sucrose solution back to its original chamber. Load the distal compartment with the 5 ml of 0.25 M sucrose solution.
5. Switch on the peristaltic pump at low/medium speed. Place the distal end of the tubing connected to the gradient maker close to the wall of the ultracentrifuge tube containing the 1.5 ml of 2.5 M sucrose solution. Open sequentially the gradient maker valve and then the outlet valve. Dispense slowly the continuous sucrose gradient into the ultracentrifuge tube lifting the end of the tubing or lowering the centrifuge tube, so the sucrose pouring out is just above the top of the liquid. Stop when the gradient reaches 1 cm from the tube top.
6. Add the T-cell exosomes (up to 1 ml) on top of the gradient (*see* **Note 8**).
7. Centrifuge at 100,000×*g* (16 h, 4 °C) in a SW41 swinging-bucket rotor (brake set at low).
8. Harvest with a p-1000 micropipettor 1 ml gradient fractions from top to bottom. Place each fraction in 1.5 ml microcentrifuge tubes pre-labeled with the fraction number, and keep them on ice. Transfer 50 μl of each gradient fraction to wells of a 96-well plate, and when the liquid reaches room temperature measure their refractive index with a refractometer. The conversion table of the refractive index into g/ml can be found at the Beckman website.

9. Calculate the amount of exosomes (based on their protein content) in the gradient fractions with a NanoDrop 2000c spectrophotometer. Collect in a 15 ml tube those gradient fractions with the highest protein content and that have a density between 1.15 and 1.19 g/ml (in general 2–3 fractions in the center of gradient). Adjust to final 11 ml of sterile PBS containing the protease inhibitor cocktail and (optional) fungizone and 0.1 % Na azide.
10. The sucrose is rinsed off the exosomes by placing the 15 ml tube in a horizontal or orbital shaker (slow motion), at least for 30 min (at 10 °C, in the fridge or cold room).
11. After 30 min (or alternatively the next day), the exosomes are transferred to a sterile Ultra-Clear™ (14 × 89 mm) Beckman tube, and pelleted by centrifugation at 100,000 × *g* (60 min, 4 °C) in a SW41 swinging-bucket rotor (brake set at low). Remove the supernatant and resuspend the exosome pellet in final 100–200 μl in a 1.5 ml RNase-free microcentrifuge tube.

    The amount of exosome protein, and exosome size, concentration, morphology, and markers are evaluated as explained in **step 6** in Subheading 3.3.1.

4 Notes

1. To prevent contamination with bovine extracellular vesicles and other debris contained in the FCS, exosome-free FCS is generated by centrifuging FCS at 100,000 × *g* overnight (4 °C). After that, harvest the cleared FCS leaving in the tube the pellet of debris and the bottom 1–2 ml of liquid. Sterilize the cleared FCS by filtering it through a 0.2 μm syringe filter. Store the exosome-free FCS at −80 °C.
2. Use a protease inhibitor cocktail that is suitable for cell culture. Addition of protease inhibitors helps to preserve the cytolytic activity of the death-inducing molecules of the TNF superfamily on the exosome surface, which are rapidly cleaved by extracellular metalloproteases.
3. Since the CTL exosomes may be used for in vitro studies, RNA analysis, or in vivo experiments, the purification of exosomes must be done in a sterile tissue culture hood. To sterilize the ultracentrifuge tubes, rinse clean tubes with sterile water, then in 70 % ethanol for 20 min, and rinse twice with sterile PBS. The lid of each Ultra-Clear™ Beckman tube holder (SW41 rotor) and the rotor lid (45Ti rotor) must be cleaned with 70 % ethanol.
4. To minimize carryover of cells and debris, harvest the supernatants gently with a 10 or 25 ml pipette, instead of pouring off

the liquid, leaving the bottom 1–2 ml of supernatant in the tubes. Pipette close to the tube wall, away from the pellet.

5. The minimum time the exosomes are centrifuged at 100,000 × *g* should be 60 min. If the time required for acceleration and de-acceleration of the ultracentrifuge is included in the 60 min, add extra 10 min (70 min total) to compensate for the loss of centrifugation time at 100,000 × *g*.
6. If the exosomes are used to analyze their intraluminal RNA content, treat the exosomes with RNase A (final concentration 2–10 ng/μl, 37 °C, 10 min) before adding the TRIzol® to remove potential cellular RNAs attached to the vesicle surface.
7. For analysis of protein composition or RNA content, exosomes are stored at −80 °C in PBS supplemented with proteases inhibitors or dissolved in Trizol, respectively. Once the exosomes are thawed, do not freeze them again. For functional studies, it is recommended not freezing the exosomes to prevent membrane breakage.
8. We recommend loading the exosomes on top of the continuous gradient, instead of loading them in the 2.5 M sucrose fraction at the bottom of the tube, as it is classically done. Thus, in case there is a problem during the preparation of the gradient, the procedure can be repeated without risk of losing the exosomes.

Acknowledgements

We thank the Research Specialists Olga A. Tkacheva and William J. Shufesky (University of Pittsburgh, Pittsburgh, PA, USA) for their comments. We also thank Dr. Lawrence P. Kane for his revisions. This work was supported by the National Institutes of Health grant AI077511 (to A.T.L.), and funds from the T.E. Starzl Transplantation Institute (to A.E.M.).

References

1. Stinchcombe JC, Griffiths GM (2003) The role of the secretory immunological synapse in killing by CD8+ CTL. Semin Immunol 15:301–305
2. Peters PJ, Geuze HJ, Van der Donk HA et al (1989) Molecules relevant for T cell-target cell interaction are present in cytolytic granules of human T lymphocytes. Eur J Immunol 19: 1469–1475
3. Monks CR, Freiberg BA, Kupfer H et al (1998) Three-dimensional segregation of supramolecular activation clusters in T cells. Nature 395:82–86
4. Stinchcombe JC, Bossi G, Booth S et al (2001) The immunological synapse of CTL contains a secretory domain and membrane bridges. Immunity 15:751–761
5. Peters PJ, Borst J, Oorschot V et al (1991) Cytotoxic T lymphocytes granules are secretory lysosomes containing both perforin and granzymes. J Exp Med 173:1099–1109
6. Bossi G, Griffiths GM (1999) Degranulation plays an essential part in regulating cells surface expression of Fas ligand in T cells and natural killer cells. Nat Med 5:90–96

7. Martinez-Lorenzo MJ, Anel A, Gamen S et al (1999) Activated human T cells release bioactive Fas ligand and APO2 ligand in microvesicles. J Immunol 163:1274–1281
8. Monleon I, Martinez-Lorenzo MJ, Monteagudo L et al (2001) Differential secretion of Fas ligand- or APO2 ligand/TNF-related apoptosis-inducing ligand-carrying microvesicles during activation-induced death of human T cells. J Immunol 167: 6736–6744
9. Lettau M, Schmidt H, Kabelitz D et al (2007) Secretory lysosomes and their cargo in T and NK cells. Immunol Lett 108:10–19
10. Blott EJ, Griffiths GM (2002) Secretory lysosomes. Nat Rev Mol Cell Biol 3:122–131
11. Stoorvogel W, Kleijmeer MJ, Geuze HJ et al (2002) The biogenesis and functions of exosomes. Traffic 3:321–330
12. Thery C, Zitvogel L, Amigorena S (2002) Exosomes: composition, biogenesis and function. Nat Rev Immunol 2:569–579
13. Buschow SI, Nolte-'tHoen ENM, Van Niel G et al (2009) MHC II in dendritic cells is targeted to lysosomes or T cell-induced exosomes via distinct multivesicular body pathways. Traffic 10:1528–1542
14. Raposo G, Stoorvogel W (2013) Extracellular vesicles: exosomes, microvesicles, and friends. J Cell Biol 200:373–383
15. Cocucci E, Racchetti G, Meldolesi J (2008) Shedding microvesicles: artefacts no more. Trends Cell Biol 19:43–51
16. Johnstone RM, Adam M, Hammond JR et al (1987) Vesicle formation during reticulocyte maturation. Association of plasma membrane activities with released vesicles (exosomes). J Biol Chem 262:9412–9420
17. Raposo G, Nijman HW, Stoorvogel W et al (1996) B lymphocytes secrete antigen-presenting vesicles. J Exp Med 183:1161–1172
18. Thery C, Regnault A, Garin J et al (1999) Molecular characterization of dendritic cell-derived exosomes. Selective accumulation of the heat shock protein hsc73. J Cell Biol 147:599–610
19. Raposo G, Tenza D, Mecheri S et al (1997) Accumulation of major histocompatibility complex class II molecules in mast cell secretory granules and their release upon degranulation. Mol Biol Cell 8:2631–2645
20. Heijnen HF, Schiel AE, Fijnheer R et al (1999) Activated platelets release two types of membrane vesicles: microvesicles by surface shedding and exosomes derived from exocytosis of multivesicular bodies and alpha-granules. Blood 94:3791–3799
21. van Niel G, Raposo G, Candalh C et al (2001) Intestinal epithelial cells secrete exosome-like vesicles. Gastroenterology 121:337–349
22. Wolfers J, Lozier A, Raposo G et al (2001) Tumor-derived exosomes are a source of shared tumor antigens for CTL cross-priming. Nat Med 7:297–303
23. Caby MP, Lankar D, Vincendeau-Scherrer C et al (2005) Exosome-like vesicles are present in human blood plasma. Int Immunol 17:879–887
24. Pisitkum T, Shen RF, Knepper MA (2004) Identification and proteomic profiling of exosomes in human urine. Proc Natl Acad Sci U S A 101:13368–13373
25. Admyre C, Grunewald J, Thyberg S et al (2003) Exosomes with major histocompatibility complex II and co-stimulatory molecules are present in human BAL fluid. Eur Respir J 22:578–583
26. Andre F, Schartz NE, Movassagh M et al (2002) Malignant effusions and immunogenic tumour-derived exosomes. Lancet 360:295–305
27. Morelli AE, Larregina AT, Shufesky WJ et al (2004) Endocytosis, intracellular sorting, and processing of exosomes by dendritic cells. Blood 104:3257–3266
28. Montecalvo A, Shufesky WJ, Beer Stolz D et al (2008) Exosomes as a short-range mechanism to spread alloantigen between dendritic cells during T-cell allorecognition. J Immunol 180:3081–3090
29. Feng D (2010) Cellular internalization of exosomes occurs through phagocytosis. Traffic 11:675–687
30. Thery C, Boussac M, Veron P et al (2001) Proteomic analysis of dendritic cell-derived exosomes: a secreted subcellular compartment distinct from apoptotic vesicles. J Immunol 166:7309–7318
31. Wubbolts R, Leckie RS, Veenhuizen PTM et al (2003) Proteomic and biochemical analyses of human B cell-derived exosomes. J Biol Chem 278:10963–10972
32. Trajkovic K, Hsu C, Chiantia S et al (2009) Ceramide triggers budding of exosome vesicles into multivesicular endosomes. Science 319:1244–1247
33. Valadi H, Ekstrom K, Bossios A et al (2007) Exosome-mediated transfer of mRNAs and microRNAs is a novel mechanism of genetic exchange between cells. Nat Cell Biol 9:654–659
34. Taylor DD, Gercel-Taylor C (2008) MicroRNA signatures of tumor-derived exosomes as diagnostic biomarkers of ovarian cancer. Gynecol Oncol 110:13–21

35. Piper Hunter M, Ismail N, Zhang X et al (2008) Detection of microRNA expression in human peripheral blood microvesicles. PLoS One 3:e3694
36. Skog J, Wurdinger T, van Rijn S et al (2008) Gliobastoma microvesicles transport RNA and proteins that promote tumour growth and provide diagnostic biomarkers. Nat Cell Biol 10:1470–1476
37. Ohshima K, Inoue K, Fujiwara A et al (2010) Let-7 microRNA family is selectively secreted into the extracellular environment via exosomes in a metastatic gastric cancer cell line. PLoS One 5:e13247
38. Thery C, Ostrowski M, Segura E (2009) Membrane vesicles as conveyors of immune responses. Nat Rev Immunol 9:581–593
39. Fevrier B, Vilette D, Archer F et al (2004) Cells release prions in association with exosomes. Proc Natl Acad Sci U S A 101: 9683–9688
40. Rajendran L, Honsho M, Zahn TR et al (2006) Alzheimer's disease β-amyloid peptides are released in association with exosomes. Proc Natl Acad Sci U S A 103:11172–11177
41. Pegtel M, Cosmopoulos K, Thorley-Lawson DA et al (2010) Functional delivery of viral miRNAs via exosomes. Proc Natl Acad Sci U S A 107:6328–6333
42. Mittelbrunn, M., Gutierrez-Vasquez, C., Villarroya-Beltri, C., et al. (2011) Unidirectional transfer of microRNA-loaded exosomes from T cells to antigen-presenting cells. *Nat Commun* **2**, 282. DOI:10:1038/ncomms1285.
43. Thery C, Duban L, Segura E et al (2002) Indirect activation of naïve CD4+ T cells by dendritic cell-derived exosomes. Nat Immunol 3:1156–1162
44. Montecalvo A, Larregina AT, Shufesky WJ et al (2012) Mechanism of transfer of functional microRNAs between mouse dendritic cells via exosomes. Blood 19:756–766
45. Muntasell A, Berger AC, Roche PA (2007) T Cell-induced secretion of MHC class II-peptide complexes on B cell exosomes. EMBO J 26:4263–4272
46. Admyre C, Bohle B, Johansson SM et al (2007) B Cell-derived exosomes can present allergen peptides and activate allergen-specific T cells to proliferate and produce Th2-like cytokines. J Allergy Clin Immunol 120:1418–1424
47. Denzer K, van Eijk M, Kleijmeer MJ et al (2000) Follicular dendritic cells carry MHC class II-expressing microvesicles at their surface. J Immunol 165:1259–1265
48. Blanchard N, Lankar D, Faure F et al (2002) TCR activation of human T cells induces the production of exosomes bearing the TCR/CD3/ζ complex. J Immunol 168: 3235–3241
49. Zitvogel L, Regnault A, Lozier A et al (1998) Eradication of established murine tumors using a novel cell-free vaccine: dendritic cell-derived exosomes. Nat Med 4:594–600
50. Del Cacho E, Gallego M, Lee SH et al (2012) Induction of protective immunity against Eimeria tenella, Eimeira maxima, and Eimeria acervulina infections using DC-derived exosomes. Infect Immun 80:1909–1916
51. Kim SH, Lechman ER, Bianco N et al (2005) Exosomes derived from IL-10-treated dendritic cells can suppress inflammation and collagen induced arthritis. J Immunol 174:6440–6448
52. Prado N, Marazuela EV, Segura E et al (2008) Exosomes from bronchoalveolar fluid of tolerized mice prevent allergic reaction. J Immunol 181:1519–1525
53. Peche H, Renaudin K, Beriou G et al (2005) Induction of tolerance by exosomes and short-term immunosuppression in a fully MHC-mismatched rat cardiac allograft model. Am J Transplant 6:1541–1550
54. Andreola G, Rivoltini L, Castelli C et al (2002) Induction of lymphocyte apoptosis by tumor cell secretion of FasL-bearing microvesicles. J Exp Med 195:1303–1316
55. Huber V, Fais S, Iero M et al (2005) Human colorectal cancer cells induced T-cell death through release of proapoptotic microvesicles: role in immune escape. Gastroenterology 128:1796–1804
56. Klibi J, Niki T, Riedel A et al (2009) Blood diffusion and Th1-suppressive effects of galectin-9-containing exosomes released by Epstein-Barr virus-infected nasopharyngeal carcinoma cells. Blood 113:1957–1966
57. Taylor DD, Gercel-Taylor C, Lyons KS et al (2003) T-cell apoptosis and suppression of T-cell receptor/CD3-zeta by Fas ligand-containing membrane vesicles shed from ovarian tumors. Clin Cancer Res 9:5113–5119
58. Valenti R, Huber V, Filipazzi P et al (2006) Human tumor-released microvesicles promote the differentiation of myeloid cells with transforming growth factor-beta-mediated suppressive activity on T lymphocytes. Cancer Res 66:9290–9298
59. Xiang X, Liu Y, Zhuang X et al (2010) TLR2-mediated expansion of MDSCs is dependent on the source of tumor exosomes. Am J Pathol 177:1606–1610

60. Mignot G, Chalmin F, Ladoire S et al (2011) Tumor exosome-mediated MDSC activation. Am J Pathol 178:1403–1404
61. Liu Y, Xiang X, Zhuang X et al (2010) Contribution of MyD88 to the tumor exosome-mediated induction of myeloid derived suppressor cells. Am J Pathol 176:2490–2499
62. Chalmin F, Ladoire S, Mignot G et al (2010) Membrane-associated Hsp72 from tumor-derived exosomes mediates STAT3-dependent immunosuppressive function of mouse and human myeloid-derived suppressor cells. J Clin Invest 120:457–471
63. Blott EJ, Bossi G, Clark R et al (2001) Fas ligand is targeted to secretory lysosomes via a proline-rich domain in its cytoplasmic tail. J Cell Sci 114:2405–2416
64. Zuccato E, Blott EJ, Holt O et al (2007) Sorting of Fas ligand to secretory lysosomes is regulated by mono-ubiquitylation and phosphorylation. J Cell Sci 120:191–199
65. Raiborg C, Stenmark H (2009) The ESCRT machinery in endosomal sorting of ubiquitylated membrane proteins. Nature 458:445–452
66. Hurley JH, Hanson PI (2010) Membrane budding and scission by the ESCRT machinery: it's all in the neck. Nat Rev Mol Cell Biol 11:556–566
67. Cai Z, Yang F, Yu L et al (2012) Activated T cell exosomes promote tumor invasion via Fas signaling pathway. J Immunol 188:5954–5961
68. Lugini L, Cecchetti S, Huber V et al (2012) Immune surveillance properties of human NK cell-derived exosomes. J Immunol 189:2833–2842
69. Munich S, Sobo-Vujanovic A, Buchser WJ et al (2012) Dendritic cell exosomes directly kill tumor cells and activate natural killer cells via TNF superfamily ligands. Oncoimmunology 1:1074–1083
70. Frangsmyr L, Baranov V, Nagaeva O et al (2005) Cytoplasmic microvesicular form of Fas ligand in human early placenta: switching the tissue immune privilege hypothesis from cellular to vesicular level. Mol Hum Reprod 11:35–41
71. Jodo S, Strehlow D, Ju S-T (2000) Bioactivities of Fas ligand-expressing retroviral particles. J Immunol 164:5062–5069
72. Jodo S, Hohlbaum AM, Xiao S et al (2000) CD95 (Fas) ligand-expressing vesicles display antibody-mediated, FcR-dependent enhancement of cytotoxicity. J Immunol 165: 5487–5494
73. Lamparski HG, Metha-Damani A, Yao J-Y et al (2002) Production and characterization of clinical grade exosomes derived from dendritic cells. J Immunol Methods 270: 211–226
74. Filipe V, Hawe A, Jiskoot W (2010) Critical evaluation of nanoparticle tracking analysis (NTA) by NanoSight for the measurement of nanoparticles and protein aggregates. Pharm Res 27:796–810
75. Thery C, Clayton A, Amigorena S et al (2006) Isolation and characterization of exosomes from cell culture supernatants and biological fluids. Current protocol in cell biology. Wiley, New York, pp 3.22.1–3.22.29

Chapter 8

Characterization of CTL by Microscopy

Giuseppe Stefano Netti

Abstract

Conventional microscopic techniques may be easily employed to detect and characterize cytotoxic T lymphocytes (CTL). Immunohistochemistry (IHC) may be effectively performed in CTL characterization to identify the location and distribution of target antigens in suspension cells or in tissues by staining with a specific antibody. The antibody may be conjugated to either a fluorescent or an enzymatic label, and the location of the label seen through a microscope approximates the position of the target antigen.

Here, immunohistochemistry and immunofluorescence for both paraffin-embedded and frozen tissues and for suspended cell are described. Moreover, specific recommendations for analysis of suspension of cells are provided.

Key words Immunohistochemistry, Immunofluorescence, Paraffin-embedded tissue, Frozen tissue, Cytospin

1 Introduction

Cytotoxic T lymphocytes (CTL) may be easily detected and characterized by several microscopic techniques. Major hallmarks of both CD4+ and CD8+ CTL are granzyme B/GZMB, granzyme A/GZMA, and perforin/PRF1, which may be analyzed with microscopy in several tissues.

Immunohistochemistry (IHC) is a widely used method which allows to detect tissue-infiltrating cells and to characterize surface cytoplasmic or nuclear antigens [1]. IHC may be effectively employed in CTL characterization to identify the location and distribution of target antigens in suspension cells or in tissues by staining with a specific antibody [2, 3]. The antibody is conjugated to either a fluorescent or an enzymatic label, and the location of the label seen through a microscope approximates the position of the target antigen [4].

Most tissues cannot be viewed under a microscope because they are too thick to allow the light to be transmitted. The tissue can be sliced into very thin sections but they should be first fixed

Elena Ranieri (ed.), *Cytotoxic T-Cells: Methods and Protocols*, Methods in Molecular Biology, vol. 1186, DOI 10.1007/978-1-4939-1158-5_8, © Springer Science+Business Media New York 2014 to prevent cell damage. To this aim the tissue is fixed with paraffin, allowing thinner section slices as compared to frozen sections. This results in better microscopic resolution and better images of subcellular structures [5].

Paraffin tissue sections are ideal for rapidly identifying cellular localization of RNA or protein. First, tissue is excised, then sectioned, and immediately fixed by formalin. After staining with the appropriate antibodies, the sections can be identified [6, 7]. In many cases a heat-based antigen unmasking technique, called antigen retrieval, is mandatory prior to immunohistochemical staining of formalin-fixed paraffin-embedded tissue sections [8].

On the other hand, frozen tissue slides are ideal for rapidly identifying cellular localization of RNA or protein. Valuable time can be saved skipping the fixation and dehydration steps required for paraffin embedding, by freezing the tissue in a modified microtome, the cryostat. In addition, frozen sections will more often retain their enzyme and antigen functions [9].

First, tissue is excised, then sectioned, immediately frozen by liquid nitrogen, and then stored at −80 °C. After staining with the appropriate antibodies localization of the target antigens can be identified [9].

Immunofluorescence is the labeling of antigens with fluorescent dyes. This technique is often used to visualize subcellular distribution of biomolecules of interest. Immunofluorescent-stained tissue sections or cells are studied using a fluorescence microscope, confocal microscopy, or flow cytometry [3, 7, 10].

The first step is cell or tissue preparation. To allow easy handling of microscope procedures the cells or the tissue are attached to a solid support. The second step is to fix and, if necessary, permeabilize the cells, to ensure free access of the antibody to its antigen. The third step of staining involves incubation with antibody. Unbound antibody is removed by washing, and the bound antibody is detected either directly (if the primary antibody itself was labeled) or indirectly, using a fluorochrome-labeled secondary reagent. Finally, the staining is evaluated using fluorescence microscopy or confocal microscopy [3, 4, 7, 10].

2 Materials

Standard equipment for histology techniques are not listed below.

2.1 Immunohistochemistry (Paraffin)

1. Fixation reagents: Formalin 10 %.
2. Dehydration and rehydration reagents: Ethanol at increasing concentrations (50, 70, 96, and 100 %).
3. Clearing agent: Xylene or other reagents (toluene, benzene, chloroform, or xylol).

4. Embedding reagents: Melted paraffin (placed in an oven at 56–58 °C).
5. Slides: Poly-L-lysine-coated slides.
6. Blocking of endogenous peroxidase activity: 3 % H_2O_2 solution in water.
7. Antigen retrieval reagents: 10 mM Sodium citrate.
8. Wash buffer: Phosphate-buffered saline (PBS).
9. Blocking buffer: 10 % Serum from host species of secondary antibody diluted in PBS, or 2 % bovine serum albumin (BSA) diluted in PBS.
10. Antibody buffer: PBS with 2 % BSA.
11. Diaminobenzidine (DAB) solution: 0.5 mg/ml Diaminobenzidine in PBS.
12. Counterstaining solution: Harris' hematoxylin.
13. Mounting solution: Organic- or aqueous-based medium.

2.2 Immunohistochemistry (Frozen)

1. Slides: Poly-L-lysine-coated superfrost slides.
2. Blocking of endogenous peroxidase activity: 3 % H_2O_2 solution in water.
3. Wash buffer: Phosphate-buffered saline (PBS).
4. Cold fixatives (+4 °C): 4 % Paraformaldehyde, acetone, methanol, ethanol.
5. Permeabilization agents: Solvents (acetone, methanol), detergents (Triton, Tween 20, Saponin, Digitonin, and Leucoperm).
6. Blocking buffer: 10 % Serum from host species of secondary antibody diluted in PBS or 2 % bovine serum albumin (BSA) diluted in PBS.
7. Primary antibody (customized).
8. Secondary antibody conjugated with appropriate enzyme.
9. Antibody controls.
10. Antibody buffer: PBS with 2 % BSA.
11. Diaminobenzidine (DAB) solution: 0.5 mg/ml Diaminobenzidine in PBS.
12. Counterstaining solution: Harris' hematoxylin.
13. Mounting solution: Organic- or aqueous-based medium.

2.3 Immunofluorescence

1. Cultured cells grown on cover slips, coupes, or cells in suspension.
2. Blocking of endogenous peroxidase activity: 3 % H_2O_2 solution in water.
3. Wash buffers: Phosphate-buffered saline (PBS), 0.05 % Tween 20 in PBS.

4. Cold fixatives (+4 °C): 4 % Paraformaldehyde, acetone, methanol, ethanol.
5. Permeabilization agents: Solvents (acetone, methanol), detergents (Triton, Tween 20, Saponin, Digitonin, and Leucoperm).
6. Primary antibody (customized).
7. Fluorochrome-labeled secondary antibody (*see* Table 1).
8. Antibody controls.
9. Aqueous mounting medium.
10. 95, 100 % Ethanol.
11. Nuclear counterstain (*see* Table 2).
12. Wash buffer: Phosphate-buffered saline (PBS).
13. Antibody buffer: 2 % Bovine serum albumin (BSA) in PBS.
14. Blocking buffer: 10 % Serum from host species of secondary antibody diluted in PBS or 2 % BSA diluted in PBS.

3 Methods

In this section the procedures for immunohistochemistry onto paraffin-embedded tissues (IHC-P) and frozen tissue (IHC-F) and for immunofluorescence (IF) are described. All the steps are summarized in Fig. 1. Carry out all procedures at room temperature unless otherwise specified. Please read **Notes 1–6** for safety and general procedures before starting.

3.1 Fixation and Paraffin Embedding of Tissue

3.1.1 Fixation Protocol

1. Tissues to be fixed and processed should be cut to a size no larger than 3 mm thick. Let tissues fix in 10 % formalin at room temperature for at least 8 h but not to exceed 24 h.
2. Rinse with running tap water for 1 h.

3.1.2 Alternative Fixation of Tissue

Many antigenic epitopes are masked or even destroyed by 10 % formalin fixation. In some cases fixation in a milder fixative such as zinc fixative for IHC is helpful to preserve the antigenic epitopes.

1. Place freshly dissected and trimmed tissues into zinc fixative and allow tissues to fix for 24–48 h at room temperature.
2. Rinse with running tap water for 30–45 min.

3.1.3 Paraffin Embedding Protocol

If tissues are to be embedded in paraffin or plastic, all traces of water must be removed because water and paraffin are immiscible. This process is called dehydration and accomplished by passing the tissue through a series of increasing alcohol concentrations.

1. The blocks are transferred sequentially to 50 % alcohol for 1 h, 70 % alcohol for 1 h, and 96 % alcohol twice for 40 min.
2. The blocks are then placed twice for about 40 min in 100 % ethanol solution to ensure that all water is removed.

Table 1
Fluorophore table

Dye	Absorbance wavelength	Emission wavelength	Visible color
Hydroxycoumarin	325	386	Blue
Methoxycoumarin	360	410	Blue
Alexa fluor 350	345	442	Blue
Aminocoumarin	350	445	Blue
Cy2	490	510	Green (dark)
FAM	495	516	Green (dark)
Alexa fluor 488	494	517	Green (light)
Fluorescein FITC	495	518	Green (light)
Alexa fluor 430	430	545	Green (light)
Alexa fluor 532	530	555	Green (light)
HEX	535	556	Green (light)
Cy3	550	570	Yellow
TRITC	547	572	Yellow
Alexa fluor 546	556	573	Yellow
Alexa fluor 555	556	573	Yellow
R-phycoerythrin (PE)	480;565	578	Yellow
Rhodamine Red-X	560	580	Orange
Tamara	565	580	Red
Cy3.5 581	581	596	Red
Rox	575	602	Red
Alexa fluor 568	578	603	Red
Red 613	480;565	613	Red
Texas Red	615	615	Red
Alexa fluor 594	590	617	Red
Alexa fluor 633	621	639	Red
Allophycocyanin	650	660	Red
Alexa fluor 633	650	668	Red
Cy5	650	670	Red
Alexa fluor 660	663	690	Red
Cy5.5	675	694	Red
TruRed	490;675	695	Red
Alexa fluor 680	679	702	Red
Cy7	743	770	Red

Table 2
Nucleic acid probes

Dye	Absorbance wavelength	Emission wavelength	Visible color
DAPI	345	455	Blue
Hoechst 33258	345	478	Blue
SYTOX blue	431	480	Blue
Hoechst 33342	343	483	Blue
YOYO-1	509	509	Green
SYTOX green	504	533	Green
TOTO 1, TO-PRO-1	509	533	Green
SYTOX orange	547	570	Yellow
Chromomycin A3	445	575	Yellow
Mithramycin	445	575	Yellow
Propidium iodide	536	617	Red
Ethidium bromide	493	620	Red

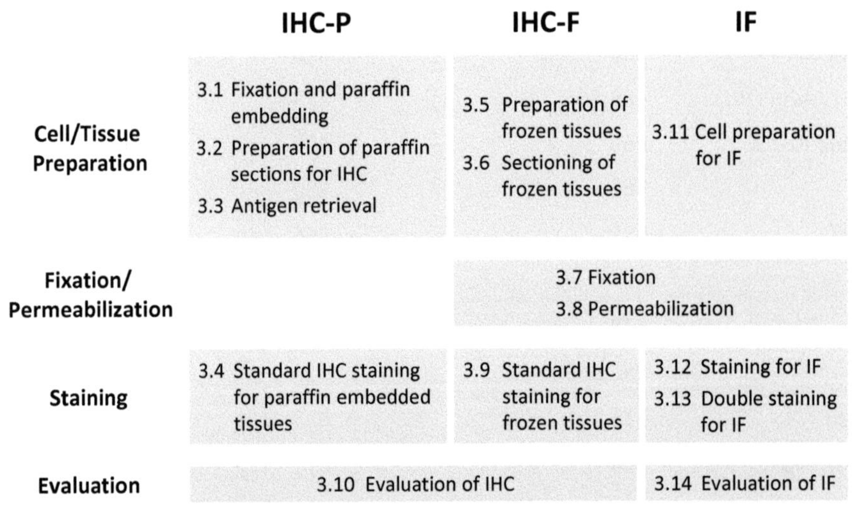

Fig. 1 Algorithm for selection of analysis methods depending on the different source samples

For paraffin embedding the tissues need to be cleared. Clearing refers to the use of an intermediate fluid that is miscible with ethanol and paraffin. The most often used clearing agents are xylene and toluene; others are benzene, chloroform, or xylol.

1. Move the blocks into pure xylene twice for about 20 min.
2. Then move the blocks in pure paraffin for 1 h.

3. Place them in an oven at 56–58 °C (the melting temperature of paraffin).
4. Transfer the blocks to pure paraffin and place in the oven for 1 h.
5. Transfer to a second pot of melted paraffin and place in oven for an additional 1–2 h.

3.2 Preparation of Paraffin Sections for Immunohistochemistry

3.2.1 Sectioning Protocol

1. Section paraffin blocks at the desired thickness (usually 4–5 μm) on a microtome and float on a 40 °C water bath containing distilled water.
2. Keep record of the orientation and sequence of the sections.
3. Transfer the sections onto a poly-L-lysine-coated slide. Allow the slides to dry overnight and store slides at room temperature until ready for use.

3.2.2 Deparaffinization and Rehydration of Tissue Slide

1. Before deparaffinization, place the slides in a 55 °C oven for 10 min to melt the paraffin.
2. Deparaffinize slides in two changes of xylene for 7–8 min each.
3. Hydrate the slides by transferring slides twice through 100 % alcohol; the two changes for 6–7 min each and transfer twice through 96 % alcohol for 2 min.
4. Wash the slides in tap water.
5. Block endogenous peroxidase activity by incubating sections in 3 % H_2O_2 solution in water. Incubate for 7–8 min at 37 °C.
6. Rinse slides 3× in PBS, 2 min each time.
7. If the antibody staining requires antigen retrieval to unmask the antigenic epitope *see* Subheading 3.3. If antigen retrieval is not required proceed to Subheading 3.4.

3.3 Antigen Retrieval

Antigen retrieval is a heat-based antigen unmasking technique that can be used prior to immunohistochemical staining of archival formalin-fixed paraffin-embedded tissue sections. While some antibodies recognize the formalin-fixed antigen, the majority of monoclonal antibodies will not stain formalin-fixed tissues. In this protocol the sodium citrate antigen retrieval method is described:

1. Place slides in a glass slide holder and fill in the rest of the rack with blank slides (ten total) to ensure even heating.
2. Place rack in 600 ml of 10 mM sodium citrate in a glass 2 L beaker. Mark a line at the top of the liquid on the beaker.
3. Microwave at 750 W for 15 min total, replacing evaporated water every 5 min.
4. Cool slides for 20 min in the beaker.
5. Wash four times in distilled water and one time in PBS.

3.4 Immunohistochemical Staining of Paraffin-Embedded Tissues

Perform all incubations in a humidified chamber and do not allow sections to dry out. Controls should also be run and must be matched to the species and isotype of each primary antibody to be tested.

1. Label slides with a solvent-resistant pen and demarcate the tissue if required.
2. Block nonspecific binding by incubating with blocking buffer for 30–60 min at room temperature in a humidified chamber (*see* **Note 7**).
3. Remove blocking buffer (*see* **Note 8**).
4. Dilute the primary antibody (i.e., granzyme B or perforin) in the antibody buffer (*see* **Notes 9** and **10**). Apply the diluted antibody to the tissue sections on the slide. Incubate for 30–60 min at room temperature or overnight at 4 °C. It is recommended to use a humidified chamber.
5. Rinse slides for three changes in PBS, 2 min each time.
6. Dilute the secondary antibody in the antibody buffer. Apply to the tissue sections on the slide and incubate for 30 min at room temperature.
7. Rinse slides for three changes in PBS, 2 min each time.
8. According to the second antibody an appropriate conjugate should be used.
9. Rinse slides for three changes in PBS, 2 min each time.
10. Prepare DAB solution. For blue stain, mix two parts DAB solution + one part 3 % $NiCl_2$. For orange-brown stain, use the DAB solution without $NiCl_2$ (*see* **Note 11**).
11. Apply the appropriate DAB solution, and allow slides to incubate for 5 min or until the desired color intensity is reached.
12. Transfer slide to a glass dish. Add ~5 µl 0.3 % H_2O_2. It may take seconds to several minutes for staining to occur, depending on the abundance of the antigen and the quality of the antibody. Observe the extent of staining under a stereomicroscope and, when the color is appropriately developed, stop the reaction by washing with several changes of PBS.
13. Counterstain in Harris' hematoxylin.
14. Dehydrate through two changes of 96 % alcohol and further two changes of 100 % alcohol.
15. Clear in three changes of xylene and cover slip using either organic- or aqueous-based medium.

3.5 Preparation of Frozen Tissues

1. Label base mold and partially fill the mold with frozen tissue matrix.
2. Remove desired tissues, and trim and cut tissue no more than 5 mm thick.

3. Place in pre-labeled base molds filled with frozen tissue matrix. Arrange tissue in the matrix near the bottom so that tissue is easily exposed when sections are cut.
4. Place a stainless steel beaker containing 2-methylbutane in liquid nitrogen and allow to cool adequately (*see* **Note 12**).
5. Place base mold with tissue into the beaker with cold 2-methylbutane and quickly immerse the block. Allow the tissue matrix to solidify completely and remove block from 2-methylbutane and place on dry ice or in the –20 °C cryostat.
6. Store blocks in the –80 °C freezer until ready for sectioning.

3.6 Sectioning of Frozen Tissues

1. Before cutting sections allow the temperature of the block to equilibrate to the temperature of the cryostat (typically –20 °C).
2. Place the tissue block on the cryostat specimen disk. Adjust the positioning of the block to align the block with the knife blade. Cut tissue block until the desired tissue is exposed.
3. Cut sections of the desired thickness (usually 5 μm), place the sections on a superfrost slide, and dry for few minutes at room temperature.
4. Fix slides by immersion in cold suitable fixative (usually acetone for 7–10 min), air-dry at room temperature, and proceed to staining.
5. Alternatively, the frozen section slides can be stored for a short period of time at –70 °C in a sealed slide box. When ready to stain, remove slides from freezer, warm to –20 °C in the cryostat or –20 °C freezer, fix for 2 min in cold fixative (acetone, 4 % paraformaldehyde, or other fixatives), and allow to come to room temperature to continue with the staining.

3.7 Fixation for IHC and ICC

Fixation should immobilize antigens while retaining cellular and subcellular structure. It should also allow for access of antibodies to all cells and subcellular compartments. The fixation method used will depend on the sensitivity of the epitope and the antibodies themselves, and may require some optimization. Remember that different fixation strategies are mutually alternative.

Fixation can be done using cross-linking reagents, such as paraformaldehyde. These are better at preserving cell structure, but may reduce the antigenicity of some cell components as the cross-linking can obstruct antibody binding. For this reason, antigen retrieval techniques may be required, particularly if there is a long fixation incubation or if a high percentage of cross-linking fixative is used. Another option is to use organic solvents. These remove lipids while dehydrating the cells. They also precipitate proteins on the cellular architecture.

3.7.1 4 % Paraformaldehyde (See **Note 13**)

1. Add 4 % paraformaldehyde to slides for 10 min only.
2. Wash with PBS or PBS with 1 % BSA.

3.7.2 Ethanol

1. Add 100–200 μl per slide of cooled 95 % ethanol and 5 % glacial acetic acid for 5–10 min.
2. Wash with PBS or PBS with 1 % BSA.

3.7.3 Methanol (See Note 14)

1. Add 100–200 μl per slide of ice-cold methanol.
2. Place at −20 °C for 10 min.
3. Wash with PBS or PBS with 1 % BSA.

3.7.4 Acetone (See Note 15)

1. Add 100–200 μl per slide of ice-cold acetone.
2. Place at −20 °C for 5–10 min.
3. Wash with PBS or PBS with 1 % BSA.

3.8 Permeabilization for IHC and ICC

Permeabilization is only required when the antibody needs access to the inside of the cells to detect the protein. These include intracellular proteins and transmembrane proteins whose epitopes are in the cytoplasmic region. The permeabilization method used will depend on the sensitivity of the epitope and the antibodies themselves, and may require some optimization. Remember that different permeabilization strategies are mutually alternative.

3.8.1 Solvents

1. Acetone fixation will also permeabilize.
2. Methanol fixation can be used to permeabilize but is not always suitable.

These reagents can be used to fix and permeabilize, or can be used after fixation with a cross-linking agent such as paraformaldehyde.

3.8.2 Detergents

1. Triton or NP-40: Use 0.1–0.2 % in PBS for 10 min only.
   These will also partially dissolve the nuclear membrane and are therefore very suitable for nuclear antigen staining. As these are harsh detergents, they will disrupt proteins when used at higher concentrations or for longer amounts of time, affecting staining results.
2. Tween 20, Saponin, Digitonin, and Leucoperm: Use 0.2–0.5 % for 10–30 min.
   These are much milder membrane solubilizers. They will give large enough pores for antibodies to go through without dissolving the plasma membrane. They are suitable for antigens in the cytoplasm or the cytoplasmic face of the plasma membrane and for soluble nuclear antigens.

3.9 Standard Immunohistochemical Staining Procedure for Frozen Sections

Perform all incubations in a humidified chamber and do not allow sections to dry out. Isotype and system controls should also be run and must be matched to the isotype of each primary antibody to be tested.

1. Label slides with a solvent-resistant pen and demarcate the tissue if required.

2. Rinse slides 3× in PBS, to remove the tissue-freezing matrix.
3. Block endogenous peroxidase activity by incubating sections in 3 % H_2O_2 solution in water. Incubate for 7–8 min at 37 °C.
4. Rinse slides 3× in PBS, 2 min each time.
5. Block nonspecific binding by incubating with blocking buffer for 30–60 min at room temperature in a humidified chamber (*see* **Note 7**).
6. Remove blocking buffer (*see* **Note 8**).
7. Dilute the primary antibody (i.e., granzyme B or perforin) in the antibody buffer (*see* **Notes 9** and **10**). Apply the diluted antibody to the tissue sections on the slide. Incubate for 30–60 min at room temperature or overnight at 4 °C. It is recommended to use a humidified chamber.
8. Rinse slides 3× in PBS, 2 min each time.
9. Dilute the secondary antibody in the antibody buffer. Apply to the tissue sections on the slide and incubate for 30 min at room temperature.
10. Rinse slides 3× in PBS, 2 min each time.
11. According to the second antibody an appropriate conjugate should be used.
12. Rinse slides 3× in PBS, 2 min each time.
13. Prepare DAB solution. For blue stain, mix two parts DAB solution + one part 3 % $NiCl_2$. For orange-brown stain, use the DAB solution without $NiCl_2$.
14. Apply the appropriate DAB solution and allow slides to incubate for 5 min or until the desired color intensity is reached.
15. Transfer slide to a glass dish. Add ~5 μl 0.3 % H_2O_2. It may take seconds to several minutes for staining to occur, depending on the abundance of the antigen and the quality of the antibody. Observe the extent of staining under a stereomicroscope and, when the color is appropriately developed, stop the reaction by washing with several changes of PBS.
16. Counterstain in Harris' hematoxylin.
17. Dehydrate through two changes of 96 % alcohol and further two changes of 100 % alcohol.
18. Clear in three changes of xylene and cover slip using either organic- or aqueous-based medium.

3.10 Evaluation of IHC

1. Examine the slides under the optical microscope with appropriate magnifications.
2. Record the results. It is recommended to photograph more significant images.

3.11 Cell Preparation for Immunofluorescence

Cell preparation can be achieved by several methods: adherent cells may be grown on microscope slides, cover slips, coupes, or an optically suitable plastic support. Suspension cells can be centrifuged onto glass slides (cytospins), bound to solid support using chemical linkers, or in some cases handled in suspension. The procedure of staining cells handled in suspension is not described here because it is a part of flow cytometry protocol. For immunofluorescence on tissues the protocols for immunohistochemistry can be used (Subheadings 3.4 and 3.9). The preparation of cell lines and cytospins is described below.

3.11.1 Cell Lines

1. Grow cultured cells on support (possibly two- or four-chamber slides) overnight at 37 °C.
2. Inspect under inverted light microscope to verify the desired appearance.
3. Wash briefly with PBS, and remove excess solution.

3.11.2 Cytospins

1. Prepare a cell suspension of not more than 0.5×10^6 cells/ml of protein-containing medium.
2. Pre-label the slides.
3. The glass slide and card are inserted/extracted from the cytospin cuvette.
4. Place empty cuvettes.
5. Load up to 200 μl of this suspension in each cuvette. Spin at 800 rpm for 3 min.
6. Extract the slide, paper, and cuvette without disarranging.
7. Carefully detach the cuvette and the paper without damaging the fresh cytospin. It is very important to hold firmly together glass slide and cuvette when extracting from metal holder.
8. Mark the area around the cytocentrifuged cells with dry point or permanent marker.
9. Proceed with either immediate fixation or air-dry at room temperature. Proceed with air-dried sample.

3.12 Staining for Immunofluorescence

Before staining for immunofluorescence, perform fixation and, possibly, permeabilization, as described in Subheadings 3.7 and 3.8. All incubations should be performed in a humidified chamber to rule out section drying. Isotype and system controls should also be run and must be matched to the isotype of each primary antibody to be tested.

1. Rinse sections twice in wash buffer for 2 min.
2. Incubate sections with blocking buffer.
3. Block for 30 min in blocking buffer to block nonspecific binding of immunoglobulin (*see* **Note 7**). Then remove blocking buffer (*see* **Note 8**).

4. Dilute primary antibody (i.e., CD4 or CD8) in antibody buffer to appropriate dilution (*see* **Notes 9**, **10**, **16**, and **17**).
5. Incubate the samples in antibody buffer with primary antibody for 30–60 min at room temperature or overnight at 4 °C. It is recommended to use a humidified chamber.
6. Wash three times (at least 5 min each) with wash buffer. Secondary antibody is applied only in indirect assays.
7. Dilute labeled secondary antibody to appropriate dilution in antibody buffer. Incubate the samples in antibody buffer with secondary antibody for 30 min at room temperature.
8. Protect the slides from light, because of the fluorescence, starting from **step** 7 to the end by covering slides with aluminum foil or black box.
9. Wash three times (at least 5 min each) with wash buffer.
10. Remove excess wash buffer.
11. Counterstain the cells with adequate nuclear probe if desired (*see* Table 2).
12. Wash in wash buffer.
13. Mount cover slip with a drop of anti-fade mounting medium (e.g., Vectashield).
14. Seal cover slip with nail polish to prevent drying and movement under microscope.
15. Store in the dark at −20 or 4 °C.

3.13 Double Immunofluorescence (Sequential Protocol)

Procedure for immunofluorescent double staining incubating the antibodies separately (i.e., CD8 and granzyme B or perforin) (Fig. 2):

1. First blocking step: Incubate cells with the first serum (10 % serum from the species that the secondary antibody was raised in) for 30 min to block unspecific binding of the antibodies (alternative blocking solution is 1 % gelatin or 1 % BSA) at room temperature.
2. Incubate cells with the first primary antibody (i.e., CD8) in 1 % BSA or 1 % serum in PBST in a humidified chamber for 30–60 min at room temperature or overnight at 4 °C depending on the concentration of the antibody and the accessibility of the antigen.
3. Decant the first primary antibody solution and wash the cells three times in PBS, 5 min each wash.
4. Incubate cells with first secondary antibody (labeled with fluorochrome-1) in 1 % BSA in PBS for 1 h at room temperature in the dark.

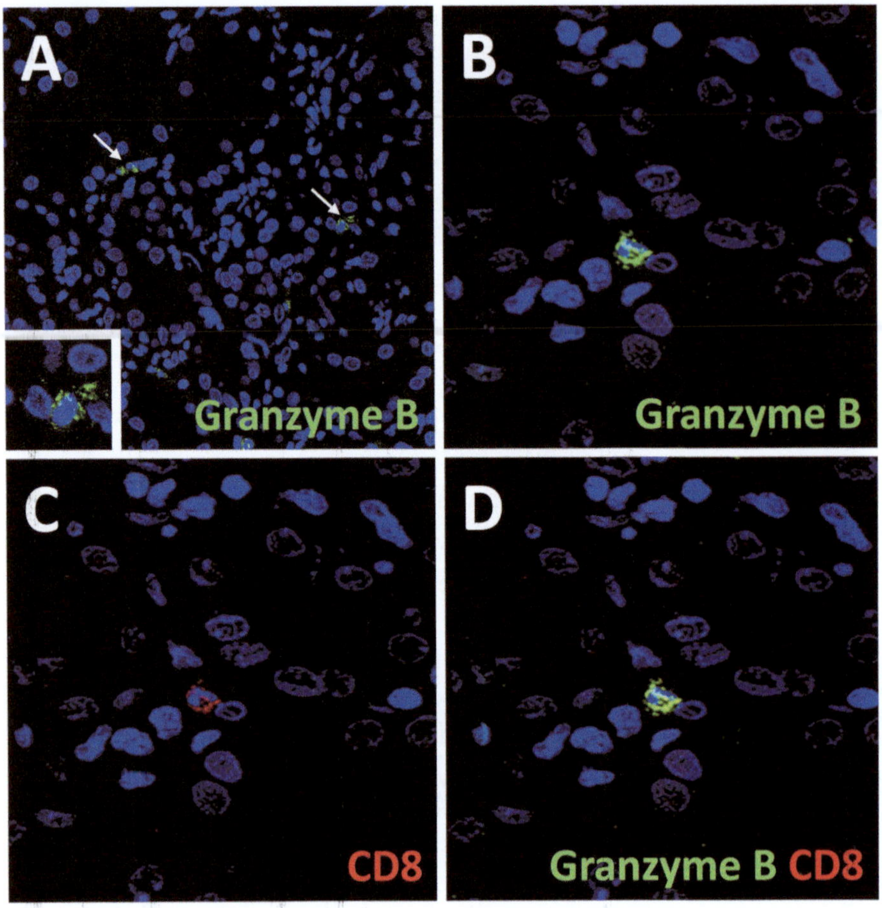

Fig. 2 Infiltrating CD8+ CTL-expressing granzyme B in renal tissue specimens during acute rejection (**A–D**)

5. Decant the first secondary antibody solution and wash three times with PBS for 5 min each in the dark.
6. Second blocking step: Incubate cells with the second serum (10 % serum from the species that the secondary antibody was raised in) for 30 min to block unspecific binding of the antibodies (alternative blocking solution is 1 % gelatin or 1 % BSA) at room temperature in the dark.
7. Incubate cells with the second primary antibody (i.e., granzyme B or perforin) in 1 % BSA in PBST in a humidified chamber in the dark for 30–60 min at room temperature or overnight at 4 °C depending on the concentration of the antibody and the accessibility of the antigen.
8. Decant the second primary antibody solution and wash the cells three times in PBS, 5 min each wash in the dark.
9. Incubate cells with second secondary antibody (labeled with fluorochrome-2) in 1 % BSA for 1 h at room temperature in the dark.

10. Decant the second secondary antibody solution and wash three times with PBS for 5 min each in the dark.
11. Counterstain the cells with adequate nuclear probe if desired (*see* Table 2).
12. Rinse with PBS in the dark.
13. Mount cover slip with a drop of anti-fade mounting medium (e.g., Vectashield).
14. Seal cover slip with nail polish to prevent drying and movement under microscope.
15. Store in the dark at −20 or 4 °C.

3.14 Evaluation of Immunofluorescence

1. Examine the slides under the fluorescent microscope or laser scanning confocal microscope with appropriate magnifications, emission, and absorption filters.
2. Record the results. It is recommended to photograph more significant images and/or stained cells.

4 Notes

1. Samples of tissue, serum, or blood origin should be handled as per guidelines for prevention of transmission of blood-borne diseases.
2. Some enzyme substrates are considered hazardous, due to potential carcinogenicity. Handle with care and refer to Material Safety Data Sheets for proper handling precautions.
3. Reagents which contain preservatives may be toxic if ingested, inhaled, or in contact with skin.
4. Formalin has been implicated as a causative agent for strong allergy reactions (contact dermatitis with prolonged exposure) and may be a carcinogen. It should be used with care and always in a well-ventilated environment.
5. Be wary of all organic solvents. Most are implicated as carcinogenic agents. Heed all precautions for the proper use of these compounds.
6. When making buffer(s) fresh before you start, there is no need to add sodium azide to the buffer.
7. Preincubation of the sample with 5 % BSA for 10 min prior to the primary antibody reaction may decrease background staining. For best results with animal tissues, use 5–10 % normal serum from the same species as the host of the secondary antibody.
8. Allow the slides to drain, shake off excess fluid with a brisk motion, and carefully wipe each slide around the sections.

9. Optimal dilutions for the primary and secondary antibodies, cell preparation, controls, as well as incubation times will need to be determined empirically and may require extensive titration. Ideally, one would use the primary antibody as recommended in the product data sheet. The antibody buffer alone may be used as a negative control. A positive control slide (a tissue known to contain the antigen under study) should also be run.
10. The appropriate negative and positive controls should always be included. The antibody buffer alone may be used as a negative control. A positive control slide (a tissue known to contain the antigen under study) should also be run.
11. Use extreme caution, DAB is a suspect carcinogen. Handle with care. Wear gloves, lab coat, and eye protection.
12. If at the preparation of the frozen tissues the block is left in 2-methylbutane too long, the block may crack.
13. Fixing in paraformaldehyde for more than 10–15 min will cross-link the proteins to the point where antigen retrieval may be required to ensure that the antibody has free access to bind and detect the protein.
14. Methanol will also permeabilize. Some epitopes are very sensitive to methanol as it can disrupt epitope structure. Acetone can be tried instead for permeabilization if required.
15. Acetone will also permeabilize. Consequently, no further permeabilization step is required.
16. It is advisable to run the appropriate negative controls. Negative controls establish background fluorescence and nonspecific staining of the primary and secondary antibodies. The negative control reagent should be isotype-matched, not specific for cells of the species being studied and of the same concentration as the test antibody. The degree of autofluorescence or negative control reagent fluorescence will vary with the type of cells under study and the sensitivity of the instrument used.
17. For fluorescent analysis of cells with Fc receptors, the use of isotype-matched negative controls is mandatory.

Acknowledgement

This work was funded by MERIT Program n. RBNE08BNL7 and by PRIN2008 Program n. 2008M9WSJX_002, both from the Italian Ministry of Education and University.

References

1. Oliver C, Jamur MC (2010) Methods in molecular biology – immunocytochemical methods and protocols. Humana, New York
2. Cavalcanti E, Gigante M, Mancini V et al (2010) JAK3/STAT5/6 pathway alterations are associated with immune deviation in CD8 T cells in renal cell carcinoma patients. J Biomed Biotechnol 2010:935764. doi:10.1155/2010/935764
3. Romagnani P, Annunziato F, Liotta F et al (2005) CD14+ CD34 low cells with stem cell phenotypic and functional features are the major source of circulating endothelial progenitors. Circ Res 97:314–322
4. Hewitson TD, Darby IA (2010) Methods in molecular biology – histology protocols. Humana, New York
5. Hewitson TD, Wigg B, Becker GJ (2010) Tissue preparation for histochemistry: fixation, embedding, and antigen retrieval for light microscopy. In: Hewitson TD, Darby IA (eds) Methods in molecular biology – histology protocols. Humana Press, New York, pp 3–18
6. Divella C, Rossini M, Loverre A et al (2010) Immunohistochemical characterization of glomerular and tubulointerstitial infiltrates in renal transplant patients with chronic allograft dysfunction. Nephrol Dial Transplant 25:4071–4077
7. Yuan H, Hsiao YH, Zhang Y et al (2013) Destructive impact of T-lymphocytes, NK and Mast cells on basal cell layers: implications for tumor invasion. BMC Cancer 13:258–272
8. Krenacs L, Krenacs T, Raffeld M (2010) Antigen retrieval for immunohistochemical reactions in routinely processed paraffin sections. In: Oliver C, Jamur MC (eds) Methods in molecular biology – immunocytochemical methods and protocols. Humana, New York, pp 85–93
9. Bratthauer GL (2010) Preparation of frozen sections for analysis. In: Oliver C, Jamur MC (eds) Methods in molecular biology – immunocytochemical methods and protocols. Humana, New York, pp 57–62
10. Gigante M, Pontrelli P, Montemurno E et al (2009) CD2AP mutations are associated with sporadic nephrotic syndrome and focal segmental glomerulosclerosis (FSGS). Nephrol Dial Transplant 24:1858–1864

Chapter 9

Intravital Imaging of Cytotoxic T Lymphocytes

Gaetano Faleo, Per-Olof Berggren, and Antonello Pileggi

Abstract

Intravital imaging approaches are proving to be essential to address new questions to better understand how the immune system operates. These approaches are especially valuable to characterize the complex organization of immune responses in vivo. Here, we examine how to take advantage of the cornea as a natural body window to apply noninvasive imaging techniques to assess cytotoxic T lymphocyte involvement in the immune rejection process in a model of intraocular allogeneic islet transplantation.

Key words In vivo imaging, CD8 T cells, Cytotoxic T lymphocytes, Immune response, Rejection, Islet transplantation, In vivo cytolabeling, Live microscopy, Anterior chamber of the eye (ACE)

1 Introduction

The latest advancements in intravital imaging have made a remarkable impact in the immunology field. In vivo imaging has emerged as an indispensable tool in biological research. Seminal work has highlighted the significance of immune cell motility and cell–cell interactions during antigen presentation [1] and lymphocyte activation in resected lymph nodes ex vivo [2, 3]. This has improved our understanding of immune cell dynamics and demonstrated their importance for successful immune regulation. However, the dynamic behavior of immune cells in target tissues during immune events in vivo remains largely unexplored. Major reasons of this knowledge gap are the limited access to target tissues in vivo and the low spatial resolution of current intravital imaging modalities. Techniques such as magnetic resonance imaging and positron emission tomography or bioluminescence [4–6] have allowed noninvasive visualization of organs/tissues deep within the body; however these techniques, although useful, cannot achieve single-cell resolution [7]. These limitations were overcome by the introduction of confocal and multiphoton fluorescence microscopy [8], which enabled high-resolution intravital imaging of cellular and subcellular dynamics in vascularized organs to maintain

Elena Ranieri (ed.), *Cytotoxic T-Cells: Methods and Protocols*, Methods in Molecular Biology, vol. 1186,
DOI 10.1007/978-1-4939-1158-5_9, © Springer Science+Business Media New York 2014

the physiology of the organ intact. Thanks to the natural transparency of the cornea, transplantation of donor tissue into the anterior chamber of the eye (ACE) bypasses many of these limitations by offering an experimental tool that enables noninvasive intravital imaging to monitor biological processes, including immune responses, longitudinally, noninvasively, and at single-cell resolution [9–18]. In particular, we describe a protocol for the study of cytotoxic T lymphocyte (CTL) involvement in the progression of the immune responses against allogeneic islet transplants [11, 12], as a paradigm of the type of immunological studies that may be pursued with intravital microscopy in the ACE. However, this experimental model is versatile and could be applied to a variety of tissues to better understand how the immune system operates in response to a tissue (i.e., transplantation and/or autoimmunity) or to assess the impact of immunotherapy.

2 Materials

Mouse strains are chosen according to the aim and the design of the study. All solutions are prepared using ultrapure water and analytical grade reagents. All reagents are prepared and stored at room temperature (unless otherwise indicated). Waste is disposed rigorously following regulations at the University of Miami.

To image CTL in vivo in a model of allogeneic transplantation, we transplanted DBA/2 mouse (H2d; Jackson Laboratories Catalog no. 000671) islets into the anterior chamber of B6.129P2-Cxcr6tm1Litt/J mice (H2b) that express green fluorescence protein (GFP) in effector and memory T lymphocytes (Jackson Laboratories Catalog no. 005693) [19]. All animal studies are conforming to national and institutional regulations. This protocol was approved by the local animal ethics committees at the University of Miami (University of Miami Animal Care and Use Committee; Animal Welfare Assurance A-3224-01, effective 12/4/02 with the Office of Laboratory Animal Welfare, National Institutes of Health, and accreditation by the *Association for Assessment and Accreditation of Laboratory Animal Care*).

2.1 Islet Transplantation into the ACE

Equipment

1. Anesthesia induction chamber (Parkland Scientific, cat. no. 9380510).
2. 0.400 Anesthesia Unit (Univentor).
3. Stereomicroscope MZ FLIII (Leica).
4. Head-holding adapter (SG-4N-S; Narishige, cat. no. SG-4N-S).
5. Gas mask (GM-4-S; Narishige, cat. no. GM-4-S).
6. UST-2 Solid Universal Joint (Narishige, cat. no. UST-2).

7. 0.5 mL Threaded plunger Hamilton gastight syringe no. 1750 (Hamilton, cat. no. 81242).
8. Heating pad.
9. 31 G Needle 3/10 cc, ×5/16″, Ultra-Fine (BD, cat. no. 328291).
10. 27 G Needle, 19 mm, 3/4″, regular bevel (BD, cat. no. 302200).
11. Polyethylene tubing 0.58 mm internal diameter (i.d.), 0.965 mm outer diameter (o.d.) (Clay Adams, cat. no. 427410).
12. Iris forceps, 10 cm long, curved 0.8 mm tips (World Precision Instruments, cat. no. 15915).
13. Blunt 27 G cannula, custom made from a 27 G needle.

Reagents

1. Isolated DBA/2 islets of Langerhans (*see* **Note 1**).
2. Isoflurane (Abbott, cat. no. B506; 1–3.5 % inhalation to effect).
3. 40 % Oxygen in 60 % nitrogen gas.
4. Phosphate-buffered saline (PBS) solution.
5. Sterile water for injection.
6. Clavamox (140 mg/L) added to the drinking water daily for 2 weeks starting on the day of transplant.
7. Buprenorphine (0.05–0.1 mg/kg, s.c.) perioperatively and BID for 2 days for invasive surgeries.
8. Viscotears (Novartis).

2.2 In Vivo Imaging of CTL and Target Killing

Equipment

1. DMLFSA upright microscope, equipped with a TCS-SP5-AOBS confocal scanner (Leica).
2. 5× Objective (Leica, cat. no. 506504).
3. Long distance water-dipping lens (Leica HXC APO 20× 0.5 W).
4. Customized microscope stage for the use of a head-holding adaptor and eye stabilizer (*see* **Note 2**).
5. Leica Confocal Software (version 2.61 or higher; Leica).
6. Volocity (Improvision; PerkinElmer).
7. Matlab (The MathWorks).

Reagents

1. CD8-FITC antibody (eBioscience, cat. no. 11-0081-81) (*see* **Note 3**).
2. Annexin V PE.
3. DAPI.

4. Xylazine (5 mg/mL) AnaSed.
5. Q-tips.
6. Phosphate-buffered saline (PBS) solution.

3 Methods

3.1 Islet Transplantation Into the ACE

While handling animals wearing appropriate personal protective equipment (PPE) is required.

1. Isolate DBA/2 mouse islets of Langerhans as previously reported [20].
2. With a P1000 pipette, collect 30–40 DBA/2 islets of Langerhans from the culture dish containing RPMI-1640 media and transfer to a media-free dish containing sterile PBS. Gather islets in the center by gently rotating the dish in small circles to favor easier islet collection (*see* **Note 4**).
3. Connect the end of the polyethylene tubing to the blunt 27 G cannula and the Hamilton syringe.
4. Aspirate islets by pulling the piston of the syringe (*see* **Note 5**).
5. Anesthetize the recipient mouse with isoflurane into the anesthesia induction chamber 2–2.5 % (vol/vol) in 40 % (vol/vol) O_2 and 60 % (vol/vol) N_2 (*see* **Note 6**).
6. Restrain mouse into the head holder under a stereomicroscope and rotate the head till the eye chosen for transplantation is facing upward.
7. With two fingers, carefully pull back the eyelids and gently place the polyethylene tubing loop of the eye stabilizer around the exposed eyeball below the corneoscleral junction (*see* **Note 7**).
8. Use a 31 G needle syringe to perform a vertical cut into the cornea close to the sclera (*see* **Note 8**).
9. Gently inject the islets into the anterior chamber by inserting the blunt cannula through the incision.
10. After islets are released from the syringe on the iris, slowly withdraw the cannula (*see* **Note 9**).
11. Apply a drop of Viscotears on the operated eye to prevent dehydration.
12. To relieve postoperative pain, inject buprenorphine (0.05 mg/kg) subcutaneously.
13. At this point, the mouse can be removed from the head holder to be transferred to a heated cage and monitored till full recovery.

3.2 In Vivo Imaging of CTL and Target Killing

Transplantation of tissue into the ACE allows serial imaging of the graft, an invaluable tool to study kinetics of the immune responses or engraftment. The frequency and the length of the imaging sessions are decided based on the study design (*see* **Note 10**).

1. Anesthetize the recipient mouse with isoflurane into the anesthesia induction chamber 2–2.5 % (vol/vol) in 40 % (vol/vol) O_2 and 60 % (vol/vol) N_2.
2. As described above, restrain mouse into the head holder and rotate upward the graft-bearing eye.
3. Pull back the eyelids and carefully place the polyethylene tubing loop of the eye stabilizer around the exposed eyeball as described earlier.
4. Place the restrained mouse under an upright microscope equipped for confocal LSM.
5. Use a low-magnification (5×) objective to assess the general status of the eye and the graft. For high-resolution pictures with LSM, water immersion dipping objectives 20 or higher should be used.
6. Apply one drop of filtered PBS to the bottom of the objective and one drop to the top of the eye, and then slowly lower the objective above the eyeball until the drop of PBS touches the eye creating a cylinder that will work as immersion liquid (*see* **Note 11**) (Fig. 1).

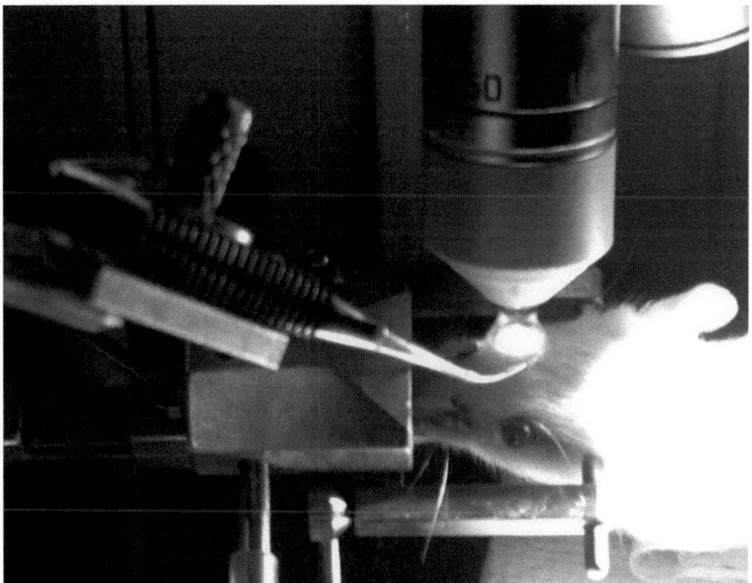

Fig. 1 Setup of the in vivo imaging experiments. The mouse head is immobilized into a customized head holder and the eyelid is kept open with forceps in order to provide adequate exposure of the cornea to the microscope objective. A cylinder of PBS between the objective and the eye serves as immersion liquid

7. The laser power used for imaging should be the minimum required to avoid damage of the tissue and bleaching of the dyes. To visualize GFP fluorescence from the T cells of the recipient animal, use a 488 nm laser and collect emission between 495 and 530 nm, islet outline can be detected by using reflected laser (backscatter) obtained by collecting emission at ±4 nm of the laser wavelength (*see* **Note 12**).
8. Acquire *Z* stacks of 512 × 512 pixels or higher with 0.5 to 3 μm *z* spacing between planes (*see* **Note 13**).
9. For analysis and image display, Volocity software and Leica confocal software can be used. The Volocity software can be used to de-noise images acquired from the in vivo imaging sessions.

4 Notes

1. After isolation, islets of Langerhans were allowed to rest overnight to let them recover from the stress caused by the isolation process.
2. The head holder and the eye stabilizer are screwed into a metal plate, which is partially covered by a heating pad to keep the animal body temperature during anesthesia.
3. The antibody should be stored at 4 °C to guarantee a longer shelf life. We find that it is best to prepare fresh antibody solution each time.
4. For imaging purposes, it is desirable to transplant a small amount of islets into the anterior chamber of the eye, to increase the possibility to keep islets scattered on the iris surface and avoid clustering. Transplantation of larger numbers (depending on the experimental model and murine strains) in diabetic animals should result in normalization of glycemic control, therefore allowing also to evaluate the metabolic function of transplanted islets.
5. The aspiration volume should be less of 1 mL to ease the following injection into the anterior chamber of the eye. To favor faster ejection with a minimal volume, islets are pelleted by gravity until injection. Aspirating a large volume into the Hamilton syringe could make the subsequent injection of islets more difficult.
6. Isoflurane levels must be cautiously controlled to ensure an adequate depth of anesthesia; notably, a shallow anesthesia could result in animal excessive movements; conversely, deep and prolonged anesthesia could cause the death of the animal. Make sure to visually monitor breathing or heart rate and to check reflexes by pinching the mouse paw regularly.

7. Be careful not to obstruct breathing while holding the mouse. The eye stabilizer is a custom-made supporting device, made of 2 cm of silicon tube looped at the tips of an iris forceps to which a screw is attached to allow fine-tuning of the loop size. The modified forceps is then placed into the UST-2 solid universal joint to anchor it to the stage. The positioning of the eye stabilizer should be done with great care. The loop should be closed around the eyeball tight enough to keep the eye still during imaging but not too tight to disrupt blood flow into the eye causing ischemia. Disruption of blood flow in the eye can be assessed by simply observing the capillaries under the microscope at low magnification.
8. This procedure might require some practice and learning curve in order to be performed satisfactorily. Damages to the cornea or the iris and excessive bleeding may result in failure of the experiment.
9. Soon after injecting islets into the ACE, maintain the cannula in place for 1 or 2 min to allow the higher pressure inside the ACE to return to normal to avoid backflow and loss of the graft.
10. Islets can be imaged under the microscope soon after transplantation. However, within the first 3 days the islets settle and adhere onto the iris where the engraftment process occurs with progressive neovasculogenesis and tissue remodeling [9, 10].
11. Dry the area surrounding the eye with Q-tips before applying PBS; otherwise the immersion liquid will not be retained in the desired area. With a transfer pipette apply one drop of PBS on top of the eye and one drop to the bottom of the objective avoiding touching the lens to prevent possible scratches.
12. A two-photon microscope can be used for the same purpose. If a transgenic mouse with fluorescent CD8 T cells is not used as recipient, alternatively CD8 T cells can be labeled in situ by injecting fluorescent antibodies commonly used for flow cytometry. Briefly, under the microscope, with a 5× objective, inject 10 μL of CD8-FITC antibody solution (2 μg/mL, eBioscience) into the ACE with a 31 G needle syringe (BD cat. no. 328438). The needle should perforate the cornea near the corneoscleral junction, making sure not to inject at an angle to avoid shear damages to the iris. Alternatively, the antibody can be injected in the posterior chamber of the eye, below the corneoscleral junction ensuring a high enough concentration of the antibody to reach the T cells infiltrating the graft. Further investigation of CTL phenotype could be done, for instance, by injecting AlexaFluor 647-conjugated anti-perforin antibodies (2 μg/mL; eBioscience).

13. The images should be acquired in the shortest possible time to avoid movements of the imaging field that will lower the image quality. The resonant scanner should be used if associated with the microscope. In the case of time-lapse acquisition, the same imaging field should be acquired with constant settings every 1 or 2 min to compile a 3D movie.

Acknowledgements

We thank the Diabetes Research Institute's Cores ("Preclinical Cell Processing and Translational Models," "Imaging," "Flow Cytometry," and "Histology Laboratory") for the invaluable technical expertise provided.

Financial support for these studies was provided by the Diabetes Research Institute Foundation (to POB and AP); the National Institute of Health (NIH) through the National Institute of Digestive and Kidney Disease (5U19AI050864-10 to AP; U01DK089538 to POB and AP; 5U42 RR016603; 1R01EB008009 to AP; F32DK083226; R56DK084321, R01DK084321, and R03DK075487, the Juvenile Diabetes Research Foundation International (4-2004-361 to POB and AP; 4-2008-811 to AP; 17-2010-5 and 17-2012-361 to AP); the American Diabetes Association (7-13-IN-32, to AP); and the Larry L. Hillblom Foundation (to GF). Additional research support was provided through funds (to POB) from Karolinska Institutet, the Swedish Research Council, the Swedish Diabetes Foundation, the Family Erling-Persson Foundation, the Family Knut and Alice Wallenberg Foundation, the Skandia Insurance Company Ltd., VIBRANT (FP7-228933-2), Strategic Research Program in Diabetes at Karolinska Institutet, the NovoNordisk Foundation, the Stichting af Jochnick Foundation, and the Berth von Kantzow's Foundation.

Disclosures: P-OB is co-founder and CEO of BioCrine AB who is using the anterior chamber of the eye in vivo imaging platform for commercial purposes.

References

1. Monks CR, Freiberg BA, Kupfer H, Sciaky N, Kupfer A (1998) Three-dimensional segregation of supramolecular activation clusters in T cells. Nature 395(6697):82–86. doi:10.1038/25764
2. Cahalan MD, Parker I (2008) Choreography of cell motility and interaction dynamics imaged by two-photon microscopy in lymphoid organs. Annu Rev Immunol 26:585–626. doi:10.1146/annurev.immunol.24.021605.090620
3. Henrickson SE, Mempel TR, Mazo IB, Liu B, Artyomov MN, Zheng H, Peixoto A, Flynn M, Senman B, Junt T, Wong HC, Chakraborty AK, von Andrian UH (2008) In vivo imaging of T cell priming. Sci Signal 1(12):pt2. doi:10.1126/stke.112pt2
4. Gordon RE, Hanley PE, Shaw D, Gadian DG, Radda GK, Styles P, Bore PJ, Chan L (1980) Localization of metabolites in animals using 31P topical magnetic resonance. Nature 287 (5784):736–738
5. Kuhl DE, Phelps ME, Kowell AP, Metter EJ, Selin C, Winter J (1980) Effects of stroke

on local cerebral metabolism and perfusion: mapping by emission computed tomography of 18FDG and 13NH3. Ann Neurol 8(1): 47–60. doi:10.1002/ana.410080108

6. Collaco AM, Geusz ME (2003) Monitoring immediate-early gene expression through firefly luciferase imaging of HRS/J hairless mice. BMC Physiol 3:8. doi:10.1186/1472-6793-3-8
7. Ntziachristos V (2010) Going deeper than microscopy: the optical imaging frontier in biology. Nat Methods 7(8):603–614. doi: 10.1038/nmeth.1483
8. Denk W, Strickler JH, Webb WW (1990) Two-photon laser scanning fluorescence microscopy. Science 248(4951):73–76
9. Speier S, Nyqvist D, Cabrera O, Yu J, Molano RD, Pileggi A, Moede T, Kohler M, Wilbertz J, Leibiger B, Ricordi C, Leibiger IB, Caicedo A, Berggren PO (2008) Noninvasive in vivo imaging of pancreatic islet cell biology. Nat Med 14(5):574–578. doi:10.1038/nm1701
10. Nyqvist D, Speier S, Rodriguez-Diaz R, Molano RD, Lipovsek S, Rupnik M, Dicker A, Ilegems E, Zahr-Akrawi E, Molina J, Lopez-Cabeza M, Villate S, Abdulreda MH, Ricordi C, Caicedo A, Pileggi A, Berggren PO (2011) Donor islet endothelial cells in pancreatic islet revascularization. Diabetes 60(10):2571–2577. doi:10.2337/db10-1711
11. Abdulreda MH, Faleo G, Molano RD, Lopez-Cabezas M, Molina J, Tan Y, Echeverria OA, Zahr-Akrawi E, Rodriguez-Diaz R, Edlund PK, Leibiger I, Bayer AL, Perez V, Ricordi C, Caicedo A, Pileggi A, Berggren PO (2011) High-resolution, noninvasive longitudinal live imaging of immune responses. Proc Natl Acad Sci U S A 108(31):12863–12868. doi:10.1073/pnas.1105002108
12. Pileggi A, Abdulreda M, Faleo G, Molano RD, Ricordi C, Caicedo A, Berggren PO (2012) The anterior chamber of the eye allows longitudinal, intravital imaging of CTLs to study islet immunobiology. J Clin Invest. doi:10.1172/JCI59285L1
13. Rodriguez-Diaz R, Speier S, Molano RD, Formoso A, Gans I, Abdulreda MH, Cabrera O, Molina J, Fachado A, Ricordi C, Leibiger I, Pileggi A, Berggren PO, Caicedo A (2012) Noninvasive in vivo model demonstrating the effects of autonomic innervation on pancreatic islet function. Proc Natl Acad Sci U S A 109 (52):21456–21461. doi:10.1073/pnas.1211659110
14. Rodriguez-Diaz R, Dando R, Huang YA, Berggren PO, Roper SD, Caicedo A (2012) Real-time detection of acetylcholine release from the human endocrine pancreas. Nat Protoc 7(6):1015–1023.doi:10.1038/nprot.2012.040
15. Abdulreda MH, Caicedo A, Berggren PO (2013) A natural body window to study human pancreatic islet cell function and survival. CellR4 1(2):111–122
16. Mojibian M, Harder B, Hurlburt A, Bruin JE, Asadi A, Kieffer TJ (2013) Implanted islets in the anterior chamber of the eye are prone to autoimmune attack in a mouse model of diabetes. Diabetologia 56(10):2213–2221. doi:10.1007/s00125-013-3004-z
17. Schmidt-Christensen A, Hansen L, Ilegems E, Fransen-Pettersson N, Dahl U, Gupta S, Larefalk A, Hannibal TD, Schulz A, Berggren PO, Holmberg D (2013) Imaging dynamics of CD11c cells and Foxp3 cells in progressive autoimmune insulitis in the NOD mouse model of type 1 diabetes. Diabetologia. doi:10.1007/s00125-013-3024-8
18. Rodriguez-Diaz R, Caicedo A (2013) Novel approaches to studying the role of innervation in the biology of pancreatic islets. Endocrinol Metab Clin North Am 42(1):39–56. doi:10.1016/j.ecl.2012.11.001
19. Unutmaz D, Xiang W, Sunshine MJ, Campbell J, Butcher E, Littman DR (2000) The primate lentiviral receptor Bonzo/STRL33 is coordinately regulated with CCR5 and its expression pattern is conserved between human and mouse. J Immunol 165(6):3284–3292
20. Pileggi A, Molano RD, Berney T, Ichii H, San Jose S, Zahr E, Poggioli R, Linetsky E, Ricordi C, Inverardi L (2005) Prolonged allogeneic islet graft survival by protoporphyrins. Cell Transplant 14(2–3):85–96

Chapter 10

The Microarray-Based Approach for the Analysis of the Transcriptome

Matteo Accetturo, Paola Pontrelli, and Loreto Gesualdo

Abstract

Microarrays play an important role in the study of the transcriptome in a variety of conditions and species. This is documented by their widespread use over the last decade in areas such as cancer, immunology, neurological disorders, renal diseases, and many others, directed towards the new frontiers of personalized medicine and drug discovery.

The following method covers a specific application of microarrays in the field of immunology, focusing on the study of antigen-induced T cell differentiation in response to viral or bacterial infection, and in the context of cancer. This protocol allows, through an "Omics" strategy, the study of the transcriptome of CTLs, concentrating only on the expression profiles of those genes more likely to be involved in CTL action. Since the biological question, in this case, is very specific, the advantage of this protocol with respect to a more traditional whole transcriptome microarray experiment is to remove the noise coming from all the genes not directly involved in the CTLs-specific pathways, highlighting weaker signals that otherwise would be hidden by the noise itself.

To address this issue we have accurately selected all the CTLs-specific pathways, extracted all the genes belonging to them, and designed a CTL-specific microarray, based on all known validated transcripts deriving from these genes. This microarray has been built for the Agilent Technologies microarray platform, the only one that, to our knowledge, at present allows autonomously designing a completely customizable microarray. We used it in the context of renal cell carcinoma (RCC), but surely it will find several more applications in many other cancers and in the context of viral and bacterial infection.

Key words Microarray design, CTLs transcriptome analysis, CTLs-specific pathways

1 Introduction

Microarray analysis has been for more than a decade the gold standard for the study of the whole transcriptome in a wide range of settings [1–9]. Now flanked by the emerging Next Generation Sequencing (NGS) ([10] and references therein), it still remains an extremely valid approach in a number of applications, especially in biomedical research, where very specific questions are often asked to the experiment, and well-established protocols and data analysis workflows are needed [11–13].

Elena Ranieri (ed.), *Cytotoxic T-Cells: Methods and Protocols*, Methods in Molecular Biology, vol. 1186,
DOI 10.1007/978-1-4939-1158-5_10, © Springer Science+Business Media New York 2014

Three main microarray platforms share the market nowadays, Affymetrix, Agilent, and Illumina, profoundly different from a technical point of view and not completely overlapping in terms of applications. Due to these differences, protocols and reagents for microarray experiments are very specific and optimized for the platform you choose and generally it is not really convenient to deviate from them. Conversely, the most critical steps in a microarray experiment are all the upstream operations to the experiment itself, namely the overall design of the study and the preparation of the sample which includes all the checks for its suitability for the microarray experiment. The former is strictly dependent on the biological setting we work in, while the latter is more general and encompass all the "good practices" to minimize technical artifacts in the subsequent steps and obtain reliable results. The overall design of the study, in turn, harbors two main aspects: one regarding samples and conditions to compare on the microarray, and the other regarding the microarray itself, in terms of probes (i.e., of genes) whose expression levels have to be measured within the microarray.

For the study of CTLs, in our laboratory, we have set up a specific protocol which enables to measure by microarrays the expression level of several accurately selected genes involved in CTLs biogenesis and functions in a variety of conditions.

In this chapter we will describe how to design a gene expression microarray experiment specifically dedicated to the study of CTLs, and how to ensure that the RNA samples are technically suitable to be processed for it. For platform-dependent downstream steps (i.e., labeling procedures, hybridization conditions, and washing practices), specific protocols and reagents apply. For these, we will refer to Agilent, as this is the platform that we currently use in our laboratory, but it is noteworthy that for other platforms significant changes may apply. The design procedure is totally in silico. For it we will describe a procedure which starts from the information provided by the Ingenuity Pathway Analysis software. As this software requires a fee, see below for an alternative procedure which exploits public databases.

To date, we have applied this method to the analysis of CD8+ T cells of patients with renal cell carcinoma (RCC). We imagine this technique to be useful not only in the context of cancer, but also to study the T cell response to viral or bacterial infections. The strength of the designed chip consists in the possibility to use peripheral blood mononuclear cells (PBMC) or CD8+ T cells as starting cell population and focus only on those genes whose expression profile dynamically changes during antigen-induced T cell differentiation.

2 Materials

2.1 In Silico Design of the CTL Microarray

No particular equipment is necessary for this step, except for an average computer (2 Gb RAM processor, or higher) and a high speed internet connection. The access to systems biology-dedicated softwares such as Ingenuity Pathway Analysis (IPA, Ingenuity ® Systems, http://www.ingenuity.com/) may be of help. The majority of them requires a fee.

2.2 Checking the RNA Integrity of the Sample

1. RNeasy Kit (Qiagen).
2. Agilent RNA 6000 Nano Kit (Agilent Technologies).
3. Agilent 2100 Bioanalyzer system (Agilent Technologies).
4. RNase-free water.

2.3 Labeling, Hybridization, and Washing

1. Low Input Quick Amp Labeling Kit, one-color (Agilent Technologies).
2. RNeasy Kit (Qiagen).
3. Ethanol 96–100 % purity.
4. Gene Expression Hybridization Kit (Agilent Technologies).
5. Gene Expression Wash Buffer Kit (Agilent Technologies).
6. 100 % acetonitrile.
7. Microarray platform (rotating oven + scanner) (Agilent Technologies).
8. RNase-free water.
9. Thermal cycler or water baths.
10. Refrigerated centrifuge.
11. NanoDrop ND UV–VIS Spectrophotometer.

3 Methods

3.1 In Silico Design of the CTL Microarray

In this step some programming skills may be required since the parsing of huge files and large datasets will be necessary in order to select the information of interest. Below we will describe the procedure to design a microarray for humans. For other species and/or model organisms some modifications might be necessary.

1. Access Ingenuity Pathway Analysis (http://www.ingenuity.com/) (*see* **Note 1**).
2. From the Project Manager, on the left hand side, open Libraries —>Ingenuity Canonical Pathways—>Signaling Pathways.

3. Select the pathways of interest. Each folder contains several pathways; they are the result of the integration of several databases and the literature. Each of them should be examined singularly. In Table 1 we have summarized the pathways we have selected to study CTLs, thinking of their biogenesis and functions. Our idea was to include all the genes that, to our knowledge, may play a role or be involved in CTL responses during physiological or pathological conditions.
4. When a pathway is of interest, download the list of genes belonging to it using the Export Data button on the right upper hand side.
5. Once all data have been exported, all files that have been generated must be concatenated in a single file, in order to have a single list of genes. This will be redundant as one gene may participate in more than one pathway. Select each gene only once, by considering their NCBI Entrez Gene ID as their unambiguous gene identifier (*see* **Note 2**).
6. Associate to each gene the NCBI Accession Number of the transcripts on which you want to design the probes to fill the microarray. This information is stored in the file gene2accession.gz downloadable via ftp at the site: ftp://ftp.ncbi.nih.gov/gene/DATA/ (*see* **Note 3**). All selected Accession Numbers should be curated RefSeq records (such as those with NM_, NR_, or NP_ accession prefixes). More than one transcript may be present for each gene, corresponding to their variants and/or isoforms. Unless different indications are available, all known validated transcripts for each gene should be considered.
7. Once you have generated the list of transcripts of interests, these can be used to design the probes that will populate the microarray. Table 2 reports the list of Accession Numbers we have generated in our laboratory for the study of CTLs.
8. Customization of Agilent microarrays is straightforward. Access the site https://earray.chem.agilent.com/earray/, which is the Agilent dedicated tool to design custom microarrays for a variety of applications. It is free of charge.
9. Select on the upper right hand side, as Application Type: Expression.
10. Select: Create a Microarray Design from Target Transcripts. Proceed with the wizard and, when requested, upload the list of NCBI Accession Numbers previously generated. Follow Agilent indications for all other steps. At the end of the procedure your probes have been designed and your microarray is completed. You can proceed with the purchase.

Table 1
Pathways involved in CTL biogenesis and functions

Pathway	Genes
Apoptosis signaling	Acinus; AIF; Apafl; Apafl-Cycs; ASK1; BAD; BAK; BAX; Bcl-2; BCL-B; Bcl-XL; Bfl-1; Bid; BIM; BIRC6; c-Raf; CAD; Calpain; Caspase 12; Caspase 2; Caspase 3; Caspase 6; Caspase 7; Caspase 8/10; Caspase 9; Cdc2; cIAP; Cytochrome C; Diablo; Endo G; ERK1/2; Fodrin; Gas2; HtrA2; IκB; ICAD; IkB-NfkB; IKK; JNK1; Lamin A; MCL1; MEK1/2; MKK4/7; NF-κB; NIK; p53; p90RSK; PARP; PKC(α,ε,θ); PLCγ; Ras; ROCK1; TNF/FasL; TNFR/Fas; zVAD-FMK
Calcium-induced T-lymphocytes apoptosis	CABIN1; CALM; CAPN2; CD3; CD3-TCR; CD4; CRAC; DAG; HDAC1/2; IP3; IP3R; Lck; MEF2D; MHCII; NFAT1; Nur77; p300; PIP2; PKC; PLCγ1; SERCA; TCR
CD27 signaling in lymphocytes	AP-1; APAF1; Bcl-XL; BID; c-Fos; c-Jun; Caspase 3; Caspase 8; Caspase 9; CD27; CD27L; CytoC; IκB; IkB-NFkB; IKK; JNK; MEK; MEKK; NFκB; NIK; SIVA; TRAF2; TRAF2-TRAF5; TRAF5
Cell cycle: G1/S checkpoint regulation	Abl1; ATM/ATR; c-Myc; Cdc25A; CDK4/6; CDK2; CyclinD; CyclinE; DP-1; E2F; E2f-Tfdp1; EBP1; GSK3β; HDAC; L11; L5; Max; Max-Myc; MDM2; NRG1; Nucleostemin; p15INK4; p16INK4; p21Cip1; p27Kip1; p53; PAK1IP1; Rb; Rb-E2F transcription repression complex; SCF; SIN3A; Smad3; Smad3-Smad4; Smad4; Suv39H1; TGF-β
Cell cycle: G2/M DNA damage checkpoint regulation	14-3-3; 14-3-3σ; 14-3-3 (β,ε,ζ); 14-3-3-Cdc25; ATM; ATM/ATR; Brca1; Cdc2; Cdc2-CyclinB; Cdc2-CyclinB-Sfn; Cdc25B/C; CDK7; Cdkn2a-Mdm2; Chk1; Chk2; CKS1; CKS2; Cyclin B; DNA-PK; Ep300/Pcaf; GADD45; MDM2; Mdm2-Mdm4-Tp53; MDM4; Myt1; p19Arf; p21Cip1; p300; p53; p90RSK; PCAF; Plk1; Reprimo; SCF; Topo II; Wee1
Cell cycle control of chromosomal replication	CDC45; CDC6; CDC7; CDK; CDT1; CHK2; DBF4; DNAPol; MCM; ORC; ORC-CDC45-CDT1-MCM-RPA; ORC1; ORC2; ORC3; ORC4; ORC5; ORC6; pre-RC; RC; RPA
Cytotoxic T-lymphocytes mediated apoptosis of target cells	APAF1; Apafl-Cycs; BCL-2; BID; CAD; Caspase3/6/7; Caspase8; Caspase9; CD3; CD3-TCR; CytoC; FADD; Fas; FasL; GranzymeB; ICAD; ICAD-CAD; MHC; Perforin; TCR
CTLA4 signaling in cytotoxic T lymphocytes	AKT; AP1; AP2; CD28; CD3; CD3-TCR; CD4; CD80; CD86; Clathrin; CTLA4; Fyn; GADS; GRB2; JAK2; LAT; Lck; LYP; MHCII; PI3K; PLCγ1; PP2A; SHP1; SHP2; SLP76; Syk; TCR; TRIM; ZAP70
Cyclins and cell cycle regulation	ATM; ATR; c-Raf; CDC25A; CDK4/6; CDK1; CDK1-Cyclin A; CDK1-Cyclin B; CDK2; CDK2-Cyclin A; CDK2-CyclinE; CDK4/6-Cyclin D1; CDK7; CyclinA; CyclinB; CyclinD1; CyclinE; CyclinH; cyclin h/cdk7; DP1; DP1-E2F-Rb; E2F; GSK3β; HDAC; Myt1; p15INK4B; p16INK4A; p18INK4C; p19INK4D; p21CIP1; p27KIP1; p53; PP2A; Rb; Rb-E2F; SCF; TGFβ; Wee1
Role of cytokines in mediating communication between immune cells	G-CSF; GM-CSF; IFN-α; IFN-β1; IFN-γ; IL-1; IL-10; IL-12; IL-13; IL-15; IL-17A; IL-17 F; IL-18; IL-2; IL-20; IL-21; IL-22; IL-23; IL-24; IL-25; IL-26; IL-27; IL-29; IL-3; IL-32; IL-4; IL-5; IL-6; IL-8; TGF-β1; TNF-α

(continued)

Table 1
(continued)

Pathway	Genes
DNA methylation and transcriptional repression signaling	DNMT1; DNMT3A; DNMT3B; HDAC1; HDAC2; Histone; MBD2; MBD3; MECP2; Mi2; MTA1/2; Nurd complex; RbBP4; RbBP7; SAP130; SAP18; SAP180; SAP30; Sin3A; Sin3AComplex; SUDS3
Granzyme A signaling	ANP32A; APEX1; CBP/p300; GAAD; GAAD-IGAAD; GranzymeA; HistoneH1; HMG2; IGAAD; Perforin; ROS; SET
Granzyme B signaling	APAF1; BID; CAD; Caspase3; Caspase8; Caspase9; CytoC; Cytochrome C-APAF1-Caspase 9; DFF; DNA-PK; EndoG; GranzymeB; ICAD; Lamin B; NUMA; PARP; Perforin
Interferon gamma signaling	Bak; Bax; Bcl-2; IFI35; IFITM1; IFNγ; IFNγRα; IFNγRβ; IRF1; IRF9; JAK1; JAK2; NF-κBp65; PIAS1; PSMB8; SOCS1; STAT1; Stat1 dimer; TAP1; TC-PTP
IL2 signaling	AP-1; BCL10; Bcl10-Card11-Malt1; BIMP3; c-Fos; c-Jun; c-Raf; Calcineurin; CALM; CD28; CD3; CD3-TCR; CD80; Elk1; ERK1/2; Fyn; GRB2; IκB; IKK; IL-2; IP3; JNK; LAT; MALT1; MEK1/2; MEK4/7; MEKK1; NF-κB; NFAT; NfkB-Nfkbia; PIP2; PLCγ; Rac; Ras; SMAD2; Smad2-Smad4; SMAD2-SMAD4-TOB; SMAD3; Smad3-Smad4; SMAD3-SMAD4-TOB; SMAD4; SOS; TCR; TGF-β; TGFBR; TOB; Vav; ZAP70
Primary immunodeficiency signaling	λ5; ADA; AID; AIRE; Artemis; BLNK; BTK; CD19; CD3δ; CD3ε; CD4; CD40; CD40L; CD45; CD8; CIITA; ICOS; Igα; IgA; IgD; IgE; IgG; IgM; IKKγ; IL-7R; IL2Rγ; JAK3; LCK; RAG-1; RAG-2; RFX5; RFXANK; RFXAP; TACI; TAP-1; TAP-2; TNFRSF13C; UNG; ZAP-70
Jak/stat signaling	AKT; Bcl-XL; c-Fos; c-Raf; CCK2R; CIS; ERK1/2; Gαq; Gastrin; GRB2; IL-6; JAK; JAK2; MEK1/2; mTOR; p21Cip1; PI3K; PIAS; PTP1B; Ras; SHC; SHP1; SHP2; SOCS; SOS; STAT; Stat dimer; STAT3; Stat3 dimer
Role of NFAT in regulation of immune response	AKAP79; AKT; AP-1; ATF2; BCR; BTK; c-Fos; c-Jun; c-Raf; Ca2+; CABIN1; Calcineurin; CALM; CD28; CD3; CD3-TCR; CD4; CD80; CD86; CK1; CRAC; CSP; Cyclosporin A; DAG; ERK1/2; FcεRI; FcγR; Fyn; G alpha-G beta-G gamma; Gα; Gβ; Gγ; GATA4; GRB2; GRB2-SOS; GSK3; GTP; IκB; IkB-NFkB; IKK; Importin; IP3; IP3R; ITK; LAT; Lck; Lyn; MEF2; MEK1/2; MHC-II; NFκB; NFAT; PI3K; PIP2; PKCθ; PLCβ; PLCγ; Ras; SLP65; SLP76; SOS; Syk; TCR; XPO1; ZAP70
PKCΘ signaling in T lymphocytes	AP-1; BCL10; Bcl10-Card11-Malt1; BIMP3; c-Fos; c-Jun; Ca2+; CaCN; Calcineurin; CAMK2; CD28; CD3; CD3-TCR; CD4; CD80; CD86; DAG; ERK1/2; Fyn; GADS; GRB2; IκB; IkB-NfkB; IKK; IL-2; IP3; JNK1; LAT; Lck; MALT1; MEKK; MHCII; MKK4; NF-κB; NFAT; Oct1; PI3K; PIP2; PKCθ; PLCγ; PMA; Rac; Ras; SLP76; SOS; TCR; Vav; ZAP70
Cell cycle regulation by BTG family proteins	BTG1; BTG2; CCRN4L; CDC2-CDK4-BTG1-CNOT7; CDK2; CDK4; CNOT7; Cyclin D1; Cyclin E; Cyclin D1-CDK4; CyclinE-CDK2; E2F; HOXB9; PP2A; PRMT1; Rb

(continued)

Table 1 (continued)

Pathway	Genes
Signaling in T lymphocytes	4-1BB; 4-1BBL; ASK1; ATF2; c-Jun; ERK1/2; IκB; IkB-NFkB; IKK; JNK; MEK1/2; NFκB; NIK; p38MAPK; TRAF1; TRAF2
T cell receptor signaling	Bcl-10; Bcl10-Card11-Malt1; BIMP3; c-Fos; c-Jun; c-Raf; Ca2+; CaM; Cbl; CD28; CD3; CD4; CD45; CD8; CSK; CTLA4; DAG; Elk-1; ERK1/2; Fyn; GADS; GRB2; IκBα; IKK; IP3; ITK; JNK1; LAT; LCK; MALT1; MEK1/2; MEKK1; MKK4; NF-κB; NFATc; NfkB-Nfkbia; PAG; PI3K; PIP2; PIP3; PKCθ; PLCγ1; PP2B; PTPN7; Rac1; Ras; RasGAP; Ras GRP; SAP-1; SHB; SLP76; SOS; TCRα; TCRβ; TEC; Tra@-Trb@; Vav; Zap70
CD28 signaling in T Helper Cells	AKT; AP-1; ARP2/3; Bcl10; c-Fos; c-Jun; Ca2+; Calcineurin; CALM; CARMA1; CD28; CD3; CD3-TCR; CD4; CD45; CD80; CD86; Cdc42; CSK; CTLA4; DAG; Fyn; GADS; GRB2; IκB; IkB-NFkB; IKK; IL-2; IP3; IP3R; ITK; JNK; LAT; Lck; MALT1; MEK1/2; MEKK1; MHCII; NFκB; NFAT; PAK1; PDK1; PI3K; PIP2; PIP3; PKCθ; PLCγ1; Rac; SHP; SLP76; Syk; TCR; Vav1; WASP; ZAP70
Cdc42 signaling	ACK1; AP-1; APC; aPKC; ARHGEF6; ARP2/3; ATF2; c-Fos; c-Jun; c-Raf; CD3; CD3-TCR; Cdc42; Cdc42-GDP; Cdc42-GTP; CEP2/5; CLIP170; CLIP170-IQGAP; Cofilin; DIAPH1; DRF3; EXO70; EXO84; Exocyst; FGD1/3; GDP; GSK3β; GTP; Integrin; IQGAP; IRSp53; ITK; JNK; LIMK; LLGL; MHC; MLC; MLCK; MLK3; MRCK; MyosinPPTase; p38 MAPK; PAK1; PAK2; PAK3; PAK4; PAR3; PAR3-PAR6-aPKC; PAR6; RalA; RASGAP; SEC10; SEC15; SEC3; SEC5; SEC6; SEC8; SPEC1; Src; TCR; TOCA1; Vav1; Vav2; WAS; WASL; WASL-WIP; WIP
Death receptor signaling	Apafl; Apafl-Cycs; APO2L; APO3L; ASK1; Bcl-2; Bid; Caspase 2; Caspase 3; Caspase 6; Caspase 7; Caspase 8/10; Caspase 9; cIAP; Cytochrome C; Daxx; Diablo; DR3; DR4/5; DR6; FADD; Fas; FasL; FLIP; HSP27; HtrA2; IκB; IkB-NfkB; IKK; JNK1; MKK4/7; NF-κB; NIK; RAIDD; RIP; TANK; TBK1; TL1; TNF-R1; TNF-R2; TNF α; TRADD; TRAF2
IL15 signaling in T lymphocytes	AKT; IL-15; IL-17; IL15α; IL15R; IL2Rγ; IL2Rβ; JAK1; JAK3; NFkB; PI3K; STAT3; STAT5
Lymphotoxin beta receptor signaling	AKT; APAF1; Apafl-Cycs; Bcl-XL; Caspase 3; Caspase 9; CBP; cIAP1; CXCL1; CytoC; Diablo; ERK1/2; IκBα; IκBα-p50-RelA; IκBδ; IκBγ-p52-RelB; IKK; IKKα; LIGHT; LTα1β2; LTβ; LTβR; NIK; p300; p300-CBP; p50; p50-relA; p52; p52-RelB; PDK1; PI3K; PIP2; PIP3; RelA; RelB; TRAF; TRAF2; TRAF2-TRAF3; TRAF3; VCAM1
Myc mediated apoptosis signaling	14-3-3; AKT; APAF1; APAF1-Caspase 9-CytoC; ARF; BAD; BAX; BCL2; BID; c-Myc; Caspase3; Caspase8; Caspase9; CytoC; FADD; Fas; FasL; GRB2; IGF-1; IGF1R; JNK; p53; PI3K; Ras; SHC; SOS
Nur77 signaling in T lymphocytes	APAF1; Bcl2; Ca2+; Cabin1; Cabin1-HDAC1/2-MEF2D-MITR-Sin3; Cabin1-HDAC1/2-Sin3; Calcineurin; CALM; Calmodulin-Ca2+; Caspase3; Caspase9; CD28; CD3; CD3-TCR; CD80; CD86; CytoC; Cytochrome C-APAF1-Caspase 9; ERK5; HDAC1/2; MEF2D; MEF2D-NFAT2-p300; MEK5; MEKK2/3; MHCII; MITR; NFAT2; Nur77; Nur77-RXRα; p300; RXRα; Sin3; TCR

(continued)

Table 1 (continued)

Pathway	Genes
PTEN signaling	14-3-3η; AKT; BAD; Bcl-2; Bcl-XL; BIM; c-Raf; CAS; Caspase 3; Caspase 9; Cbl; Cdc42; CK2; cyclin D1; ERK1/2; FAK; FasL; FOXO; GRB2; Growth Factor Receptor; GSK3; IKK; ILK; Integrin; MAGI; Magi-Pten; MAST2; MEK1/2; MSP58; NF-κB; p21Cip1; p27Kip1; p70 S6K; PDK1; PI3K p101; PI3K p110γ; PI3K p110; PI3K p85; PIP2; PIP3; PKCζ; PREX2; PTEN; Rac; Ras; SHC; SHIP; SIPL1; SOS
SAPK/JNK signaling	ASK1; ATF-2; c-Jun; Cdc42; CRK; CRKL; Daxx; DLK; DUSP8; Elk-1; FADD; Gα12/13; Gβγ; GAB1; GADD45; GCKs; GRB2; HNRPK; HPK1; IRS1; JIP1/2/3; JNK; Jnk dimer; LAD; LCK; LZK; MEKK1; MEKK2; MEKK3; MEKK4; MKK4/7; MKP2/5; MLK1/2/3; NFAT4; NFATc1; NO; p53; PI3K; PI3Kγ; Rac; Ras; RIP; SHC; SOS; TAB1; TAK1; TCR; TRADD; TRAF2; ZAK
Apoptosis in toxicity pathway	Acinus; AIF; Apaf1; Apaf1-Cycs; ASK1; BAD; BAK; BAX; Bcl-2; BCL-B; Bcl-XL; Bfl-1; Bid; BIM; BIRC6; c-Raf; CAD; Calpain; Caspase 12; Caspase 2; Caspase 3; Caspase 6; Caspase 7; Caspase 8/10; Caspase 9; Cdc2; cIAP; Cytochrome C; Diablo; Endo G; ERK1/2; Fodrin; Gas2; HtrA2; IκB; ICAD; IkB-NfkB; IKK; JNK1; Lamin A; MCL1; MEK1/2; MKK4/7; NF-κB; NIK; p53; p90RSK; PARP; PKC(α,ε,θ); PLCγ; Ras; ROCK1; TNF/FasL; TNFR/Fas; zVAD-FMK
CD40 signaling	A20; ACT1; AP-1; ATF1; CD40; CD40L; ERK1/2; FCER2; IκB; ICAM1; IkB-NFkB; IKK; JAK3; JNK; LTA; MAPKAPK2; MKK; NF-κB; NIK; p38 MAPK; PI3K; STAT3; Stat3 dimer; TAK1; TANK; TRAF1; TRAF2; TRAF3; TRAF5; TRAF6
CXCR4 signaling	AC; AKT; AP-1; ATP; c-Fos; c-Jun; c-Raf; Ca2+; cAMP; CAS; CD4; Crk; CXCR4; DAG; Dock180; Egr1; Elk1; Elmo; Elmo-Dock180; ERK1/2; FAK; G alpha-G beta-G gamma; Gα; Gα13; Gαi; Gβ; Gβγ; Gγ; GTP; IP3; IP3R; JNK; Lyn; MEK1/2; MLC; PAK; Paxillin; PI3K; PIP2; PKC; PLCβ; Rac; Ras; Rho; RhoGEF; ROCK; SDF1; Src
iCOS iCOSL signaling in T helper	ITK; LAT; Lck; MHCII; NF-κB; NFAT; PDK1; PI3K; PIP2; PIP3; PKCθ; PLCγ1; PTEN; Rac1; SHC; SHIP; SLP76; TAPP; TCR; TRIM; Vav1; ZAP70
IL10 signaling	ARG2; Bilirubin; Biliverdin; BLVR; c-Fos; c-Jun; CCR1; CCR5; CD14; CO; Elk-1; FCGRII; Heme; HMOX1; IκB; IkB-NFkB; IKK; IL-1; IL-10; IL-10Rα; IL-10Rβ; IL-4Rα; IL-6; IL1R; JAK1; JNK1; LBP; Lbp-lipopolysaccharide; LPS; MKK3/6; MKK4; NF-κB; NIK; p38MAPK; SOCS3; SP1; STAT3; Stat3 dimer; TAB1; TAK1; TNF; TRAF6; TYK2
IL17 signaling	ACT-1; AKT; ATF2; c-Jun; C/EBPβ; COX2; CRP; CXCL1; CXCL5; Elk-1; Eotaxin-1; ERK1/2; GSK3β; HBD-2; I-TAC; IL-17A; IL-17A dimer; IL-17 F; IL-19; IL-6; IL-8; IL17RA; IL17RC; IL17A-IL17F; IL17R; iNOS; IP-10; JAK1/2; JAK2; JNK; JNK1; MAPKAPK2; MCP-1; MKK1/2; MKK3/6; MMP3; MUC5B; NIK; p38MAPK β; p38 MAPK; p50; PI3K; Ras; RELA; RELA-p50; TAK1; TIMP1; TRAF6

(continued)

Table 1
(continued)

Pathway	Genes
IL4 signaling	AKT; CD23; Corticosteroid; CR; GRB2; HMG(I)Y; IgE; IL-13Rα; IL-2Rγ; IL-4; IL-4Rα; IRF4; IRS1; JAK1; JAK2; JAK3; MHC II; mTOR; NFAT; p70 S6K; PI3K; PIP2; PIP3; Ras; SHC; SHIP; SHP1; SOCS1; SOS; STAT6; Stat6 dimer; TYK2
IL6 signaling	A2M; AKT; c-Fos; c-Jun; c-Raf; CD14; CK2; Collagen type I; CRP; CYP19; Elk-1; ERK1/2; GP130; GRB2; HSP27; IκB; IkB-NfkB; IKK; IL-1; IL-1R; IL-6; IL-6R; IL-8; JAK2; JNK; LBP; Lbp-lipopolysaccharide; LPS; MAPKAPK2; MCL1; MDR1; MEK1/2; MKK3/6; MKK4/7; NF-κB; NF-IL6; NIK; p38MAPK; PI3K; Ras; SHC; SHP2; SOCS1; SOCS3; SOS; SRF; STAT3; Stat3 dimer; TAB1; TAK1; TNF-α; TNFR; TRAF2; TRAF6; TSG6; VEGF
IL8 signaling	β-Arrestin 2; 4E-BP1; AG1478; AKT; Ang-1; Ang-2; AP-1; Bax; Bcl-2; Bcl-XL; C3botulinumtoxin; Cadherin E; CAP37; CathepsinB; CD11b; CD11c; CD35; Cox-2; CXCL1; CXCR1; CXCR1/R2; CXCR2; CyclinD; DAG; EGFR; ERK1/2; FAK; Gα12/13; Gαi; Gβi; Gγi; G-protein α-β-γ; G-protein β-γ; HB-EGF; HNP-1; IκB; ICAM-1; IkB-NFkB1-RelA; IKK; IL-8; Integrinαvβ3; IP3; IQGAP1; IRAK; Iressa; JNK; LASP-1; LIMkinase; Mac-1; MEK1/2; MMP2; MMP9; MPO; mTOR; Myosin IIRLC; NADPHoxidase; NFkB1-RelA; NIK; p50NFκB; p65NFκB; p70S6K; PAK2; PI3K; PI3Kγ; PIP2; PKC; PLCβ2; PLD; pro-HB-EGF; PYK2; RAB11FIP2; Rac; Raf; Ras; Repertaxin; Rho; RhoA; ROCK; Src; Staurosporine; SU6656; TIE-2; TRAF6; VASP; VCAM-1; VEGF; VEGFR; Y-27632
Interferon signaling	Bak; Bax; Bcl-2; DRIP150; GIP2; GIP3; Glucocorticoid; IFI35; IFIT1; IFIT3; IFITM1; IFNα/β; IFNγ; IFNγRα; IFNγRβ; IFNAR1; IFNAR2; IRF1; IRF9; ISGF3; JAK1; JAK2; MX1; NF-κBp65; OAS1; PIAS1; PSMB8; SOCS1; STAT1; Stat1 dimer; Stat1-Stat2; STAT2; TAP1; TC-PTP; TYK2
Natural killer cell signaling	2B4; 3BP2; AIRM1; AKT; c-Raf; Ca2+; CD247 dimer; CD247-Fcer1g; CD3z; CD94; DAG; DAP10; DAP12; EAT-2; ERK1/2; FCER1; Fcer1g dimer; FCGR3; Fyn; GRB2; Hcst dimer; IP3; IRp60; KIR-S; KIR-L; Klra1 dimer; Klrc1-Klrd1; LAIR1; LAT; LCK/Fyn; LILRB1; Ly49d; MEK1/2; NCK; NKG2A; NKG2C; NKG2D; NKG2E; NKP30; NKP44; NKP46; NKR-P1; PAK; PI3K; PIP2; PIP3; PKC; PLCγ; Rac; Ras; SAP; SHC; SHIP; SHP; SLP76; SOS; Syk/Zap70; Tyrobp dimer; Vav
NFkB signaling	β-TrCP; A20; ABIN-1; AKT; BAFF; Bcl10; Bcl10-Card10-Malt1; BIMP1; BMP2/4; BR3; CARD11; Caspase8; CBP/p300; CD40; CD40L; Chuk-Ikbkb-Ikbkg; CK2; Cot; EGF; GH; Growth factor receptor; GSK-3β; HDAC1/2; IκB; IkB-NfkB1-RelA; IkB-NfkB2-RelA; IKKα; IKKβ; IKKγ; IL-1; IL-1R/TLR; Insulin; IRAK1/4; IRAK-M; JNK1; LCK; LTA; LTBR; MALT1; MEKK3/NIK; MKK6/7; MYD88; NAK; NAP1; NF-κB p50/p52; NF-κB1; NF-κB2 p100; NfkB-RelA; NfkB1-RelA; NfkB2(p52)-RelB; NGF; NIK; p65/RelA; PI3K; PKAc; PKC(β,θ); PKCζ; PKR; PLCγ2; RANKL; Ras; RelB; RIP; TAB1; TAB2/3; TAK1; TANK; TCR; TGF-α; TIRAP; TNF-α; TNFR; TRAF2/3/5; TRAF5/6; TRAF2; TRAF6; TTRAP; UBE2N; Ube2n-Ube2v1; UBE2V1; Zap70

(continued)

Table 1 (continued)

Pathway	Genes
OX40 signaling pathway	Bcl-XL; Bcl2; c-Jun; CD3; CD3-TCR; CD4; IκB; IkB-NfkB; IL-2; JNK; MHC; NF-κB; OX40; OX40L; TCR; TRAF2; TRAF3; TRAF5
p38 MAPK signaling	ASK1; ATF-1; ATF-2; c-Myc; Cdc25B; CHOP; cPLA2; CREB; Daxx; eEF2K; Elk-1; FADD; HistoneH3; HMG-14; HPK1; HSP27; IL-1; IL-1R; IRAK; MAPKAPK2/3; Max; MEF2; MKK3; MKK4; MKK6; MKP1/5; MNK1/2, MSK1/2; p38MAPK α; p38MAPK β; p38MAPK δ; p38MAPK γ; p53; PRAK; RSK; SRF; Stat1; TAB1; TAB2; TAK1; TAU; TGF-β; TIFA; TNF/FasL; TNFR/Fas; TRADD; TRAF2; TRAF6; Type I/Type II receptor
Role of BDCA1 in DNA damage response	ATF1; ATM; ATR; ATRIP; BACH1; BARD1; BASC; BLM; BRCA1; BRCA1-BARD1; BRCA1-BARD1-BRCA2-Rad51-FANCD2; BRCA2; BRCC36; CCDC98; Chk1; Chk2; CTIP; E2F; FA; FANCA; FANCC; FANCE; FANCF; FANCG; FANCD2; GADD45; MDC1; MLH1; MRE11; MSH2; MSH6; NBS1; OCT-1; p21CIP1; p53; PLK1; Rad50; Rad51; RAP80; Rb; RFC; STAT1; SWI/SNF
HIF1alpha signaling	AKT; ARD1; ARNT; Arnt-Hif1a; c-Jun; Cul2; Elongin-B; Elongin-C; EPO; ET-1; GLUT; HIF1α; HIF1α-VHL-Cul2-Elongin-RBX1; HSP90; HSP90-HIF1α; Jab1; Lactate; LDH; MAPK; MDM2; Mdm2-Tp53; MMPs; NOS; p300/CBP; p53; PHD; PI3K; Pyruvate; Ras; RBX1; Ref1; SRC-1; VEGF; VHL; VHL-Cul2-Elongin-RBX1
Chemokine signaling	c-Fos; c-Jun; c-Raf; Ca2+; CaM; CAMK; CCR3; CCR5; Cofilin; CXCR4; DAG; EOTAXIN; EOTAXIN-2; ERK1/2; FAK; Fos-Jun; G-αi; G-αq; IP3; JNK1; LIMK; Mcp-1; MCP-3; MCP-4; MEK1/2; Mip-1β; MLC2; MLCP; NOX1; p38 MAPK; PI3Kγ; PIP2; PKC (α,β); PLCβ; PLCγ; PYK2; RANTES; Ras; RhoA; ROCK2; SDF-1; Src
Antigen presentation pathway	B2m-Mhc1a; B2m-Mhc1a-peptide fragment; CALR; CD74-Mhc2a-Mhc2b; CIITA; CLIP; CNX; IFNγ; LMP2; LMP7; LMPX; LMPY; MHC I-α; MHC I-β; MHC II-α; MHC II-β; Mhc2a-Mhc2b-peptide fragment; NLRC5; PDIA3; peptide-Tap1-Tap2; Psmb5-Psmb6-Psmb8-Psmb9; TAP1; TAP2; TPN
TGFbeta signaling	Activins/Inhibins; AP-1; Bcl-2; BMP2/4/7; c-Jun; c-Raf; CBP; ERK1/2; FoxH1; GRB2; GSC; HDAC1; Hoxc8; HPK1; JNK1/2; MEK1/2; MIS; MKK3/6; MKK4; Nkx2.5; Nodal; OAZ; p38MAPK; PAI-1; PIASγ; PITX2; Ras; Runx2; Runx3; SARA; SKI; Smad1/5/8; Smad2/3; Smad1/5/8-Smad4; Smad2/3-Smad4; Smad4; Smad6; Smad7; Smurf1; Smurf2; SOS; TAB1; TAK1; TCF; TFE3; TGF-β; TGIF; TLX2; TRAF6; Type IBMPR; Type IReceptor; Type I BMP receptor-Type II BMP receptor; Type I Receptor-Type II Receptor; Type IIBMPR; Type IIReceptor; VDR
Sphingosie-1-phosphate signaling	AC; AKT; ASAH; Caspase; Ceramide; ERK1/2; FAK; Gα12/13; Gαi; Gαq; PDGF; PDGFR; PI3K; PLC; Rac; Rho; S-1P; S1PR1; S1PR2; S1PR3; S1PR4; S1PR5; SMPD; Sphingomyelin; Sphingosine; SPHK

(continued)

Table 1 (continued)

Pathway	Genes
Dendritic cell maturation	AKT; ATF2; CCR7; CD1; CD1a; CD205; CD32; CD40; CD40L; CD58; CD80; CD83; CD86; Collagen; CpGDNA; CREB; DAP12; DDR1; ERK1/2; Fascin; FcγRII; FcγR; GM-CSF; HLADR; IκB; ICAM-1; ICSBP; IFNα/β; IFNβ; IFNAR1; IgG; IkB-NFkB; IKK; IL-1; IL-1β; IL-10; IL-12; IL-12p40; IL-15; IL-1 F8; IL-1 F9; IL-23p19; IL-32; IL-6; IL1RRP2; Immunecomplex; JAK2; JNK; LEPR; Leptin; lipopeptide; LPS; LTα1β2; LTβR; MHCI; MHCII; MonoacylMDP; MYD88; NFκB; NFκBp52; NfkB2-RelB; NIK; p38MAPK; p38MAPK-α; PI3K; PLC; Poly I:CRNA; RelB; SEB; STAT1; Stat1-Stat2; STAT2; STAT4; TAB1β; TCR; TLR2/3/4/9; TLR2/4; TLR2/3/4; TLR4; TNF-α; TNFR; TRAF6; TREM2
LPS-stimulated MAPK signaling	AP-1; ASK1; ATF1; ATF2; ATF2-Jun; c-Fos; c-Jun; c-Raf; CD14; CDC42; CREB; CREB-ATF1; Elk1; ERK1/2; IκB; IkB-NFkB; IKK; JNK; LBP; LPS; MEK1/2; MKK1/4; MKK3/4/6; NFκB-p50; NFκB-p65; NF-kB; NIK; p38 MAPK; PAK1; PC-PLC; PI3K; PKC; Rac1; Ras; SRF; SRF-Elk1; TAK1; TLR4
April mediated signaling	AP-1; APRIL; BCMA; c-Fos; c-Jun; Elk1; IκB; IκB-NFκB; IKK; JNK; MEKK1; MKK7; NF-κB; NFAT; NIK; p38 MAPK; SEK1; TACI; TRAF1; TRAF1-TRAF2-TRAF3; TRAF2; TRAF2-TRAF5-TRAF6; TRAF3; TRAF5; TRAF6
TWEAK signaling	APAF1; BID; Caspase3, 6, 7; Caspase8; Caspase9; CIAP; CytoC; Cytochrome C-APAF1-Caspase 9; DR3; FADD; FN14; IκB; IkB-NfkB; IKK; NF-κB; NIK; RIP; SODD; TRADD; TRAF1; TRAF2; TRAF3; TWEAK
Tool-like receptor signaling	A20; c-Fos; c-Jun; CD14; CD14-Myd88-Tlr2-Tlr6; Chuk-Ikbkb-Ikbkg; Elk-1; IκBα; IKKα; IKKβ; IKKγ; IRAK; JNK1; LBP; Lipopolysaccharide; Mannans; Map3k7-Map3k7ip1-Map3k7ip2; MD-2; MEKK1; MKK3/6; MKK4; MycobacterialLipoprotein; MYD88; Myd88-Tlr1-Tlr2; NF-κB; NIK; p38 MAPK; PKR; PPARα; SIGIRR; SITPEC; ST2L; TAB1; TAB2; TAK1; TICAM1; TICAM2; TIRAP; TLR1; TLR10; TLR2; TLR3; TLR4; TLR5; TLR6; TLR7; TLR8; TLR9; TOLLIP; TRAF1; TRAF4; TRAF6
TNFR1 signaling	A20; AP-1; APAF1; c-Fos; c-Jun; Caspase2; Caspase3,6,7; Caspase9; Cdc42; cIAP; CytoC; Cytochrome C-APAF1-Caspase 9; FADD; GCK; IκB; I-TRAF; IkB-NfkB; IKK; JNK1; MADD; MEKK1; MKK4; NF-κB; NIK; PAK; Procaspase8; RAIDD; RIP; tBID; TNF-α; TNFR1; TRADD; TRAF2
TNFR2 signaling	A20; AP-1; c-Fos; c-Jun; cIAP; IκB; IkB-NfkB; IKK; JNK1; MEKK1; MKK4; NF-κB; NIK; TANK; TBK1; TNFα/β; TNFR2; TRAF1; TRAF2
FAK signaling	α-Actin; AKT; ARHGEF6/7; ASAP1; c-Raf; Calpain; CAS; CAS-Crk; CAS-Crk-DOCK 180; Crk; Crk-DOCK 180-Paxillin; Crk-Paxillin; CSK; DOCK180; EGF; EGFR; ERK1/2; F-Actin; FAK; FAK-Src; Fyn; GRAF; GRB2; Hyaluronan; Integrin; MEK1/2; PAK; Paxillin; PDK1; PI3K; PIP2; PIP3; PKL; PLCγ; PTEN; Rac; Ras; RHAMM; SOS; Src; Talin; Tensin; Vinculin; WAS

(continued)

Table 1
(continued)

Pathway	Genes
Wnt/beta-catenin signaling	β-catenin; β-TrCP; AKT; APC; APPL; Axin; Axin-2; Bcl-9; Bcl9-Cbp/p300-Ctnnb1-Lef/Tcf; Beta-catenin-LEF/TCF; c-Jun; c-Myc; Cadherin(E,N,P,VE); CBP; CD44; CK1; CK1/2; CX43; Cyclin D1; DKK; DKK1; Dsh; Dsh-Frat1; Frizzled; Gαq/o; GBP; Groucho; GSK3; HDAC1; HPK1; ILK; KREMEN; LEF/TCF; LRH-1; LRP1/5/6; MDM2; MMP7; NLK; OCT-4; p14ARF; p53; PAR-1; PIN1; PP2A; PPARδ; RA; RAR; Reptin; SFRP; SFRP1; SOX; Src; TAB1; TAK1; TCF1; TCF4; TGF-β; TGFBR; Ub; WIF1; Wnt
mTOR signaling	40SRibosome; 40S Ribosome-eIF3-mRNA-eIF4A-eIF4B-eIF4E-eIF4G; 4EBP; 4EBP-eIF4E; AKT; AMP; AMPK; ATG13; DAG; DGKζ; eIF3; eIF4A; eIF4A-eIF4B-eIF4E-eIF4G; eIF4B; eIF4E; eIF4G; ERK1/2; FKBP1; GBL; HIF1α; INSR; Insulin; IRS1; LKB1; mTOR; mTORC1; mTORC2; p70S6K; PA; PC; PDK1; PI3K; PIP2; PIP3; PKC; PKCα; PLD; PMA; PP2A; PRAS40; Protor; Rac; Rapamycin; Raptor; Ras; Redd1; Rheb; Rho; Rictor; RPS6; RSK; SIN1; TSC1; Tsc1-Tsc2; TSC2; ULK1; VEGF
Antiproliferative role of TOB in T cell signaling	CDK2; CyclinA; CyclinE; ERK2; IL-2; p27KIP1; p90S6K; PABP1; PABP4; Rb; SCF SKP2; SMAD2; Smad2-Smad4; SMAD2-SMAD4-TOB; SMAD3; Smad3-Smad4; SMAD3-SMAD4-TOB; SMAD4; TGF-β; TGFBR; TOB; TSG

Genes belonging to each pathway are reported with their gene symbol in order to be as much self-explainable as possible

3.2 RNA Integrity Control of the Sample

Total RNA integrity, in principle, could also be checked by a conventional electrophoretic run on a 1.5 % denaturing agarose gel. In this case, for a good quality RNA, 28S and 18S rRNA bands should clearly be seen, and the intensity of the former should be approximately twice as the intensity of the latter. In our laboratory we prefer to assess RNA integrity by using Agilent Bioanalyzer, as it gives more precise and standardized results and requires less amounts of RNA. Moreover a quantitative estimate of the RNA integrity is expressed by the R.I.N. (RNA Integrity Number), a number between 0 (which means completely degraded RNA) and 10 (which means completely intact RNA). R.I.N. allows direct comparison between samples from different experiments.

Always use RNase-free equipment when dealing with RNA.

1. Isolate total RNA from CD8+ cells or PBMC as indicated by the RNeasy Kit.
2. Determine its concentration. Agilent recommends, for a concentration between 25 and 500 ng/μl, using 1 μl to check for RNA integrity on 2100 Agilent Bioanalyzer. Actually, also at 10 ng/μl, 1 μl can be sufficient. It is always convenient to prepare an appropriately diluted working solution for downstream steps (*see* **Note 4**).

Table 2
Genes and corresponding transcripts used to design the CTL microarray probes

Gene symbol	Entrez gene ID for human	Entrez gene name	Accession number(s)	Gene symbol	Entrez gene ID for human	Entrez gene name	Accession number(s)
p38MAPKγ	6300	Mitogen-activated protein kinase 12	NM_002969.3	eIF4B	1975	Eukaryotic translation initiation factor 4B	NM_001417.4
IL-13Rα	3597	Interleukin 13 receptor, alpha 1	NM_001560.2	Caspase 6	839	Caspase 6, apoptosis-related cysteine peptidase	NM_032992.2, NM_001226.3
EOTAXIN-2	6369	Chemokine (C-C motif) ligand 24	NM_002991.2	TFE3	7030	Transcription factor binding to IGHM enhancer 3	NM_006521.4
LMP7	5696	Proteasome (prosome, macropain) subunit, beta type, 8	NM_004159.4, NM_148919.3	Leptin	3952	Leptin	NM_000230.2
TGIF	7050	TGFB-induced factor homeobox 1	NM_173208.1, NM_173211.1, NM_173207.1, NM_003244.2, NM_173210.1, NM_173209.1, NM_174886.1, NM_170695.2	DGKzeta	8525	Diacylglycerol kinase, zeta	NM_001105540.1, NM_001199266.1, NM_201532.2, NM_003646.3, NM_001199267.1, NM_201533.3, NM_001199268.1
BCMA	608	Tumor necrosis factor receptor superfamily, member 17	NM_001192.2	Rac	5879	Ras-related C3 botulinum toxin substrate 1 (rho family, small GTP binding protein Rac1)	NM_006908.4, NM_018890.3

(continued)

Table 2
(continued)

Gene symbol	Entrez gene ID for human	Entrez gene name	Accession number(s)	Gene symbol	Entrez gene ID for human	Entrez gene name	Accession number(s)
Elongin-C	6921	Transcription elongation factor B (SIII), polypeptide 1 (15 kDa, elongin C)	NM_001204859.1, NM_001204863.1, NM_001204858.1, NM_001204860.1, NM_001204857.1, NM_001204861.1, NM_001204862.1, NM_001204864.1, NM_005648.3	IL-8	3576	Interleukin 8	NM_000584.3
Smad7	4092	SMAD family member 7	NM_001190823.1, NM_005904.3, NM_001190821.1, NM_001190822.1	LIGHT	8740	Tumor necrosis factor (ligand) superfamily, member 14	NM_003807.3, NM_172014.2
TSG	57045	Twisted gastrulation homolog 1 (Drosophila)	NM_020648.5	MITR	9734	Histone deacetylase 9	NM_001204148.1, NM_001204145.1, NM_058176.2, NM_178423.1, NM_001204146.1, NM_001204147.1, NM_001204144.1, NM_178425.2, NM_014707.1
3BP2	6452	SH3-domain binding protein 2	NM_001145855.1, NM_001122681.1, NM_001145856.1, NM_003023.4	SITPEC	51295	ECSIT homolog (Drosophila)	NM_016581.4, NM_001142465.2, NM_001243204.1, NM_001142464.2

PAK1	5058	p21 protein (Cdc42/Rac)-activated kinase 1	NM_002576.4, NM_001128620.1	BLNK	29760	B-cell linker	NM_001258442.1, NM_013314.3, NR_047681.1, NM_001258441.1, NM_001258440.1, NR_047680.1, NM_001114094.1, NR_047683.1, NR_047682.1
NFAT1	4773	Nuclear factor of activated T-cells, cytoplasmic, calcineurin-dependent 2	NM_173091.3, NM_001136021.2, NM_001258296.1, NM_001258295.1, NM_012340.4, NM_001258292.1, NM_001258294.1, NM_001258297.1	IL-4	3565	Interleukin 4	NM_000589.3, NM_172348.2
PAG	55824	Phosphoprotein associated with glycosphingolipid microdomains 1	NM_018440.3	IL-10	3586	Interleukin 10	NM_000572.2
ATF1	466	Activating transcription factor 1	NM_005171.4	Cot	1326	Mitogen-activated protein kinase kinase kinase 8	NM_005204.3, NM_001244134.1
S1PR4	8698	Sphingosine-1-phosphate receptor 4	NM_003775.3	IL1RRP2	8808	Interleukin 1 receptor-like 2	NM_003854.2
c-Raf	5894	v-raf-1 murine leukemia viral oncogene homolog 1	NM_002880.3	CD3ε	916	CD3e molecule, epsilon (CD3-TCR complex)	NM_000733.3
HMG2	3148	High mobility group box 2	NM_001130688.1, NM_002129.3, NM_001130689.1	Abl1	25	c-abl oncogene 1, non-receptor tyrosine kinase	NM_005157.4, NM_007313.2

(continued)

Table 2
(continued)

Gene symbol	Entrez gene ID for human	Entrez gene name	Accession number(s)	Gene symbol	Entrez gene ID for human	Entrez gene name	Accession number(s)
IL-26	55801	Interleukin 26	NM_018402.1	LASP-1	3927	LIM and SH3 protein 1	NM_001271608.1, NR_073384.1, NM_006148.3
SP1	6667	Sp1 transcription factor	NM_001251825.1, NM_003109.1, NM_138473.2	PDIA3	2923	Protein disulfide isomerase family A, member 3	NM_005313.4
WIF1	11197	WNT inhibitory factor 1	NM_007191.4	p15INK4	1030	Cyclin-dependent kinase inhibitor 2B (p15, inhibits CDK4)	NM_078487.2, NM_004936.3
CTLA4	1493	Cytotoxic T-lymphocyte-associated protein 4	NM_001037631.2, NM_005214.4	Hoxc8	3225	Homeobox C9	NM_006897.1
TRAF3	7187	TNF receptor-associated factor 3	NM_001199427.1, NM_145726.2, NM_003300.3, NM_145725.2	CAP37	566	Azurocidin 1	NM_001700.3
IP-10	3627	Chemokine (C-X-C motif) ligand 10	NM_001565.3	Paxillin	5829	Paxillin	NM_001243756.1, NM_002859.3, NM_025157.4, NM_001080855.2
RHAMM	3161	Hyaluronan-mediated motility receptor (RHAMM)	NM_012484.2, NM_001142557.1, NM_012485.2, NM_001142556.1	STAT4	6775	Signal transducer and activator of transcription 4	NM_003151.3, NM_001243835.1

PRMT1	3276	Protein arginine methyltransferase 1	NR_033397.4, NM_001536.5, NM_198318.4, NM_001207042.2	NIK	9448	Mitogen-activated protein kinase kinase kinase kinase 4	NM_001242560.1, NM_004834.4, NM_001242559.1, NM_145687.3, NM_145686.3
NUMA	4926	Nuclear mitotic apparatus protein 1	NM_006185.2	MADD	8567	MAP-kinase activating death domain	NM_130476.2, NM_130471.2, NM_001135944.1, NM_130474.2, NM_003682.3, NM_130470.2, NM_130472.2, NM_001135943.1, NM_130473.2, NM_130475.2
DBF4	10926	DBF4 homolog (*S. cerevisiae*)	NM_006716.3	MDC1	9656	Mediator of DNA-damage checkpoint 1	NM_014641.2
GAAD	4830	NME/NM23 nucleoside diphosphate kinase 1	NM_000269.2, NM_198175.1	SFRP1	6422	Secreted frizzled-related protein 1	NM_003012.4
S1PR3	1903	Sphingosine-1-phosphate receptor 3	NM_005226.3	BRCA2	675	Breast cancer 2, early onset	NM_000059.3
TPN	6892	TAP binding protein (tapasin)	NM_172208.2, NM_003190.4, NM_172209.2	FANCD2	2177	Fanconi anemia, complementation group D2	NM_001018115.1, NM_033084.3
NCK	4690	NCK adaptor protein 1	NM_006153.4, NM_001190796.1	TREM2	54209	Triggering receptor expressed on myeloid cells 2	NM_018965.3, NM_001271821.1
ASAP1	50807	ArfGAP with SH3 domain, ankyrin repeat, and PH domain 1	NM_018482.3, NM_001247996.1	Rad50	10111	RAD50 homolog (S. cerevisiae)	NM_005732.3

(continued)

Table 2
(continued)

Gene symbol	Entrez gene ID for human	Entrez gene name	Accession number(s)	Gene symbol	Entrez gene ID for human	Entrez gene name	Accession number(s)
CD80	941	CD80 molecule	NM_005191.3	TNF-R2	7133	Tumor necrosis factor receptor superfamily, member 1B	NM_001066.2
CRAC	84876	ORAI calcium release-activated calcium modulator 1	NM_032790.3	NFAT2	4772	Nuclear factor of activated T-cells, cytoplasmic, calcineurin-dependent 1	NM_006162.3, NM_172387.1, NM_172390.1, NM_172389.1, NM_172388.1
SODD	9530	BCL2-associated athanogene 4	NM_001204878.1, NM_004874.3	NLRC5	84166	NLR family, CARD domain containing 5	NM_032206.4
ASK1	4217	Mitogen-activated protein kinase kinase kinase 5	NM_005923.3	ZAK	51776	Sterile alpha motif and leucine zipper containing kinase AZK	NM_133646.2, NM_016653.2
HtrA2	27429	HtrA serine peptidase 2	NM_145074.2, NM_013247.4	RANTES	6352	Chemokine (C-C motif) ligand 5	NM_002985.2
GH	2688	Growth hormone 1	NM_022562.2, NM_022561.2, NM_022559.2, NM_000515.3, NM_022560.2	Brca1	672	Breast cancer 1, early onset	NR_027676.1, NM_007298.3, NM_007294.3, NM_007297.3, NM_007299.3, NM_007300.3

Caspase 8	841	Caspase 8, apoptosis-related cysteine peptidase	NM_001080124.1, NM_033356.3, NM_033355.3, NM_001080125.1, NM_033358.3, NM_001228.4	4-Oct	5460	POU class 5 homeobox 1	NM_002701.4, NM_203289.4, NM_001173531.1
RhoGEF	9826	Rho guanine nucleotide exchange factor (GEF) 11	NM_014784.3, NM_198236.2	TLR9	54106	Toll-like receptor 9	NM_017442.3
Bcl10	8915	B-cell CLL/lymphoma 10	NM_003921.4	Daxx	1616	Death-domain-associated protein	NM_001141970.1, NM_001254717.1, NM_001350.4, NM_001141969.1
CDC7	8317	Cell division cycle 7	NM_001134419.1, NM_003503.3, NM_001134420.1	TAP1	6890	Transporter 1, ATP-binding cassette, subfamily B (MDR/TAP)	NM_000593.5
NLK	51701	Nemo-like kinase	NM_016231.4	c-Fos	2353	FBJ murine osteosarcoma viral oncogene homolog	NM_005252.3
Apafl	317	Apoptotic peptidase activating factor 1	NM_181861.1, NM_013229.2, NM_181869.1, NM_001160.2, NM_181868.1	MAPKAPK2	9261	Mitogen-activated protein kinase-activated protein kinase 2	NM_004759.4, NM_032960.3
PREX2	80243	Phosphatidylinositol-3,4,5-trisphosphate-dependent Rac exchange factor 2	NM_024870.2, NM_025170.4	Bfl-1	597	BCL2-related protein A1	NM_004049.3, NM_001114735.1

(continued)

Table 2
(continued)

Gene symbol	Entrez gene ID for human	Entrez gene name	Accession number(s)	Gene symbol	Entrez gene ID for human	Entrez gene name	Accession number(s)
PIN1	5300	Peptidylprolyl cis/trans isomerase, NIMA-interacting 1	NR_038422.2, NR_038830.1, NM_006221.3	Acinus	22985	Apoptotic chromatin condensation inducer 1	NM_001164815.1, NM_001164816.1, NM_014977.3, NM_001164817.1, NM_001164814.1
NAP1	64343	5-azacytidine induced 2	NM_022461.4, NM_001271650.1, NM_001134433.1, NM_001134432.1	RIP	8737	Receptor (TNFRSF)-interacting serine-threonine kinase 1	NM_003804.3
FCER1	2207	Fc fragment of IgE, high affinity I, receptor for; gamma polypeptide	NM_004106.1	Nodal	4838	Nodal growth differentiation factor	NM_018055.4
TLR8	51311	Toll-like receptor 8	NM_138636.4	VDR	7421	Vitamin D (1,25-dihydroxyvitamin D3) receptor	NM_001017536.1, NM_000376.2, NM_001017535.1
CCR7	1236	Chemokine (C-C motif) receptor 7	NM_001838.3	NKP44	9436	Natural cytotoxicity triggering receptor 2	NM_001199510.1, NM_001199509.1, NM_004828.3
IL-2	3558	Interleukin 2	NM_000586.3	PAK2	5062	p21 protein (Cdc42/Rac)-activated kinase 2	NM_002577.4
IFN-β1	3456	Interferon, beta 1, fibroblast	NM_002176.2	DNMT3A	1788	DNA (cytosine-5-)-methyltransferase 3 alpha	NM_022552.4, NM_153759.3, NM_175629.2, NM_175630.1

DR3	8718	Tumor necrosis factor receptor superfamily, member 25	NM_003790.2, NM_001039664.1, NM_148966.1, NM_148967.1, NM_148965.1, NM_148970.1	RbBP7	5931	Retinoblastoma binding protein 7	NM_002893.3, NM_001198719.1
RelB	5971	v-rel reticuloendotheliosis viral oncogene homolog B	NM_006509.3	Rictor	253260	RPTOR independent companion of MTOR, complex 2	NM_152756.3
RASGAP	5921	RAS p21 protein activator (GTPase activating protein) 1	NM_022650.2, NM_002890.2	MEKK1	4214	Mitogen-activated protein kinase kinase kinase 1, E3 ubiquitin protein ligase	NM_005921.1
CYP19	1588	Cytochrome P450, family 19, subfamily A, polypeptide 1	NM_031226.2, NM_000103.3	NKG2E	3823	Killer cell lectin-like receptor subfamily C, member 3	NM_007333.2, NM_002261.2
CD94	3824	Killer cell lectin-like receptor subfamily D, member 1	NM_001114396.1, NM_002262.3, NM_007334.2	NF-IL6	1051	CCAAT/enhancer binding protein (C/EBP), beta	NM_005194.3
SMAD4	4089	SMAD family member 4	NM_005359.5	CXCL5	6374	Chemokine (C-X-C motif) ligand 5	NM_002994.4
MSP58	10445	Microspherule protein 1	NM_001278341.1, NM_006337.4, NM_001012300.1	IGF1R	3480	Insulin-like growth factor 1 receptor	NM_000875.3
TIE-2	7010	TEK tyrosine kinase, endothelial	NM_000459.3	GranzymeB	3002	Granzyme B (granzyme 2, cytotoxic T-lymphocyte-associated serine esterase 1)	NM_004131.4

(continued)

Table 2
(continued)

Gene symbol	Entrez gene ID for human	Entrez gene name	Accession number(s)	Gene symbol	Entrez gene ID for human	Entrez gene name	Accession number(s)
TCF	3172	Hepatocyte nuclear factor 4, alpha	NM_175914.4, NM_178849.2, NM_001030003.2, NM_001258355.1, NM_000457.4, NM_178850.2, NM_001030004.2	LAT	27040	Linker for activation of T cells	NM_001014988.1, NM_014387.3, NM_001014989.1, NM_001014987.1
Rad51	5888	RAD51 homolog (S. cerevisiae)	NM_133487.3, NM_001164270.1, NM_002875.4, NM_001164269.1	CNX	821	Calnexin	NM_001024649.1, NM_001746.3
FANCA	2175	Fanconi anemia, complementation group A	NM_001018112.1, NM_000135.2	HIF1α	3091	Hypoxia inducible factor 1, alpha subunit (basic helix-locp-helix transcription factor)	NM_001243084.1, NM_181054.2, NM_001530.3
TIRAP	114609	Toll-interleukin 1 receptor (TIR) domain containing adaptor protein	NM_148910.2, NM_001039661.1	IGAAD	6418	SET nuclear oncogene	NM_001248000.1, NM_001248001.1, NM_003011.3, NM_001122821.1
ARHGEF6	9459	Rac/Cdc42 guanine nucleotide exchange factor (GEF) 6	NM_004840.2	MBD3	53615	Methyl-CpG binding domain protein 3	NM_003926.5

CAS	9564	Breast cancer anti-estrogen resistance 1	NM_001170714.1, NM_014567.3, NM_001170715.1, NM_001170719.1, NM_001170721.1, NM_001170716.1, NM_001170720.1, NM_001170717.1, NM_001170718.1	CDK2	1017	Cyclin-dependent kinase 2	NM_052827.2, NM_001798.3
TIMP1	7076	TIMP metallopeptidase inhibitor 1	NM_003254.2	UBE2N	7334	Ubiquitin-conjugating enzyme E2N	NM_003348.3
RAP80	51720	Ubiquitin interaction motif containing 1	NM_001199298.1, NM_016290.4, NM_001199297.1	FLIP	8837	CASP8 and FADD-like apoptosis regulator	NM_001127184.2, NM_003879.5, NM_001202515.1, NM_001202516.1, NM_001202519.1, NM_001202517.1, NM_001202518.1, NM_001127183.2
AIF	9131	Apoptosis-inducing factor, mitochondrion-associated, 1	NM_145813.2, NM_004208.3, NM_145812.2, NM_001130846.2, NM_001130847.3	CX43	2697	Gap junction protein, alpha 1, 43 kDa	NM_000165.3
CBP	1387	CREB binding protein	NM_004380.2, NM_001079846.1	MLC2	4633	Myosin, light chain 2, regulatory, cardiac, slow	NM_000432.3
Lck	3932	Lymphocyte-specific protein tyrosine kinase	NM_001042771.1, NM_005356.3	MLK3	4296	Mitogen-activated protein kinase kinase kinase 11	NM_002419.3

(continued)

Table 2 (continued)

Gene symbol	Entrez gene ID for human	Entrez gene name	Accession number(s)	Gene symbol	Entrez gene ID for human	Entrez gene name	Accession number(s)
CD40	958	CD40 molecule, TNF receptor superfamily member 5	NM_001250.4, NM_152854.2	Reptin	10856	RuvB-like 2 (*E. coli*)	NM_006666.1
IRF9	10379	Interferon regulatory factor 9	NM_006084.4	IL-12p40	3593	Interleukin 12B (natural killer cell stimulatory factor 2, cytotoxic lymphocyte maturation factor 2, p40)	NM_002187.2
TOB	10140	Transducer of ERBB2, 1	NM_001243885.1, NM_001243877.1, NM_005749.3	CAD	1677	DNA fragmentation factor, 40 kDa, beta polypeptide (caspase-activated DNase)	NM_004402.2
eIF4E	1977	Eukaryotic translation initiation factor 4E	NM_001130679.1, NM_001130678.1, NM_001968.3	DIAPH1	1729	Diaphanous homolog 1 (Drosophila)	NM_001079812.2, NM_005219.4
APO2L	8743	Tumor necrosis factor (ligand) superfamily, member 10	NR_033994.1, NM_003810.3, NM_001190943.1, NM_001190942.1	IL-17	3605	Interleukin 17A	NM_002190.2
IL-1 F9	56300	Interleukin 36, gamma	NM_019618.2	IRp60	11314	CD300a molecule	NM_001256841.1, NM_007261.3
FKBP1	2280	FK506 binding protein 1A, 12 kDa	NM_000801.4, NM_054014.3, NM_001199786.1	CD40L	959	CD40 ligand	NM_000074.2

MIS	268	Anti-Mullerian hormone	NM_000479.3	Ras GRP	10125	RAS guanyl releasing protein 1 (calcium and DAG-regulated)	NM_005739.3, NM_001128602.1
ORC6	23594	Origin recognition complex, subunit 6	NR_037620.1, NM_014321.3	p38MAPKα	1432	Mitogen-activated protein kinase 14	NM_139012.2, NM_001315.2, NM_139014.2, NM_139013.2
PABP4	8761	Poly(A) binding protein, cytoplasmic 4 (inducible form)	NM_003819.3, NM_001135654.1, NM_001135653.1	CD35	1380	Complement component (3d/Epstein Barr virus) receptor 2	NM_001877.4, NM_001006658.2
BIMP1	29775	Caspase recruitment domain family, member 10	NM_014550.3	PAR6	50855	Par-6 partitioning defective 6 homolog alpha (*C. elegans*)	NM_016948.2, NM_001037281.1
LYP	26191	Protein tyrosine phosphatase, non-receptor type 22 (lymphoid)	NM_001193431.1, NM_015967.5, NM_012411.4	IQGAP1	8826	IQ motif containing GTPase activating protein 1	NM_003870.3
Src	6714	v-src sarcoma (Schmidt-Ruppin A-2) viral oncogene homolog (avian)	NM_198291.1, NM_005417.3	GRAF	23092	Rho GTPase activating protein 26	NM_001135608.1, NM_015071.4
GAB1	2549	GRB2-associated binding protein 1	NM_002039.3, NM_207123.2	ATF2	1386	Activating transcription factor 2	NM_001880.3, NM_001256091.1, NM_001256094.1, NR_045773.1, NM_001256093.1, NR_045774.1, NM_001256092.1, NR_045770.1, NR_045769.1, NR_045771.1, NM_001256090.1, NR_045772.1, NR_045768.1

(continued)

Table 2
(continued)

Gene symbol	Entrez gene ID for human	Entrez gene name	Accession number(s)	Gene symbol	Entrez gene ID for human	Entrez gene name	Accession number(s)
IFNγRα	3459	Interferon gamma receptor 1	NM_000416.2	CHOP	1649	DNA-damage-inducible transcript 3	NM_001195054.1, NM_004083.5, NM_001195055.1, NM_001195056.1, NM_001195057.1, NM_001195053.1
Chk2	11200	Checkpoint kinase 2	NM_001257387.1, NM_145862.2, NM_007194.3, NM_001005735.1	Bid	637	BH3-interacting domain death agonist	NM_001244567.1, NM_001244572.1, NM_001196.3, NM_001244570.1, NM_197966.2, NM_001244569.1, NM_197967.2
IRSp53	10458	BAI1-associated protein 2	NM_017451.2, NM_001144888.1, NM_017450.2, NM_006340.2	SAP130	79595	Sin3A-associated protein, 130 kDa	NM_024545.3, NM_001145928.1
ICosL	23308	Inducible T-cell co-stimulator ligand	NM_015259.4	EXO70	23265	Exocyst complex component 7	NM_001145298.2, NR_028133.1, NM_001013839.2, NM_015219.3, NM_001145297.2, NM_001145299.2
MSH6	2956	mutS homolog 6 (E. coli)	NM_000179.2	IkBα	4792	Nuclear factor of kappa light polypeptide gene enhancer in B-cells inhibitor, alpha	NM_020529.2

FANCF	2188	Fanconi anemia, complementation group F	NM_022725.3	EGFR	1956	Epidermal growth factor receptor	NM_201284.1, NM_005228.3, NM_201282.1, NM_201283.1
MEKK4	4216	Mitogen-activated protein kinase kinase kinase 4	NM_005922.2, NM_006724.2	MMP9	4318	Matrix metallopeptidase 9 (gelatinase B, 92 kDa gelatinase, 92 kDa type IV collagenase)	NM_004994.2
JAK3	3718	Janus kinase 3	NM_000215.3	Cofilin	1072	Cofilin 1 (non-muscle)	NM_005507.2
PRAS40	84335	AKT1 substrate 1 (proline-rich)	NM_001098633.3, NM_001278160.1, NM_001098632.2, NM_001278159.1, NM_032375.5	PPARδ	5467	Peroxisome proliferator-activated receptor delta	NM_001171819.1, NM_006238.4, NM_001171820.1, NM_177435.2, NM_001171818.1
MKK7	5609	Mitogen-activated protein kinase kinase 7	NM_145185.2	ET-1	1906	Endothelin 1	NM_001168319.1, NM_001955.4
IL-25	64806	Interleukin 25	NM_022789.3, NM_172314.1	PKL	9815	G protein-coupled receptor kinase-interacting ArfGAP 2	NM_057169.3, NM_001135214.1, NM_057170.3, NM_139201.2, NM_014776.3, NM_001135213.1
GADS	9402	GRB2-related adaptor protein 2	NM_004810.2	L5	6125	Ribosomal protein L5	NM_000969.3
HOXB9	3219	Homeobox B9	NM_024017.4	RFXAP	5994	Regulatory factor X-associated protein	NM_000538.3
MMP3	4314	Matrix metallopeptidase 3 (stromelysin 1, progelatinase)	NM_002422.3	Nkx2.5	1482	NK2 homeobox 5	NM_001166176.1, NM_004387.3, NM_001166175.1

(continued)

Table 2
(continued)

Gene symbol	Entrez gene ID for human	Entrez gene name	Accession number(s)	Gene symbol	Entrez gene ID for human	Entrez gene name	Accession number(s)
IFNAR1	3454	Interferon (alpha, beta, and omega) receptor 1	NM_000629.2	ULK1	8408	unc-51-like kinase 1 (*C. elegans*)	NM_003565.2
IRF1	3659	Interferon regulatory factor 1	NM_002198.2	MD-2	23643	Lymphocyte antigen 96	NM_001195797.1, NM_015364.4
CD11c	3687	Integrin, alpha X (complement component 3 receptor 4 subunit)	NM_000887.3	TRAF5	7188	TNF receptor-associated factor 5	NM_001033910.2, NM_145759.2, NM_004619.3
CathepsinB	1476	Cystatin B (stefin B)	NM_000100.3	iNOS	4843	Nitric oxide synthase 2, inducible	NM_000625.4
ATRIP	84126	ATR-interacting protein	NM_001271022.1, NM_032166.3, NM_130384.2, NM_001271023.1	Cul2	8453	Cullin 2	NM_001198777.1, NM_003591.3, NM_001198778.1, NM_001198779.1
RAB11FIP2	22841	RAB11 family-interacting protein 2 (class I)	NM_014904.2	NBS1	4683	Nibrin	NM_002485.4
CD27	939	CD27 molecule	NM_001242.4	POU2F1	5451	POU class 2 homeobox 1	NR_037163.1, NM_002697.3, NM_001198786.1, NM_001198783.1
14-3-3 σ	2810	Stratifin	NM_006142.3	LMP2	5698	Proteasome (prosome, macropain) subunit, beta type, 9	NM_002800.4
BRCC36	79184	BRCA1/BRCA2-containing complex, subunit 3	NM_001018055.2, NM_024332.3, NM_001242640.1	IL-3	3562	Interleukin 3 (colony-stimulating factor, multiple)	NM_000588.3

Rheb	6009	Ras homolog enriched in brain	NM_005614.3	IL-21	59067	Interleukin 21	NM_021803.3, NM_001207006.2
IL-2Rγ	3561	Interleukin 2 receptor, gamma	NM_000206.2	OAS1	4938	2′–5′-oligoadenylate synthetase 1, 40/46 kDa	NM_002534.2, NM_016816.2, NM_001032409.1
Cytochrome C	54205	Cytochrome c, somatic	NM_018947.5	PYK2	2185	Protein tyrosine kinase 2 beta	NM_004103.4, NM_173174.2, NM_173176.2, NM_173175.2
HDAC2	3066	Histone deacetylase 2	NM_001527.3, NR_033441.1, NR_073443.1	CCR3	1232	Chemokine (C–C motif) receptor 3	NM_001837.3, NM_178329.2, NM_001164680.1, NM_178328.1
HSP90	3320	Heat shock protein 90 kDa alpha (cytosolic), class A member 1	NM_001017963.2, NM_005348.3	NKP46	9437	Natural cytotoxicity triggering receptor 1	NM_004829.5, NM_001242356.1, NM_001145457.1, NM_001242357.1, NM_001145458.1
BAFF	10673	Tumor necrosis factor (ligand) superfamily, member 13b	NM_001145645.2, NM_006573.4	MYD88	4615	Myeloid differentiation primary response 88	NM_001172568.1, NM_001172566.1, NM_001172569.1, NM_001172567.1, NM_002468.4
A20	7128	Tumor necrosis factor, alpha-induced protein 3	NM_001270508.1, NM_006290.3, NM_001270507.1	CD83	9308	CD83 molecule	NM_004233.3, NM_001251901.1, NM_001040280.1
CLIP	972	CD74 molecule, major histocompatibility complex, class II invariant chain	NM_004355.3, NM_001025158.2, NM_001025159.2	PLCβ2	5330	Phospholipase C, beta 2	NM_004573.2

(continued)

Table 2
(continued)

Gene symbol	Entrez gene ID for human	Entrez gene name	Accession number(s)	Gene symbol	Entrez gene ID for human	Entrez gene name	Accession number(s)
Ang-2	285	Angiopoietin 2	NM_001118887.1, NM_001147.2, NM_001118888.1	SEC10	10640	Exocyst complex component 5	NM_006544.3
GP130	3572	Interleukin 6 signal transducer (gp130, oncostatin M receptor)	NM_175767.2, NM_001190981.1, NM_002184.3	ACT-1	10758	TRAF3-interacting protein 2	NM_147686.3, NM_001164281.2, NR_028338.2, NM_001164283.2
IL-13	3596	Interleukin 13	NM_002188.2	ANP32A	8125	Acidic (leucine-rich) nuclear phosphoprotein 32 family, member A	NM_006305.3
EOTAXIN	6356	Chemokine (C–C motif) ligand 11	NM_002986.2	TOCA1	54874	Formin binding protein 1-like	NM_017737.4, NM_001164473.2, NM_001024948.2
CXCR1	3577	Chemokine (C–X–C motif) receptor 1	NM_000634.2	HMOX1	3162	Heme oxygenase (decycling) 1	NM_002133.2
TSC2	7249	Tuberous sclerosis 2	NM_001077183.1, NM_001114382.1, NM_000548.3	CCDC98	84142	Family with sequence similarity 175, member A	NM_139076.2
STAT6	6778	Signal transducer and activator of transcription 6, interleukin-4 induced	NM_003153.4, NM_001178079.1, NM_001178078.1, NM_001178080.1, NM_001178081.1, NR_033659.1	SRC-1	8648	Nuclear receptor coactivator 1	NM_003743.4, NM_147223.2, NM_147233.2

L11	6135	Ribosomal protein L11	NM_001199802.1, NM_000975.3	LKB1	6794	Serine/threonine kinase 11	NM_000455.4
SHP2	5781	Protein tyrosine phosphatase, non-receptor type 11	NM_002834.3, NM_080601.1	MMP2	4313	Matrix metallopeptidase 2 (gelatinase A, 72 kDa gelatinase, 72 kDa type IV collagenase)	NM_001127891.1, NM_004530.4
ACK1	10188	Tyrosine kinase, non-receptor, 2	NM_001010938.1, NM_005781.4	Mcp-1	6347	Chemokine (C–C motif) ligand 2	NM_002982.3
CXCR2	3579	Chemokine (C–X–C motif) receptor 2	NM_001168298.1, NM_001557.3	Bcl-XL	598	BCL2-like 1	NM_001191.2, NM_138578.1
TICAM2	353376	Toll-like receptor adaptor molecule 2	NM_021649.6	NRG1	3084	Neuregulin 1	NM_001160001.1, NM_013956.3, NM_013964.3, NM_013957.3, NM_013958.3, NM_001159999.1, NM_013962.2, NM_001160005.1, NM_004495.3, NM_001160002.1, NM_001160007.1, NM_001159995.1, NM_013960.3, NM_013959.3, NM_001159996.1, NM_001160004.1, NM_001160008.1
SPEC1	56882	CDC42 small effector 1	NM_020239.3, NM_001038707.1	MUC5B	727897	Mucin 5B, oligomeric mucus/gel-forming	NM_002458.2
Perforin	5551	Perforin 1 (pore forming protein)	NM_001083116.1, NM_005041.4	LTA	4049	lymphotoxin alpha (TNF superfamily, member 1)	NM_000595.3, NM_001159740.2

(continued)

Table 2
(continued)

Gene symbol	Entrez gene ID for human	Entrez gene name	Accession number(s)	Gene symbol	Entrez gene ID for human	Entrez gene name	Accession number(s)
IL-20	50604	Interleukin 20	NM_018724.3	NOX1	27035	NADPH oxidase 1	NM_013955.2, NM_007052.4, NM_001271815.1
BTG1	694	B-cell translocation gene 1, anti-proliferative	NM_001731.2	Fas	355	Fas (TNF receptor superfamily, member 6)	NR_028036.2, NR_028035.2, NR_028034.2, NM_000043.4, NM_152871.2, NR_028033.2, NM_152872.2
Cyclin D1	595	Cyclin D1	NM_053056.2	BAD	572	BCL2-associated agonist of cell death	NM_032989.2, NM_004322.3
Dock180	1793	Dedicator of cytokinesis 1	NM_001380.3	DAP10	10870	Hematopoietic cell signal transducer	NM_014266.3, NM_001007469.1
Bcl-2	596	B-cell CLL/lymphoma 2	NM_000657.2, NM_000633.2	PLCγ1	5335	Phospholipase C, gamma 1	NM_002660.2, NM_182811.1
β-Arrestin 2	409	Arrestin, beta 2	NM_001257329.1, NM_001257328.1, NM_001257331.1, NM_001257330.1, NR_047516.1, NM_004313.3, NM_199004.1	CD14	929	CD14 molecule	NM_000591.3, NM_001174105.1, NM_001174104.1, NM_001040021.2
S1PR5	53637	Sphingosine-1-phosphate receptor 5	NM_030760.4, NM_001166215.1	SOCS1	8651	Suppressor of cytokine signaling 1	NM_003745.1

Syk	6850	Spleen tyrosine kinase	NM_003177.5, NM_001135052.2, NM_001174168.1, NM_001174167.1	MEKK2	10746	Mitogen-activated protein kinase kinase kinase 2	NM_006609.4
RbBP4	5928	Retinoblastoma binding protein 4	NM_001135255.1, NM_005610.2, NM_001135256.1	ARD1	8260	*N*(alpha)-acetyltransferase 10, NatA catalytic subunit	NM_001256119.1, NM_003491.3, NM_001256120.1
Jab1	10987	COP9 signalosome subunit 5	NM_006837.2	PAR-1	2011	MAP/microtubule affinity-regulating kinase 2	NM_017490.3, NM_001039469.2, NM_001163297.1, NM_004954.4, NM_001163296.1
CD205	4065	Lymphocyte antigen 75	NM_002349.3	RFX5	5993	Regulatory factor X, 5 (influences HLA class II expression)	NM_001025603.1, NM_000449.3
CD8	925	CD8a molecule	NM_001768.6, NR_027353.1, NM_001145873.1, NM_171827.3	AIRE	326	Autoimmune regulator	NM_000383.3
DDR1	780	Discoidin domain receptor tyrosine kinase 1	NM_001202522.1, NM_001202523.1, NM_001202521.1, NM_013993.2, NM_001954.4, NM_013994.2	STAT1	6772	Signal transducer and activator of transcription 1, 91 kDa	NM_139266.2, NM_007315.3
Lamin A	4000	Lamin A/C	NR_047544.1, NM_005572.3, NM_170708.3, NR_047545.1, NM_170707.3, NM_001257374.1	DR6	27242	Tumor necrosis factor receptor superfamily, member 21	NM_014452.3

(continued)

Table 2
(continued)

Gene symbol	Entrez gene ID for human	Entrez gene name	Accession number(s)	Gene symbol	Entrez gene ID for human	Entrez gene name	Accession number(s)
SMAD3	4088	SMAD family member 3	NM_001145103.1, NM_005902.3, NM_001145104.1, NM_001145102.1	SIPL1	81858	SHANK-associated RH domain interactor	NR_038270.1, NM_030974.3
IL-17F	112744	Interleukin 17F	NM_052872.3	I-TAC	6373	Chemokine (C–X–C motif) ligand 11	NM_005409.4
LMPX	5693	Proteasome (prosome, macropain) subunit, beta type, 5	NM_001130725.1, NM_001144932.1, NM_002797.3	p70S6K	6198	Ribosomal protein S6 kinase, 70 kDa, polypeptide 1	NM_001272043.1, NM_001272042.1, NM_001272060.1, NM_003161.3, NM_001272044.1
CD3delta	915	CD3d molecule, delta (CD3-TCR complex)	NM_000732.4, NM_001040651.1	RhoA	387	Ras homolog family member A	NM_001664.2
TLR1	7096	Toll-like receptor 1	NM_003263.3	GAB2	9846	GRB2-associated binding protein 2	NM_080491.2, NM_012296.3
Vav1	7409	Vav 1 guanine nucleotide exchange factor	NM_005428.3, NM_001258207.1, NM_001258206.1	RPS6	6194	Ribosomal protein S6	NM_001010.2
Diablo	56616	Diablo, IAP-binding mitochondrial protein	NM_001278304.1, NM_138930.3, NR_024600.1, NM_001278302.1, NM_001278342.1, NM_019887.5, NM_001278303.1, NR_024601.1	SAP18	10284	Sin3A-associated protein, 18 kDa	NM_005870.4

MPO	4353	Myeloperoxidase	NM_000250.1	SHB	6461	Src homology 2 domain containing adaptor protein B	NM_003028.2
TLX2	3196	T-cell leukemia homeobox 2	NM_016170.4	Redd1	54541	DNA-damage-inducible transcript 4	NM_019058.2
PKCα	5578	Protein kinase C, alpha	NM_002737.2	CDC6	990	Cell division cycle 6	NM_001254.3
p53	7157	Tumor protein p53	NM_001276699.1, NM_001276696.1, NM_001276697.1, NM_001126118.1, NM_001126115.1, NM_001126112.2, NM_001276760.1, NM_000546.5, NM_001276761.1, NM_001126116.1, NM_001126114.2, NM_001276698.1, NM_001126113.2, NM_001126117.1, NM_001276695.1	Gas2	2620	Growth arrest-specific 2	NM_177553.2, NM_005256.3, NM_001143830.1
Nucleostemin	26354	Guanine nucleotide binding protein-like 3 (nucleolar)	NM_014366.4, NM_206826.1, NM_206825.1	MEKK3	4215	Mitogen-activated protein kinase kinase kinase 3	NM_203351.1, NM_002401.3
Caspase 7	840	Caspase 7, apoptosis-related cysteine peptidase	NM_001227.4, NM_001267057.1, NM_033338.5, NM_001267056.1, NM_001267058.1, NM_033340.3, NM_033339.4	p21Cip1	1026	Cyclin-dependent kinase inhibitor 1A (p21, Cip1)	NM_001220777.1, NM_078467.2, NM_000389.4, NM_001220778.1

(continued)

Table 2
(continued)

Gene symbol	Entrez gene ID for human	Entrez gene name	Accession number(s)	Gene symbol	Entrez gene ID for human	Entrez gene name	Accession number(s)
Axin	8312	Axin 1	NM_181050.2, NM_003502.3	SOCS3	9021	Suppressor of cytokine signaling 3	NM_003955.3
RAIDD	8738	CASP2 and RIPK1 domain containing adaptor with death domain	NM_003805.3	STAT2	6773	Signal transducer and activator of transcription 2, 113 kDa	NM_198332.1, NM_005419.3
Elk1	2002	ELK1, member of ETS oncogene family	NM_001257168.1, NM_001114123.2, NM_005229.4	TAU	4137	Microtubule-associated protein tau	NM_016835.4, NM_005910.5, NM_001123067.3, NM_016841.4, NM_001203251.1, NM_016834.4, NM_001123066.3, NM_001203252.1
MKK6	5608	Mitogen-activated protein kinase kinase 6	NM_002758.3	EAT-2	117157	SH2 domain containing 1B	NM_053282.4
EXO84	149371	Exocyst complex component 8	NM_175876.3	TLR5	7100	Toll-like receptor 5	NM_003268.5
CCR1	1230	Chemokine (C-C motif) receptor 1	NM_001295.2	MDM4	4194	Mdm4 p53 binding protein homolog (mouse)	NM_002393.4, NM_001204171.1, NM_001204172.1, NR_024171.2
Rb	5925	Retinoblastoma 1	NM_000321.2	TRAF1	7185	TNF receptor-associated factor 1	NM_001190947.1, NM_005658.4, NM_001190945.1

β-TrCP	8945	Beta-transducin repeat containing E3 ubiquitin protein ligase	NM_001256856.1, NM_003939.4, NM_033637.3	IL-1β	3553	Interleukin 1, beta	NM_000576.2
BACH1	83990	BRCA1-interacting protein C-terminal helicase 1	NM_032043.2	2B4	51744	CD244 molecule, natural killer cell receptor 2B4	NM_016382.3, NM_001166663.1, NM_001166664.1
IL-1 F8	27177	Interleukin 36, beta	NM_173178.1, NM_014438.3	IkBβ	4793	Nuclear factor of kappa light polypeptide gene enhancer in B-cells inhibitor, beta	NM_001243116.1, NR_040515.1, NM_002503.4
TBK1	29110	TANK-binding kinase 1	NM_013254.3	CTIP	5932	Retinoblastoma binding protein 8	NM_203292.1, NM_002894.2, NM_203291.1
PARP	142	Poly (ADP-ribose) polymerase 1	NM_001618.3	CCRN4L	25819	CCR4 carbon catabolite repression 4-like (*S. cerevisiae*)	NM_012118.2
Cdc42	998	Cell division cycle 42	NM_001039802.1, NM_044472.2, NM_001791.3	VASP	7408	Vasodilator-stimulated phosphoprotein	NM_003370.3
Raptor	57521	Regulatory-associated protein of MTOR, complex 1	NM_020761.2, NM_001163034.1	ROCK1	6093	Rho-associated, coiled-coil containing protein kinase 1	NM_005406.2
CD86	942	CD86 molecule	NM_006889.4, NM_001206924.1, NM_176892.1, NM_175862.4, NM_001206925.1	4-1BBL	8744	Tumor necrosis factor (ligand) superfamily, member 9	NM_003811.3
MCP-4	6357	Chemokine (C-C motif) ligand 13	NM_005408.2	c-Myc	4609	v-myc myelocytomatosis viral oncogene homolog (avian)	NM_002467.4

(continued)

Table 2
(continued)

Gene symbol	Entrez gene ID for human	Entrez gene name	Accession number(s)	Gene symbol	Entrez gene ID for human	Entrez gene name	Accession number(s)
HMG-14	3150	High mobility group nucleosome binding domain 1	NM_004965.6	Caspase 2	835	Caspase 2, apoptosis-related cysteine peptidase	NM_032982.3, NM_001224.4, NM_032983.3
HMG(I)Y	3159	High mobility group AT-hook 1	NM_145901.2, NM_002131.3, NM_145905.2, NM_145902.2, NM_145903.2, NM_145899.2	GADD45	1647	Growth arrest and DNA-damage-inducible, alpha	NM_001924.3, NM_001199741.1, NM_001199742.1
ERK5	5598	Mitogen-activated protein kinase 7	NM_139033.2, NM_139032.2, NM_139034.2, NM_002749.3	DUSP8	1850	Dual specificity phosphatase 8	NM_004420.2
NFAT4	4775	Nuclear factor of activated T-cells, cytoplasmic, calcineurin-dependent 3	NM_004555.3, NM_173163.2, NM_173165.2	IFIT1	3434	Interferon-induced protein with tetratricopeptide repeats 1	NM_001270928.1, NM_001548.4, NM_001270930.1, NM_001270929.1, NM_001270927.1
p90S6K	6195	Ribosomal protein S6 kinase, 90 kDa, polypeptide 1	NM_001006665.1, NM_002953.3	Bcl-9	607	B-cell CLL/lymphoma 9	NM_004326.2
SAP-1	5794	Protein tyrosine phosphatase, receptor type, H	NM_001161440.1, NM_002842.3	CXCL1	2919	Chemokine (C–X–C motif) ligand 1 (melanoma growth stimulating activity, alpha)	NM_001511.3, NR_046035.1
PCAF	8850	K(lysine) acetyltransferase 2B	NM_003884.4	c-Jun	3725	Jun proto-oncogene	NM_002228.3

Runx2	860	Runt-related transcription factor 2	NM_001015051.3, NR_103533.1, NM_001278478.1, NM_001024630.3, NR_103532.1	ADA	100	Adenosine deaminase	NM_000022.2
CD44	960	CD44 molecule (Indian blood group)	NM_001202555.1, NM_001001390.1, NM_001001389.1, NM_001202556.1, NM_000610.3, NM_001001392.1, NM_001202557.1, NM_001001391.1	MMP7	4316	Matrix metallopeptidase 7 (matrilysin, uterine)	NM_002423.3
ICAD	1676	DNA fragmentation factor, 45 kDa, alpha polypeptide	NM_004401.2, NM_213566.1	PTP1B	5770	Protein tyrosine phosphatase, non-receptor type 1	NM_002827.2
PTPN7	5778	Protein tyrosine phosphatase, non-receptor type 7	NR_037664.1, NM_002832.3, NM_001199797.1, NM_080588.2, NR_037663.1	IFNγRβ	3460	Interferon gamma receptor 2 (interferon gamma transducer 1)	NM_005534.3
Gα13	10672	Guanine nucleotide binding protein (G protein), alpha 13	NM_006572.4	BAX	581	BCL2-associated X protein	NR_027882.1, NM_138764.4, NM_004324.3, NM_138761.3, NM_138763.3
Cox-2	5743	Prostaglandin-endoperoxide synthase 2 (prostaglandin G/H synthase and cyclooxygenase)	NM_000963.2	WASL	8976	Wiskott–Aldrich syndrome-like	NM_003941.2

(continued)

Table 2
(continued)

Gene symbol	Entrez gene ID for human	Entrez gene name	Accession number(s)	Gene symbol	Entrez gene ID for human	Entrez gene name	Accession number(s)
MEK5	5607	Mitogen-activated protein kinase kinase 5	NM_002757.3, NM_145160.2, NM_001206804.1	CRP	1401	C-reactive protein, pentraxin-related	NM_000567.2
SIN1	79109	Mitogen-activated protein kinase-associated protein 1	NM_001006620.1, NM_001006619.1, NM_001006618.1, NM_024117.3, NM_001006617.1, NM_001006621.1	ERK2	5594	Mitogen-activated protein kinase 1	NM_002745.4, NM_138957.2
Smurf1	57154	SMAD specific E3 ubiquitin protein ligase 1	NM_181349.2, NM_020429.2, NM_001199847.1	Cadherin E	999	Cadherin 1, type 1, E-cadherin (epithelial)	NM_004360.3
PITX2	5308	Paired-like homeodomain 2	NM_153427.2, NM_001204399.1, NM_153426.2, NM_001204397.1, NM_001204398.1, NM_000325.5	TNF-α	7124	Tumor necrosis factor	NM_000594.3
IL-19	29949	Interleukin 19	NM_013371.3, NM_153758.2	CD4	920	CD4 molecule	NM_001195016.2, NM_001195017.2, NM_000616.4, NM_001195014.2, NM_001195015.2
Igα	973	CD79a molecule, immunoglobulin-associated alpha	NM_001783.3, NM_021601.3	ICos	29851	Inducible T-cell co-stimulator	NM_012092.3

NIK	9020	Mitogen-activated protein kinase kinase kinase 14	NM_003954.3	IL15Rα	3601	Interleukin 15 receptor, alpha	NM_002189.3, NM_172200.2, NR_046362.1, NM_001243539.1, NM_001256765.1
IL-7R	3575	Interleukin 7 receptor	NM_002185.3	SHP1	5777	Protein tyrosine phosphatase, non-receptor type 6	NM_080548.4, NM_002831.5, NM_080549.3
Vav2	7410	Vav 2 guanine nucleotide exchange factor	NM_003371.3, NM_001134398.1	TSG6	7130	Tumor necrosis factor, alpha-induced protein 6	NM_007115.3
Myt1	9088	Protein kinase, membrane associated tyrosine/threonine 1	NM_182687.2, NM_001258451.1, NM_001258450.1, NM_004203.4	TTRAP	51567	Tyrosyl-DNA phosphodiesterase 2	NM_016614.2
TICAM1	148022	Toll-like receptor adaptor molecule 1	NM_182919.3	ORC2	4999	Origin recognition complex, subunit 2	NR_033915.1, NM_006190.4
IL2Rβ	3560	Interleukin 2 receptor, beta	NM_000878.3	MSH2	4436	mutS homolog 2, colon cancer, nonpolyposis type 1 (*E. coli*)	NM_001258281.1, NM_000251.2
14-3-3epsilon	7533	Tyrosine 3-monooxygenase/tryptophan 5-monooxygenase activation protein, eta polypeptide	NM_003405.3	IKKγ	8517	Inhibitor of kappa light polypeptide gene enhancer in B-cells, kinase gamma	NM_001099857.1, NM_003639.3, NM_001099856.2, NM_001145255.1
CDT1	81620	Chromatin licensing and DNA replication factor 1	NM_030928.3	LILRB1	10859	Leukocyte immunoglobulin-like receptor, subfamily B (with TM and ITIM domains), member 1	NM_001081637.1, NM_001081638.2, NR_103518.1, NM_001278399.1, NM_001081639.2, NM_001278398.1, NM_006669.5

(continued)

Table 2
(continued)

Gene symbol	Entrez gene ID for human	Entrez gene name	Accession number(s)	Gene symbol	Entrez gene ID for human	Entrez gene name	Accession number(s)
BIRC6	57448	Baculoviral IAP repeat containing 6	NM_016252.3	Elongin-B	6923	Transcription elongation factor B (SIII), polypeptide 2 (18 kDa, elongin B)	NM_207013.2, NM_007108.3
LEPR	3953	Leptin receptor	NM_001198689.1, NM_001198688.1, NM_001198687.1, NM_002303.5, NM_001003679.3, NM_001003680.3	DRF3	81624	Diaphanous homolog 3 (Drosophila)	NM_001258370.1, NM_001258368.1, NM_030932.3, NM_001258369.1, NM_001258367.1, NM_001258366.1, NM_001042517.1
IL-32	9235	Interleukin 32	NM_001012634.1, NM_004221.4, NM_001012636.1, NM_001012635.1, NM_001012632.1, NM_001012631.1, NM_001012718.1, NM_001012633.1	TAB2	23118	TGF-beta activated kinase 1/MAP3K7 binding protein 2	NM_015093.4
IL-27	246778	Interleukin 27	NM_145659.3	CCK2R	887	Cholecystokinin B receptor	NM_176875.3
FAK	5747	Protein tyrosine kinase 2	NM_005607.4, NM_001199649.1, NM_153831.3	Mip-1β	6351	Chemokine (C–C motif) ligand 4	NM_002984.2

SIVA	10572	SIVA1, apoptosis-inducing factor	NM_021709.2, NM_006427.3	Max	4149	MYC-associated factor X	NM_145113.2, NM_001271069.1, NM_145112.2, NR_073138.1, NR_073137.1, NM_001271068.1, NM_197957.3, NM_002382.4, NM_145114.2
Fyn	2534	FYN oncogene related to SRC, FGR, YES	NM_153047.3, NM_153048.3, NM_002037.5	RAG-2	5897	Recombination activating gene 2	NM_001243786.1, NM_001243785.1, NM_000536.3
Runx3	864	Runt-related transcription factor 3	NM_004350.2, NM_001031680.2	GRB2	2885	Growth factor receptor-bound protein 2	NM_203506.2, NM_002086.4
NKR-P1	3820	Killer cell lectin-like receptor subfamily B, member 1	NM_002258.2	MX1	4599	Myxovirus (influenza virus) resistance 1, interferon-inducible protein p78 (mouse)	NM_002462.3, NM_001178046.1, NM_001144925.1
Wee1	7465	WEE1 homolog (*S. pombe*)	NM_001143976.1, NM_003390.3	EPO	2056	Erythropoietin	NM_000799.2
MECP2	4204	Methyl CpG binding protein 2 (Rett syndrome)	NM_001110792.1, NM_004992.3	UNG	7374	Uracil-DNA glycosylase	NM_003362.3, NM_080911.2
TLR10	81793	Toll-like receptor 10	NM_001195107.1, NM_001017388.2, NM_001195108.1, NM_030956.3, NM_001195106.1	DP-1	7027	Transcription factor Dp-1	NM_007111.4, NR_026580.1
JAK1	3716	Janus kinase 1	NM_002227.2	PRAK	8550	Mitogen-activated protein kinase-activated protein kinase 5	NM_139078.2, NM_003668.3

(continued)

Table 2 (continued)

Gene symbol	Entrez gene ID for human	Entrez gene name	Accession number(s)	Gene symbol	Entrez gene ID for human	Entrez gene name	Accession number(s)
IKKβ	3551	Inhibitor of kappa light polypeptide gene enhancer in B-cells, kinase beta	NR_033818.1, NM_001556.2, NM_001190720.2, NR_040009.1, NM_001242778.1, NR_033819.1	GranzymeA	3001	Granzyme A (granzyme 1, cytotoxic T-lymphocyte-associated serine esterase 3)	NM_006144.3
IL-5	3567	Interleukin 5 (colony-stimulating factor, eosinophil)	NM_000879.2	IGF-1	3479	Insulin-like growth factor 1 (somatomedin C)	NM_001111284.1, NM_000618.3, NM_001111283.1, NM_001111285.1
APO3L	8742	Tumor necrosis factor (ligand) superfamily, member 12	NR_037146.1, NM_003809.2	PAI-1	5054	Serpin peptidase inhibitor, clade E (nexin, plasminogen activator inhibitor type 1), member 1	NM_000602.4
CD45	5788	Protein tyrosine phosphatase, receptor type, C	NR_052021.1, NM_002838.4, NM_080921.3, NM_001267798.1	MHC I-β	567	Beta-2-microglobulin	NM_004048.2
IFITM1	8519	Interferon induced transmembrane protein 1	NM_003641.3	ATR	545	Ataxia telangiectasia and Rad3 related	NM_001184.3
OX40L	7292	Tumor necrosis factor (ligand) superfamily, member 4	NM_003326.3	MDM2	4193	MDM2 oncogene, E3 ubiquitin protein ligase	NM_001145340.2, NM_001145337.2, NM_001278462.1, NM_001145339.2, NM_002392.5

PKCθ	5588	Protein kinase C, theta	NM_006257.3, NM_001242413.1	RXRα	6256	Retinoid X receptor, alpha	NM_002957.4
GM-CSF	1437	Colony-stimulating factor 2 (granulocyte-macrophage)	NM_000758.3	IRF4	3662	Interferon regulatory factor 4	NR_046000.1, NM_001195286.1, NM_002460.3
PPARα	5465	Peroxisome proliferator-activated receptor alpha	NM_005036.4, NM_001001928.2	SHIP	3635	Inositol polyphosphate-5-phosphatase, 145 kDa	NM_005541.3, NM_001017915.1
p27KIP1	1027	Cyclin-dependent kinase inhibitor 1B (p27, Kip1)	NM_004064.3	MLCK	4638	Myosin light chain kinase	NM_053028.3, NM_053025.3, NM_053032.2, NM_053031.2, NM_053027.3, NM_053026.3
HNRPK	3190	Heterogeneous nuclear ribonucleoprotein K	NM_031262.2, NM_002140.3, NM_031263.2	OAZ	23090	Zinc finger protein 423	NM_001271620.1, NM_015069.3
ICAM1	3383	Intercellular adhesion molecule 1	NM_000201.2	β-catenin	1499	Catenin (cadherin-associated protein), beta 1, 88 kDa	NM_001098210.1, NM_001904.3, NM_001098209.1
CDC45	8318	Cell division cycle 45	NM_001178011.1, NM_003504.3, NM_001178010.1	LMPY	5694	Proteasome (prosome, macropain) subunit, beta type, 6	NM_002798.2, NM_001270481.1
CIITA	4261	Class II, major histocompatibility complex, transactivator	NM_000246.3	CSK	1445	c-src tyrosine kinase	NM_004383.2, NM_001127190.1
SLP76	3937	Lymphocyte cytosolic protein 2 (SH2 domain containing leukocyte protein of 76 kDa)	NM_005565.3	HPK1	11184	Mitogen-activated protein kinase kinase kinase kinase 1	NM_001042600.1, NM_007181.4

(continued)

Table 2
(continued)

Gene symbol	Entrez gene ID for human	Entrez gene name	Accession number(s)	Gene symbol	Entrez gene ID for human	Entrez gene name	Accession number(s)
TNFRSF13C	115650	Tumor necrosis factor receptor superfamily, member 13C	NM_052945.3	S1PR1	1901	Sphingosine-1-phosphate receptor 1	NM_001400.4
Axin-2	8313	Axin 2	NM_004655.3	FANCC	2176	Fanconi anemia, complementation group C	NM_000136.2, NM_001243744.1, NM_001243743.1
CABIN1	23523	Calcineurin binding protein 1	NM_001201429.1, NM_012295.3, NM_001199281.1	NKP30	259197	Natural cytotoxicity triggering receptor 3	NM_001145467.1, NM_001145466.1, NM_147130.2
CCR5	1234	Chemokine (C–C motif) receptor 5 (gene/ pseudogene)	NM_000579.3, NM_001100168.1	LAD	9047	SH2 domain containing 2A	NM_001161442.1, NM_001161441.1, NM_001161444.1, NM_001161443.1, NM_003975.3
Gastrin	2520	Gastrin	NM_000805.4	Fodrin	6709	Spectrin, alpha, non-erythrocytic 1	NM_001130438.2, NM_001195532.1, NM_003127.3
ATG13	9776	Autophagy related 13	NM_001205120.1, NM_001205121.1, NM_014741.4, NM_001142673.2, NM_001205122.1, NM_001205119.1	RANKL	8600	Tumor necrosis factor (ligand) superfamily, member 11	NM_003701.3, NM_033012.3
CRKL	1399	v-crk sarcoma virus CT10 oncogene homolog (avian)-like	NM_005207.3	JNK1	5599	Mitogen-activated protein kinase 8	NM_139046.1, NM_002750.2, NM_139049.1, NM_139047.1

EBP1	5036	Proliferation-associated 2G4, 38 kDa	NM_006191.2	TRAF2	7186	TNF receptor-associated factor 2	NM_021138.3
CD3z	919	CD247 molecule	NM_198053.2, NM_000734.3	Caspase 12	100506742	Caspase 12 (gene/ pseudogene)	NR_034066.1, NR_034061.1, NR_034065.1, NM_001191016.1, NR_034068.1, NR_034063.1, NR_034067.1, NR_034070.1, NR_034064.1, NR_034071.1
ORC3	23595	Origin recognition complex, subunit 3	NM_181837.2, NM_012381.3, NM_001197259.1	Smurf2	64750	SMAD specific E3 ubiquitin protein ligase 2	NM_022739.3
PI3K p101	23533	Phosphoinositide-3-kinase, regulatory subunit 5	NM_001251855.1, NM_001251852.1, NM_001142633.2, NM_014308.3, NM_001251851.1, NM_001251853.1	INSR	3643	Insulin receptor	NM_000208.2, NM_001079817.1
p38MAPKβ	5600	Mitogen-activated protein kinase 11	NM_002751.5	MALT1	10892	Mucosa-associated lymphoid tissue lymphoma translocation gene 1	NM_173844.1, NM_006785.2
SAP30	8819	Sin3A-associated protein, 30 kDa	NM_003864.3	CyclinH	902	Cyclin H	NM_001199189.1, NM_001239.3
GBL	64223	MTOR-associated protein, LST8 homolog (S. cerevisiae)	NM_001199175.1, NM_022372.4, NM_001199173.1, NM_001199174.1	XPO1	7514	Exportin 1 (CRM1 homolog, yeast)	NM_003400.3

(continued)

Table 2
(continued)

Gene symbol	Entrez gene ID for human	Entrez gene name	Accession number(s)	Gene symbol	Entrez gene ID for human	Entrez gene name	Accession number(s)
ILK	3611	Integrin-linked kinase	NM_001014794.2, NM_001278441.1, NM_001278442.1, NM_004517.3, NM_001014795.2	ABIN-1	10318	TNFAIP3-interacting protein 1	NM_001258456.1, NM_001258454.1, NM_001252385.1, NM_001252391.1, NM_006058.4, NM_001252392.1, NM_001252386.1, NM_001252390.1, NM_001258455.1, NM_001252393.1
eEF2K	29904	Eukaryotic elongation factor-2 kinase	NM_013302.3	IL-6R	3570	Interleukin 6 receptor	NM_181359.2, NM_000565.3, NM_001206866.1
A2M	2	Alpha-2-macroglobulin	NM_000014.4	TRIM	50852	T cell receptor-associated transmembrane adaptor 1	NM_016388.2
G-CSF	1440	Colony-stimulating factor 3 (granulocyte)	NM_001178147.1, NM_000759.3, NM_172219.2, NM_172220.2, NR_033662.1	TCF1	6927	HNF1 homeobox A	NM_000545.5
SAP180	51742	AT rich interactive domain 4B (RBP1-like)	NM_031371.3, NM_001206794.1, NM_016374.5	TANK	10010	TRAF family member-associated NFKB activator	NM_133484.1, NM_004180.2, NM_001199135.1
TYK2	7297	Tyrosine kinase 2	NM_003331.4	pro-HB-EGF	1839	Heparin-binding EGF-like growth factor	NM_001945.2

CAPN2	824	Calpain 2, (m/II) large subunit	NM_001748.4, NM_001146068.1	AIRM1	27036	Sialic acid binding Ig-like lectin 7	NM_014385.3, NM_001277201.1, NR_102350.1, NM_016543.3
SUDS3	64426	Suppressor of defective silencing 3 homolog (*S. cerevisiae*)	NM_022491.2	CARMA1	84433	Caspase recruitment domain family, member 11	NM_032415.4
FN14	51330	Tumor necrosis factor receptor superfamily, member 12A	NM_016639.2	SDF-1	6387	Chemokine (C–X–C motif) ligand 12	NM_000609.6, NM_199168.3, NM_001033886.2, NM_001178134.1, NM_001277990.1
BTK	695	Bruton agammaglobulinemia tyrosine kinase	NM_000061.2	PLCγ2	5336	Phospholipase C, gamma 2 (phosphatidylinositol-specific)	NM_002661.3
PIAS1	8554	Protein inhibitor of activated STAT, 1	NM_016166.1	OX40	7293	Tumor necrosis factor receptor superfamily, member 4	NM_003327.3
FANCG	2189	Fanconi anemia, complementation group G	NM_004629.1	ARNT	405	Aryl hydrocarbon receptor nuclear translocator	NM_001668.3, NM_178427.2, NM_001197325.1
FANCE	2178	Fanconi anemia, complementation group E	NM_021922.2	IL-10Rβ	3588	Interleukin 10 receptor, beta	NM_000628.4
ATM	472	Ataxia telangiectasia mutated	NM_000051.3	p38MAPKδ	5603	Mitogen-activated protein kinase 13	NR_072996.1, NM_002754.4
Endo G	2021	Endonuclease G	NM_004435.2	FADD	8772	Fas (TNFRSF6)-associated via death domain	NM_003824.3

(continued)

Table 2
(continued)

Gene symbol	Entrez gene ID for human	Entrez gene name	Accession number(s)	Gene symbol	Entrez gene ID for human	Entrez gene name	Accession number(s)
MLH1	4292	mutL homolog 1, colon cancer, nonpolyposis type 2 (*E. coli*)	NM_001167618.1, NM_001258274.1, NM_001258271.1, NM_001258273.1, NM_001167617.1, NM_000249.3, NM_001167619.1	GBP	10023	Frequently rearranged in advanced T-cell lymphomas	NM_005479.3
IL17RC	84818	Interleukin 17 receptor C	NR_037807.1, NM_001203263.1, NM_153460.3, NM_153461.3, NM_001203264.1, NM_001203265.1, NM_032732.5	NF-kBp65	5970	v-rel reticuloendotheliosis viral oncogene homolog A (avian)	NM_001145138.1, NM_001243984.1, NM_021975.3, NM_001243985.1
IFNγ	3458	Interferon, gamma	NM_000619.2	PTEN	5728	Phosphatase and tensin homolog	NM_000314.4
ZAP70	7535	Zeta-chain (TCR) associated protein kinase 70 kDa	NM_207519.1, NM_001079.3	IL-29	282618	Interferon, lambda 1	NM_172140.1
DNMT3B	1789	DNA (cytosine-5-)-methyltransferase 3 beta	NM_175850.2, NM_006892.3, NM_175849.1, NM_001207055.1, NM_001207056.1, NM_175848.1	LZK	9175	Mitogen-activated protein kinase kinase kinase 13	NM_004721.4, NM_001242314.1, NR_038322.1, NM_001242317.1
CDK7	1022	Cyclin-dependent kinase 7	NM_001799.3	IL-22	50616	Interleukin 22	NM_020525.4

Lyn	4067	v-yes-1 Yamaguchi sarcoma viral related oncogene homolog	NM_001111097.2, NM_002350.3	SKI	6497	v-ski sarcoma viral oncogene homolog (avian)	NM_003036.3
IL-24	11009	Interleukin 24	NM_006850.3, NM_001185157.1, NM_001185158.1, NM_001185156.1	DKK1	22943	Dickkopf 1 homolog (Xenopus laevis)	NM_012242.2
LBP	3929	Lipopolysaccharide binding protein	NM_004139.3	NFkBp52	4791	Nuclear factor of kappa light polypeptide gene enhancer in B-cells 2 (p49/p100)	NR_048560.1, NM_001077494.2, NM_001261403.1, NM_002502.4
Caspase 3	836	Caspase 3, apoptosis-related cysteine peptidase	NM_004346.3, NM_032991.2	TRAF4	9618	TNF receptor-associated factor 4	NM_004295.3
CDK4	1019	Cyclin-dependent kinase 4	NM_000075.3	RalA	5898	v-ral simian leukemia viral oncogene homolog A (ras related)	NM_005402.3
MEF2D	4209	Myocyte enhancer factor 2D	NM_005920.3, NM_001271629.1	IL-4Rα	3566	Interleukin 4 receptor	NM_001257406.1, NM_000418.3, NM_001257407.1, NM_001257997.1
SPHK	8877	Sphingosine kinase 1	NM_001142602.1, NM_021972.3, NM_182965.2, NM_001142601.1	WIP	7456	WAS/WASL-interacting protein family, member 1	NM_003387.4, NM_001077269.1
p16INK4	1029	Cyclin-dependent kinase inhibitor 2A	NM_058195.3, NM_058197.4, NM_001195132.1, NM_000077.4	ICSBP	3394	Interferon regulatory factor 8	NM_002163.2

(continued)

Table 2
(continued)

Gene symbol	Entrez gene ID for human	Entrez gene name	Accession number(s)	Gene symbol	Entrez gene ID for human	Entrez gene name	Accession number(s)
4E-BP1	1978	Eukaryotic translation initiation factor 4E binding protein 1	NM_004095.3	IL-10Rα	3587	Interleukin 10 receptor, alpha	NM_001558.3, NR_026691.1
PI3K p110γ	5294	Phosphatidylinositol-4,5-bisphosphate 3-kinase, catalytic subunit gamma	NM_002649.2	AID	57379	Activation-induced cytidine deaminase	NM_020661.2
TGF-α	7039	Transforming growth factor, alpha	NM_001099691.2, NM_003236.3	CD28	940	CD28 molecule	NM_001243077.1, NM_006139.3, NM_001243078.1
CD27L	970	CD70 molecule	NM_001252.3	Egr1	1958	Early growth response 1	NM_001964.2
LRH-1	2494	Nuclear receptor subfamily 5, group A, member 2	NM_003822.4, NM_001276464.1, NM_205860.2	CREB	1385	cAMP responsive element binding protein 1	NM_004379.3, NM_134442.3
TL1	9966	Tumor necrosis factor (ligand) superfamily, member 15	NM_005118.3, NM_001204344.1	TACI	23495	Tumor necrosis factor receptor superfamily, member 13B	NM_012452.2
ORC5	5001	Origin recognition complex, subunit 5	NM_002553.3, NM_181747.3	RFXANK	8625	Regulatory factor X-associated ankyrin-containing protein	NM_134440.1, NM_003721.2
p300	2033	E1A binding protein p300	NM_001429.3	CLIP170	6249	CAP-GLY domain containing linker protein 1	NM_001247997.1, NM_198240.1, NM_002956.2
TLR2	7097	Toll-like receptor 2	NM_003264.3	BTG2	7832	BTG family, member 2	NM_006763.2

SHC	6464	SHC (Src homology 2 domain containing) transforming protein 1	NM_183001.4, NM_003029.4, NM_001130040.1, NM_001130041.1, NM_001202859.1	G-αq	2776	Guanine nucleotide binding protein (G protein), q polypeptide	NM_002072.3
STAT3	6774	Signal transducer and activator of transcription 3 (acute-phase response factor)	NM_213662.1, NM_139276.2, NM_003150.3	S1PR2	9294	Sphingosine-1-phosphate receptor 2	NM_004230.3
BCL-B	10017	BCL2-like 10 (apoptosis facilitator)	NM_020396.2	LAIR1	3903	Leukocyte-associated immunoglobulin-like receptor 1	NM_002287.3, NM_021706.2
SAP	4068	SH2 domain containing 1A	NM_002351.4, NM_001114937.2	IL-6	3569	Interleukin 6 (interferon, beta 2)	NM_000600.3
Collagen type I	1277	Collagen, type I, alpha 1	NM_000088.3	TAP2	6891	Transporter 2, ATP-binding cassette, subfamily B (MDR/TAP)	NM_000544.3, NM_018833.2
RAG-1	5896	Recombination activating gene 1	NM_000448.2	CD11b	3684	Integrin, alpha M (complement component 3 receptor 3 subunit)	NM_000632.3, NM_001145808.1
VCAM-1	7412	Vascular cell adhesion molecule 1	NM_001078.3, NM_001199834.1, NM_080682.2	CNOT7	29883	CCR4-NOT transcription complex, subunit 7	NM_013354.5, NM_054026.2
TCRβ	6957	T cell receptor beta locus	NG_001333.2	p19INK4D	1032	Cyclin-dependent kinase inhibitor 2D (p19, inhibits CDK4)	NM_001800.3, NM_079421.2
Ang-1	284	Angiopoietin 1	NM_001146.3, NM_001199859.1	MCL1	4170	Myeloid cell leukemia sequence 1 (BCL2-related)	NM_021960.4, NM_001197320.1, NM_182763.2

(continued)

Table 2
(continued)

Gene symbol	Entrez gene ID for human	Entrez gene name	Accession number(s)	Gene symbol	Entrez gene ID for human	Entrez gene name	Accession number(s)
NKG2A	3821	Killer cell lectin-like receptor subfamily C, member 1	NM_213657.2, NM_002259.4, NM_007328.3, NM_213658.2	PKCz	5590	Protein kinase C, zeta	NM_001033581.1, NM_002744.4, NM_001242874.1, NM_001033582.1
TRAF6	7189	TNF receptor-associated factor 6, E3 ubiquitin protein ligase	NM_004620.3, NM_145803.2	CXCR4	7852	Chemokine (C–X–C motif) receptor 4	NM_003467.2, NM_001008540.1
ORC1	4998	Origin recognition complex, subunit 1	NM_001190819.1, NM_001190818.1, NM_004153.3	ITK	3702	IL2-inducible T-cell kinase	NM_005546.3
TNF-R1	7132	Tumor necrosis factor receptor superfamily, member 1A	NM_001065.3	PKR	5610	Eukaryotic translation initiation factor 2-alpha kinase 2	NM_001135651.2, NM_002759.3, NM_001135652.2
IFI35	3430	Interferon-induced protein 35	NM_005533.4	p50NFkB	4790	Nuclear factor of kappa light polypeptide gene enhancer in B-cells 1	NM_001165412.1, NM_003998.3
TLR4	7099	Toll-like receptor 4	NM_138557.2, NM_003266.3, NM_138554.4	LTβR	4055	Lymphotoxin beta receptor (TNFR superfamily, member 3)	NM_001270987.1, NM_002342.2
PAK1IP1	55003	PAK1-interacting protein 1	NM_017906.2	ROCK2	9475	Rho-associated, coiled-coil containing protein kinase 2	NM_004850.3
IRS1	3667	Insulin receptor substrate 1	NM_005544.2	BAK	578	BCL2-antagonist/killer 1	NM_001188.3
TGF-β1	7040	Transforming growth factor, beta 1	NM_000660.4	DRIP150	9282	Mediator complex subunit 14	NM_004229.3

PDK1	5170	3-phosphoinositide dependent protein kinase-1	NM_002613.4, NM_031268.5, NM_001261816.1	CD1a	909	CD1a molecule	NM_001763.2
TIFA	92610	TRAF-interacting protein with forkhead-associated domain	NM_052864.2	Cdc25B	994	Cell division cycle 25B	NM_004358.3, NM_021873.2, NM_021872.2
GSK3beta	2932	Glycogen synthase kinase 3 beta	NM_001146156.1, NM_002093.3	SEC5	55770	Exocyst complex component 2	NM_018303.5, NR_073064.1
PAR3	56288	Par-3 partitioning defective 3 homolog (*C. elegans*)	NM_001184792.1, NM_001184787.1, NM_001184793.1, NM_001184788.1, NM_019619.3, NM_001184785.1, NM_001184794.1, NM_001184790.1, NM_001184789.1, NM_001184791.1, NM_001184786.1	TLR7	51284	Toll-like receptor 7	NM_016562.3
TLR6	10333	Toll-like receptor 6	NM_006068.4	BARD1	580	BRCA1-associated RING domain 1	NM_000465.2
SEK1	6416	Mitogen-activated protein kinase kinase 4	NM_003010.2	mTOR	2475	Mechanistic target of rapamycin (serine/threonine kinase)	NM_004958.3
DAP12	7305	TYRO protein tyrosine kinase binding protein	NR_033390.1, NM_001173514.1, NM_001173515.1, NM_003332.3, NM_198125.2	GSC	145258	Goosecoid homeobox	NM_173849.2

(continued)

Table 2
(continued)

Gene symbol	Entrez gene ID for human	Entrez gene name	Accession number(s)	Gene symbol	Entrez gene ID for human	Entrez gene name	Accession number(s)
IFNAR2	3455	Interferon (alpha, beta, and omega) receptor 2	NM_207585.1, NM_207584.1, NM_000874.3	FasL	356	Fas ligand (TNF superfamily, member 6)	NM_000639.1
IL-18	3606	Interleukin 18 (interferon-gamma-inducing factor)	NM_001562.3, NM_001243211.1	Chk1	1111	Checkpoint kinase 1	NM_001244846.1, NM_001114121.2, NR_045205.1, NR_045204.1, NM_001114122.2, NM_001274.5
TC-PTP	5771	Protein tyrosine phosphatase, non-receptor type 2	NM_080423.2, NM_001207013.1, NM_080422.2, NM_002828.3	PABP1	26986	Poly(A) binding protein, cytoplasmic 1	NM_002568.3
IL17RA	23765	Interleukin 17 receptor A	NM_014339.6	LTβ	4050	Lymphotoxin beta (TNF superfamily, member 3)	NM_002341.1, NM_009588.1
MRCK	8476	CDC42 binding protein kinase alpha (DMPK-like)	NM_003607.3, NM_014826.4	SARA	9372	Zinc finger, FYVE domain containing 9	NM_007324.3, NM_004799.3
ARG2	384	Arginase, type II	NM_001172.3	DNMT1	1786	DNA (cytosine-5-)-methyltransferase 1	NM_001379.2, NM_001130823.1
APEX1	328	APEX nuclease (multifunctional DNA repair enzyme) 1	NM_080649.2, NM_001244249.1, NM_001641.3, NM_080648.2	p18INK4C	1031	Cyclin-dependent kinase inhibitor 2C (p18, inhibits CDK4)	NM_001262.2, NM_078626.2

IKKα	1147	Conserved helix-loop-helix ubiquitous kinase	NM_001278.3	CD32	2213	Fc fragment of IgG, low affinity IIb, receptor (CD32)	NM_001002275.2, NM_001190828.1, NM_004001.4, NM_001002273.2, NM_001002274.2
Smad6	4091	SMAD family member 6	NR_027654.1, NM_005585.4, NM_001142861.2	AKAP79	9495	A kinase (PRKA) anchor protein 5	NM_004857.3
DNA-PK	5591	Protein kinase, DNA-activated, catalytic polypeptide	NM_001081640.1, NM_006904.6	PAK4	10298	p21 protein (Cdc42/Rac)-activated kinase 4	NM_001014831.2, NM_001014835.1, NM_001014832.1, NM_005884.3, NM_001014834.2
MBD2	8932	Methyl-CpG binding domain protein 2	NM_015832.4, NM_003927.4	Nur77	3164	Nuclear receptor subfamily 4, group A, member 1	NM_002135.4, NM_001202233.1, NM_173157.2
GCK	5871	Mitogen-activated protein kinase kinase kinase kinase 2	NM_004579.3	SIGIRR	59307	Single immunoglobulin and toll-interleukin 1 receptor (TIR) domain	NM_021805.2, NM_001135054.1, NM_001135053.1
SRF	6722	Serum response factor (c-fos serum response element-binding transcription factor)	NM_003131.2	TAB1	10454	TGF-beta activated kinase 1/MAP3K7 binding protein 1	NM_153497.2, NM_006116.2
SIN3A	25942	SIN3 transcription regulator homolog A (yeast)	NM_001145358.1, NM_015477.2, NM_001145357.1	IRAK-M	11213	Interleukin-1 receptor-associated kinase 3	NM_001142523.1, NM_007199.2
Artemis	64421	DNA cross-link repair 1C	NM_001033858.1, NM_001033857.1, NM_001033855.1, NM_022487.2	VHL	7428	von Hippel-Lindau tumor suppressor, E3 ubiquitin protein ligase	NM_198156.2, NM_000551.3

(continued)

Table 2
(continued)

Gene symbol	Entrez gene ID for human	Entrez gene name	Accession number(s)	Gene symbol	Entrez gene ID for human	Entrez gene name	Accession number(s)
JAK2	3717	Janus kinase 2	NM_004972.3	VEGF	7422	Vascular endothelial growth factor A	NM_001204385.1, NM_001171623.1, NM_001025370.2, NM_001204384.1, NM_001171627.1, NM_003376.5, NM_001171629.1, NM_001025367.2, NM_001025369.2, NM_001171622.1, NM_001033756.2, NM_001171628.1, NM_001025368.2, NM_001171625.1, NM_001171630.1, NM_001171626.1, NM_001025366.2, NM_001171624.1
FoxH1	8928	Forkhead box H1	NM_003923.2	CKS1	1163	CDC28 protein kinase regulatory subunit 1B	NM_001826.2, NR_024163.1
IFIT3	3437	Interferon-induced protein with tetratricopeptide repeats 3	NM_001031683.2, NM_001549.4	Reprimo	56475	Reprimo, TP53 dependent G2 arrest mediator candidate	NM_019845.2

BIM	10018	BCL2-like 11 (apoptosis facilitator)	NM_207003.2, NM_138626.3, NM_138627.3, NM_001204107.1, NM_001204113.1, NM_001204108.1, NM_207002.3, NM_138625.3, NM_138621.4, NM_138624.3, NM_001204106.1, NM_006538.4, NM_138623.3, NM_001204112.1, NM_001204111.1, NM_138622.3, NM_001204109.1, NM_001204110.1	Cdc25A	993	Cell division cycle 25A	NM_001789.2, NM_201567.1
TRADD	8717	TNFRSF1A-associated via death domain	NM_003789.3	IL-23p19	51561	Interleukin 23, alpha subunit p19	NM_016584.2
UBE2V1	7335	Ubiquitin-conjugating enzyme E2 variant 1	NM_001257397.1, NM_001257394.1, NM_021988.5, NM_001257396.1, NM_022442.5, NM_199144.2, NM_001032288.2, NM_001257393.1, NM_001257398.1, NR_047556.1, NM_001257395.1, NR_047554.1, NR_047553.1, NR_047555.1, NM_001257399.1	4-1BB	3604	Tumor necrosis factor receptor superfamily, member 9	NM_001561.5

(continued)

Table 2
(continued)

Gene symbol	Entrez gene ID for human	Entrez gene name	Accession number(s)	Gene symbol	Entrez gene ID for human	Entrez gene name	Accession number(s)
Tensin	7145	Tensin 1	NM_022648.4	MDR1	5243	ATP-binding cassette, subfamily B (MDR/TAP), member 1	NM_000927.4
TOLLIP	54472	Toll-interacting protein	NM_019009.3	ORC4	5000	Origin recognition complex, subunit 4	NM_001190882.2, NM_181741.3, NM_002552.4, NM_001190879.2, NM_181742.3, NM_001190881.2
SEC6	11336	Exocyst complex component 3	NM_007277.4	SEC3	55763	Exocyst complex component 1	NM_018261.3, NM_178237.2, NM_001024924.1
NKG2C	3822	Killer cell lectin-like receptor subfamily C, member 2	NM_002260.3	CD58	965	CD58 molecule	NM_001779.2, NM_001144822.1, NR_026665.1
SEC8	60412	Exocyst complex component 4	NM_021807.3, NM_001037126.1	MAST2	23139	Microtubule-associated serine/threonine kinase 2	NM_015112.2
NGF	4803	Nerve growth factor (beta polypeptide)	NM_002506.2	TSC1	7248	Tuberous sclerosis 1	NM_001162427.1, NM_001162426.1, NM_000368.4

TCF4	6925	Transcription factor 4	NM_001243232.1, NM_003199.2, NM_001083962.1, NM_001243226.1, NM_001243233.1, NM_001243228.1, NM_001243231.1, NM_001243234.1, NM_001243227.1, NM_001243230.1, NM_001243236.1, NM_001243235.1	WASP	7454	Wiskott–Aldrich syndrome	NM_000377.2
SEC15	54536	Exocyst complex component 6	NM_001013848.2, NM_019053.4	APRIL	8741	Tumor necrosis factor (ligand) superfamily, member 13	NM_172088.2, NM_172087.2, NM_001198624.1, NM_001198623.1, NM_001198622.1, NR_073490.2, NM_003808.3
HDAC1	3065	Histone deacetylase 1	NM_004964.2	SMAD2	4087	SMAD family member 2	NM_005901.5, NM_001135937.2, NM_001003652.3
CALR	811	Calreticulin	NM_004343.3	Caspase 9	842	Caspase 9, apoptosis-related cysteine peptidase	NR_102732.1, NM_032996.3, NM_001278054.1, NM_001229.4, NR_102733.1
Cbl	867	Cbl proto-oncogene, E3 ubiquitin protein ligase	NM_005188.3	TLR3	7098	Toll-like receptor 3	NM_003265.2
IL-15	3600	Interleukin 15	NM_172175.2, NR_037840.2, NM_000585.4	GATA4	2626	GATA binding protein 4	NM_002052.3

(continued)

Table 2
(continued)

Gene symbol	Entrez gene ID for human	Entrez gene name	Accession number(s)	Gene symbol	Entrez gene ID for human	Entrez gene name	Accession number(s)
BLM	641	Bloom syndrome, RecQ helicase-like	NM_000057.2	cIAP1	329	Baculoviral IAP repeat containing 2	NM_001256163.1, NM_001166.4, NM_001256166.1
CIS	1154	Cytokine inducible SH2-containing protein	NM_145071.2, NM_013324.5				
DLK	7786	Mitogen-activated protein kinase kinase kinase 12	NM_001193511.1, NM_006301.3				
CD19	930	CD19 molecule	NM_001178098.1, NM_001770.5				
Suv39H1	6839	Suppressor of variegation 3-9 homolog 1 (Drosophila)	NM_003173.2				
Crk	1398	v-crk sarcoma virus CT10 oncogene homolog (avian)	NM_005206.4, NM_016823.3				
Vinculin	7414	Vinculin	NM_014000.2, NM_003373.3				
Myt1	4661	Myelin transcription factor 1	NM_004535.2				
CKS2	1164	CDC28 protein kinase regulatory subunit 2	NM_001827.1				
MKK3	5606	Mitogen-activated protein kinase kinase 3	NM_002756.4, NM_145109.2				

TAK1	6885	Mitogen-activated protein kinase kinase kinase 7	NM_145331.2, NM_145332.2, NM_003188.3, NM_145333.2
EGF	1950	Epidermal growth factor	NM_001963.4, NM_001178130.1, NM_001178131.1
Cdc2	983	Cyclin-dependent kinase 1	NM_001170407.1, NM_033379.4, NM_001170406.1, NM_001786.4
FCER2	2208	Fc fragment of IgE, low affinity II, receptor for (CD23)	NM_002002.4, NM_001207019.2, NM_001220500.1
TCRα	6955	T cell receptor alpha locus	NG_001332.2
MCP-3	6354	Chemokine (C–C motif) ligand 7	NM_006273.3
RBX1	9978	Ring-box 1, E3 ubiquitin protein ligase	NM_014248.3
PAK3	5063	p21 protein (Cdc42/Rac)-activated kinase 3	NM_001128173.1, NM_001128166.1, NM_001128167.1, NM_001128168.1, NM_002578.3, NM_001128172.1

Each gene is described by the corresponding gene symbol and Entrez Gene description and indicated unambiguously by their Entrez Gene ID. Accession numbers are from NCBI database

3. Decontaminate the electrodes of the instrument as follows: slowly fill one of the wells of an electrode cleaner with 350 μl RNaseZAP, place the electrode cleaner in the Bioanalyzer, and close the lid for 1 min; slowly fill one of the wells of another electrode cleaner with 350 μl RNase-free water, place the electrode cleaner in the Bioanalyzer, and close the lid for 10 s. Wait another 10 s for the water on the electrodes to evaporate before closing the lid.
4. Prepare the gel by placing 550 μl of Agilent RNA 6000 Nano gel matrix into the spin filter supplied with the kit and spin for 10 min at 1,100 × *g*.
5. Prepare the gel-dye Mix by adding 1 μl of dye and 65 μl of filtered gel and spin the tube for 10 min at room temperature at 13,100 × *g*.
6. Load 9.0 μl of the gel-dye mix at the bottom of the well in the chip marked with a G.
7. Perform the priming of the chip as indicated by the RNA 6000 Nano kit. This is one of the key steps of the assay (*see* **Note 5** for details).
8. Add 5 μl of the RNA 6000 Nano marker into the well marked with the ladder symbol and each of the 12 sample wells.
9. Load the ladder and samples by adding 1 μl of the RNA ladder into the well marked with the ladder symbol, and 1 μl of each sample into each of the 12 sample wells. Both the ladder and samples should be heat denatured before loading. This is another key point of the assay (*see* **Note 6** for details).
10. Run the assay as indicated in the RNA 6000 Nano kit guide.
11. Consider samples suitable for a gene expression microarray experiment, those presenting a R.I.N ≥ 7. Figure 1 shows how a good quality RNA should appear (R.I.N. = 10). As degradation increases the two major peaks will progressively broaden and reduce in height, while the baseline will increase. Figure 2 shows a degraded RNA (R.I.N. = 5).

3.3 Labeling, Hybridization, and Washing

This last step refers entirely to Agilent One-Color Microarray-Based Gene Expression Analysis protocol, which is already very detailed and optimized for the use of the Agilent Low Input Quick Amp Labeling kit. As previously indicated in the introduction this is a strictly platform-dependent step; therefore it is not convenient to apply substantial adjustments to this protocol. To our knowledge, at present the possibility to autonomously design a completely customizable-by-the-user microarray chip, at no additional charge, is only offered by Agilent. The choice of Agilent platform for our CTL microarray is therefore straightforward. Below we will

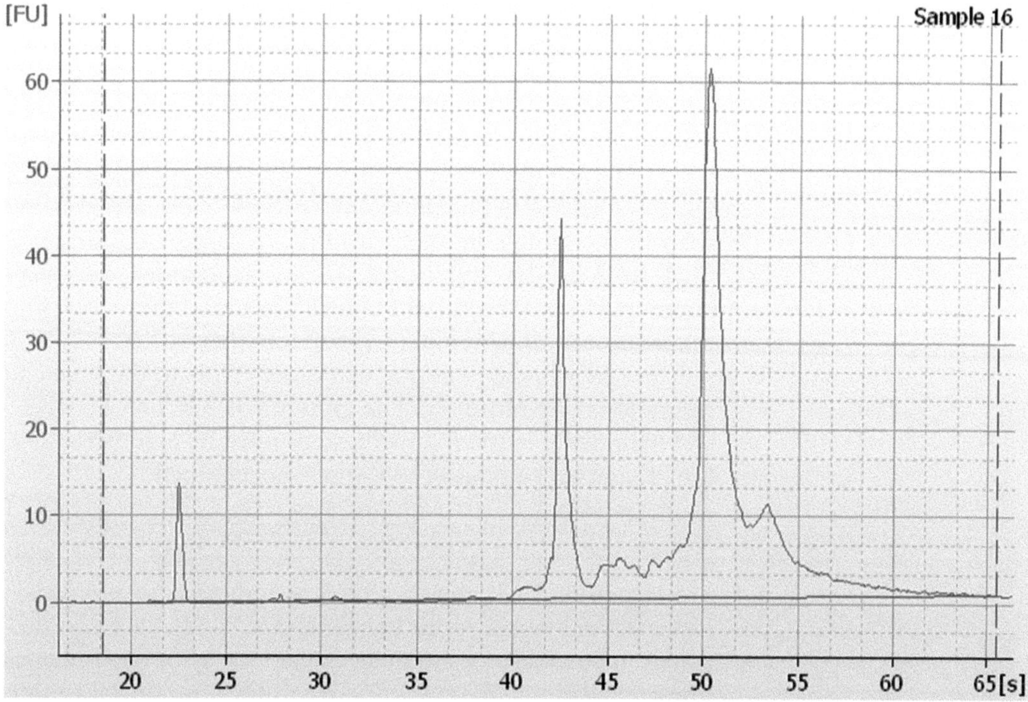

Fig. 1 Good quality RNA with a R.I.N. = 10. The two main peaks of 18S rRNA (between 40 and 45 s) and 28S rRNA (at approximately 50 s) are clearly distinguishable. The baseline is flat

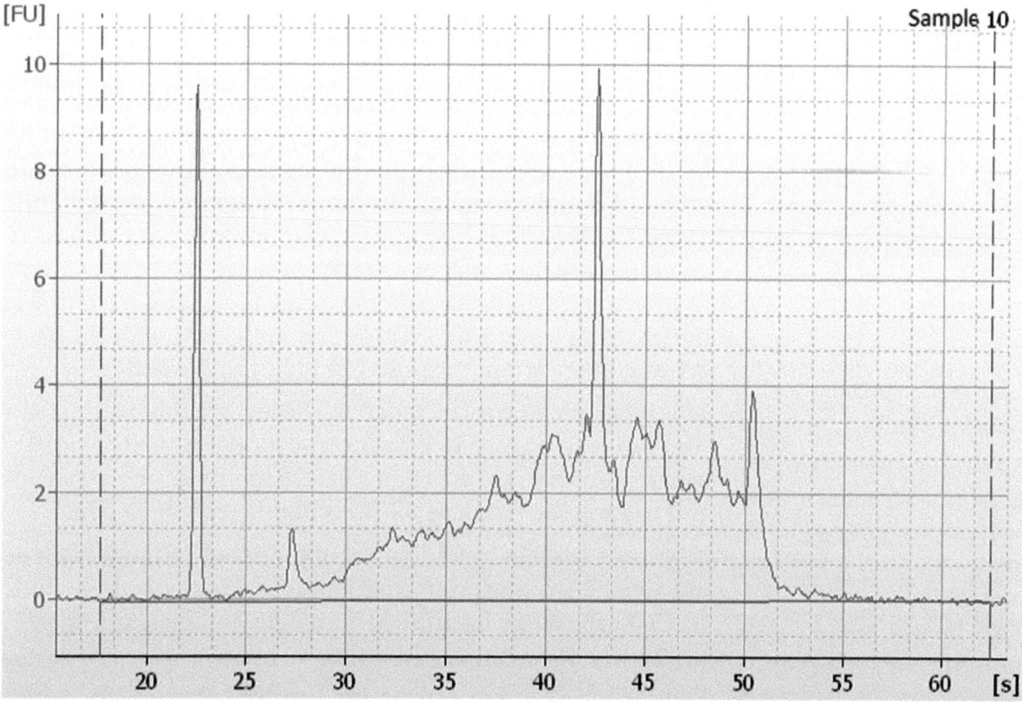

Fig. 2 A moderately degraded RNA with a R.I.N. = 5.18S and 28S peaks is almost undistinguishable due to the numerous non-rRNA fragments present

summarize the different steps of the Agilent One-Color protocol, commenting some key points when necessary.

1. For all steps involving water baths, a thermal cycler can alternatively be used with no issues. The overall procedure requires 2 or 3 days. In our laboratory we usually take advantage of one of the available stopping points and conduct this step in 3 days.
2. Prepare the sample immediately prior to use by diluting your total RNA to 10–200 ng/μl. In our laboratory we usually dilute to 25 or 50 ng/μl, the choice depends on the stock solution concentration, as pipetting too low amounts of volume to prepare the working solution can cause errors to the final concentrations (*see* **Note 7**). The amount of RNA to be labeled and hybridized in the following steps must be exactly the same for all samples belonging to the same experiment.
3. Add the RNA sample to the Spike-In mix solution previously prepared according to the One-Color RNA Spike-In kit guide.
4. Produce your Cy3-labeled cRNA as indicated in the Agilent Low Input Quick Amp Labeling Kit, one-color protocol. Briefly, it consists of a simultaneous at least 100-fold amplification and labeling of the starting total RNA, passing through a cDNA intermediate. Both at the end of the cDNA production and the labeled cRNA production, a stopping point is available, where the samples can be stored at −80 °C. It can be useful to take advantage of one of these in order to arrange the subsequent 17-h hybridization step overnight.
5. Purify the Cy3-labeled cRNA on Qiagen RNeasy mini spin columns and quantify by NanoDrop Spectrophotometer, as indicated in the Agilent Low Input Quick Amp Labeling Kit, one-color protocol. Also in this case no deviation from the protocol is recommended. In our laboratory during the purification we also always perform the additional extra spin of the columns with no buffer at 4 °C for 30 s before the final elution of the samples, in order to remove any remaining trace of RPE buffer. Samples can be kept on ice until used with no issues, provided they are not exposed to light (*see* **Note 8**).
6. 10× Blocking Agent (included in the kit) for the hybridization step can be prepared in advance and stored at −20 °C up to 2 months. In this case vortexing before use must be very strong, and heating for 5 min at 37 °C is highly recommended.
7. Fragment samples by adding the appropriate volumes (depending on the microarray format) of 25× Fragmentation Buffer and 10× Blocking Agent to the samples and incubate at 60 °C for exactly 30 min. (*see* **Note 9**).
8. Load samples onto the array and incubate at 65 °C for 17 h in the rotating oven. Incubation time can also be increased up to

18–19 h, not more. It is important, however, to maintain the same incubation time for all samples belonging to the same project (and that therefore will presumably be compared to each other).

9. Wash the arrays using Wash Buffers 1 and 2 (Gene Expression Wash Buffer Kit) for 1 min each. Use separate and dedicated wash dishes. Add a magnetic stir bar at moderate speed. Very slowly extract microarrays from wash buffers, in order to keep them clean and dry (*see* **Note 10**). Perform an additional acetonitrile wash by plunging for 5–10 s the microarray in 100 % acetonitrile.
10. Immediately cover the microarray with an ozone barrier (*see* **Note 11**) and scan.
11. Proceed with feature extraction and selection of differentially expressed genes by appropriate statistical tests.

4 Notes

1. IPA requires a fee. With a little additional effort, however, the same information can be gathered free of charge from public databases. A good collection of annotated gene sets is provided by the Molecular Signatures Database (MSigDB) [14] (http://www.broadinstitute.org/gsea/msigdb/index.jsp) maintained by the Broad Institute of MIT and Harvard. Among the C2 (curated gene sets) Collections, the CP (Canonical pathways) offers a list of canonical pathways compiled by domain experts. For each pathway all genes belonging to it are provided. Even though pathway names can differ from those reported in Table 1, this type of information is perfectly analogous to that selected through IPA and therefore can be used to design our CTL microarray as well.
2. Unfortunately, not only synonyms are widespread throughout the list, but also the same gene symbol is often written in different ways.
3. *gene2accession.gz* file is a huge file that contains the association between NCBI Entrez Gene IDs and Accession Numbers for all species present in NCBI. For this reason you unlikely will be able to open it with the text editors commonly installed on the computers. It can be useful to previously parse this file by selecting the rows beginning with 9606, which is the Tax ID corresponding to *Homo sapiens*, or any other Tax ID of interest if you deal with other species. Some programming skills are required for this step.
4. When high RNA yields are obtained, exact RNA quantitation is difficult to estimate due to RNA viscosity. In these cases, after

preparation of the working solution a second measurement can be convenient in order to double-check the concentration. The working solution should not be less than 100 ng/µl.

5. Chip priming consists in the loading of the gel-dye mix into the chip. This operation must be performed carefully, as the success of the subsequent electrophoretic run will depend on it. Gel-dye mix should be evenly distributed in all chip channels, without any particle or air bubble blocking them. Indeed, samples flow into the channels consecutively, all conveying in sequence (starting from sample 1 to sample 12) in a single master channel. Obstructing one channel, especially soon after the initial starting, will impair the entire electrophoretic run.
6. Sample heat denaturation (70 °C for 2 min) is essential to prevent the formation of secondary structures that could, also in this case, block or delay the entire sample flux. Immediately before loading, samples should therefore be heat denatured.
7. Samples belonging to the same project can also be run separately, especially when their number is high and requires many slides. Each slide can harbor from one to eight different samples, depending on the format chosen. In our laboratory we have designed the microarray choosing the 8x15K format that harbors eight different samples on one slide. When possible, on each slide a comparable number of samples belonging to the study group and the control group should be hybridized. It is advisable to start from the same concentrations for samples belonging to the same project and that therefore will presumably be compared to each other.
8. Cyanines are light-sensitive and their uneven degradation might invalidate all the subsequent results. When a differential expression between two samples is in fact detected, in case of uneven cyanine degradation, assigning a biological or a technical meaning becomes difficult.
9. Also in this case fragmentation must be uniform for all samples; otherwise, assigning a biological or a technical meaning to a subsequent differential expression detection becomes difficult.
10. Every visible sign on the slide will affect the quality of the scanned image, obscuring the corresponding probes and therefore loosing data.
11. Cyanines are ozone-sensitive and their uneven degradation might invalidate all the subsequent results. When a differential expression between two samples is in fact detected, in case of uneven cyanine degradation, assigning a biological or a technical meaning becomes difficult.

Acknowledgements

M.A. is supported by Ministero dell'Istruzione, dell'Università e della Ricerca (MIUR) PROGRAMMA OPERATIVO NAZIONALE (PON) RICERCA E COMPETITIVITÀ 2007-2013 PONa3_00395 "BIOSCIENZE e SALUTE (B&H).

References

1. Schadt EE, Edwards SW, GuhaThakurta D et al (2004) A comprehensive transcript index of the human genome generated using microarrays and computational approaches. Genome Biol 5:R73
2. Joshi T, Chen Y, Becker JM et al (2004) Genome-scale gene function prediction using multiple sources of high-throughput data in yeast Saccharomyces cerevisiae. OMICS 8:322–333
3. Greenberg SA (2001) DNA microarray gene expression analysis technology and its application to neurological disorders. Neurology 57:755–761
4. Grant GM, Fortney A, Gorreta F et al (2004) Microarrays in cancer research. Anticancer Res 24:441–448
5. Clarke PA, te Poele R, Workman P (2004) Gene expression microarray technologies in the development of new therapeutic agents. Eur J Cancer 40:2560–2591
6. Mocellin S, Provenzano M, Rossi CR et al (2005) DNA array-based gene profiling: from surgical specimen to the molecular portrait of cancer. Ann Surg 241:16–26, Erratum in: (2013) Ann Surg, 257, 554
7. Sausville EA, Holbeck SL (2004) Transcription profiling of gene expression in drug discovery and development: the NCI experience. Eur J Cancer 40:2544–2549
8. Hu YF, Kaplow J, He Y (2005) From traditional biomarkers to transcriptome analysis in drug development. Curr Mol Med 5:29–38
9. Searfoss GH, Ryan TP, Jolly RA (2005) The role of transcriptome analysis in pre-clinical toxicology. Curr Mol Med 5:53–64
10. Mutz KO, Heilkenbrinker A, Lönne M et al (2013) Transcriptome analysis using next-generation sequencing. Curr Opin Biotechnol 24:22–30
11. Parnell GP, Tang BM, Nalos M et al (2013) Identifying key regulatory genes in the whole blood of septic patients to monitor underlying immune dysfunctions. Shock 40:166–174
12. Abd AJ, El Faramawy Y, Quitterer U (2013) Microarray gene expression profiling reveals antioxidant-like effects of angiotensin II inhibition in atherosclerosis. Front Physiol 4:148
13. Lim HY, Sohn I, Deng S et al (2013) Prediction of disease-free survival in hepatocellular carcinoma by gene expression profiling. Ann Surg Oncol 20:3747–3753
14. Subramanian A, Tamayo P, Mootha VK et al (2005) Gene set enrichment analysis: a knowledge-based approach for interpreting genome-wide expression profiles. Proc Natl Acad Sci U S A 102:15545–15550

Chapter 11

miRNome Analysis Using Real-Time PCR

Paola Pontrelli, Matteo Accetturo, and Loreto Gesualdo

Abstract

MicroRNAs (miRNAs) are short RNA molecules that regulate gene expression in eukaryotic organisms, thus influencing physiological mechanisms such as development, cell proliferation, cell death, and cell differentiation. The importance of the gene regulatory system operated by miRNAs is emerging as a central topic in the setting of several diseases included infectious disease and cancer. The different techniques used for the study of the entire "miRNome" give the opportunity to go better inside these novel mechanisms of gene expression regulation.

In the following method we describe a protocol based on quantitative real-time PCR (qRT-PCR) with SYBR® green technology, to specifically analyze the expression levels of only those miRNAs that target genes involved in CTLs biogenesis and functions. Through an in silico approach, we designed a custom microRNA qPCR panel focused on those miRNAs relevant in regulation of CTLs-specific pathways. The panel we created was customized by EXIQON, since this company proposed a method based on the use of LNA enhanced primers, which guarantee increased affinity and specificity for each microRNA. The advantage of this protocol with respect to a whole miRNome analysis consists in the possibility to evidence weaker signals that otherwise would be secreted and remove the noise itself generated by other miRNAs not directly involved in the regulation of CTLs-specific pathways. This panel can be applicable in the study of CTLs behavior in pathological conditions such as infectious disease and cancer or can be used to characterize changes in patients' immune responsiveness after therapeutic intervention in order to understand the molecular mechanisms underlying these effects.

Key words MicroRNA, Pathway analysis, Cytotoxic T lymphocytes, Quantitative real-time PCR panels, LNA oligonucleotide primers

1 Introduction

Regulation of gene expression may be due to several mechanisms that modulate different biological processes from DNA transcription to RNA translation. In recent years the study of miRNA expression profiling represented a novel approach to provide additional understanding in cell biology. The whole set of miRNAs expression profiling, also known as the "miRNome," can be studied by diverse approach. Several high-throughput technologies have been developed over the past years to obtain sensitive profiling, such as microarray [1, 2] and quantitative real-time PCR (qPCR) [3, 4].

Elena Ranieri (ed.), *Cytotoxic T-Cells: Methods and Protocols*, Methods in Molecular Biology, vol. 1186,
DOI 10.1007/978-1-4939-1158-5_11, © Springer Science+Business Media New York 2014

miRNA Microarrays give the opportunity to detect the presence and/or regulation of a wide range of defined miRNAs. This kind of method should not be used to make quantitative statements, but to define the presence and/or the relative change in miRNAs expression between two or more conditions [5]. Different microarray platforms for miRNA profiling are commercially available, with diverse technical procedures to maximize sensitivity and specificity in the analysis of miRNA expression levels [2].

Reverse transcription-quantitative polymerase chain reaction (qRT-PCR) is the most commonly used method to study mature miRNA levels [6]. Several RT-qPCR-based miRNA quantitation methods have been developed in the last decade [3], and also a combination of methods have been proposed to help in passing over the limits linked to miRNA sequence characteristics and abundance and to the different technical approaches [7]. Other than technical and biological problems linked to extraction protocols or differences in transcriptional activity, another important point in RT-qPCR-based miRNA quantitation methods is represented by the choice of the normalization strategy [8]: the "good practices" indicate that, when setting up a new experiment, several normalization strategies should be compared to find the optimal one with the appropriate controls or reference miRNAs for the dataset in consideration.

In the following method we describe some key aspects of miRNA isolation and a workflow that we developed to specifically analyze miRNA signature in CTLs through a qRT-PCR approach using SYBR green. Starting from a list of specific pathways that, according to our knowledge, are involved into the CTLs biogenesis and functions, we have designed a microRNA qPCR panel containing only those miRNAs involved in the regulation of the selected pathways and therefore important in CTLs functional behavior. Diverse company allows the generation of custom Real-time PCR plates based on both SYBR green assays and TaqMan® assays. We generated custom panels from EXIQON since this company offers microRNA detection systems using LNA-primers technology, thus increasing sensitivity and specificity of each assay, and reducing background.

The strength of the method consists in the possibility to use peripheral blood mononuclear cells (PBMC) or CD8+ T cells as starting cell population and focus only on those miRNAs whose profile can change dynamically during antigen-induced T cell differentiation. This strategy should remove the noise coming from other miRNAs not directly involved in the regulation of CTLs-specific pathways, emphasizing weaker signals that otherwise might be secreted. We imagine this approach to be useful in the context of cancer, but also to study the T cell response to viral or bacterial infections or to observe the molecular mechanisms leading to changes in the immune response in patients undergoing therapeutic intervention.

2 Materials

2.1 In Silico Design of the CTLs miRNA PCR Panels

1. Computer (2 Gb RAM processor, or higher).
2. High speed internet connection.

2.2 PBMC Isolation and miRNA Extraction

1. Ficoll-Hypaque density gradient solution (GE Healthcare).
2. Phosphate Buffered Saline (PBS).
3. miRNeasy Mini Kit (Qiagen).
4. Spectrophotometer.

2.3 qRT-PCR

1. Pick-&-Mix 384-well custom designed microRNA qPCR plates (EXIQON).
2. Universal cDNA Synthesis Kit II (EXIQON).
3. ExiLENT SYBR® Green master mix (EXIQON).
4. ROX solution (SIGMA).
5. Quantitative Real-Time PCR system with a 384-Well block module.
6. Thermocycler.
7. Centrifuge for 384-well plates.
8. Sealing foils for plates.

3 Methods

3.1 In Silico Design of the CTLs miRNA PCR Panels

This step requires some programming ability for the management of large datasets and the selection of the information of interest.

To identify specific miRNAs for the study of CTLs, we started with the selection of the Canonical Pathways that, according to our knowledge, are involved into the CTLs biogenesis and functions. To this purpose we used the canonical pathways included into the libraries of the Ingenuity Pathway analysis (IPA) software (http://www.ingenuity.com/) (*see* **Note 1**) (Table 1). *All the genes included into the selected pathways were used to generate a list in which each gene was associated to its NCBI Entrez Gene ID, as unique gene identifier, and subsequently to the NCBI Accession Number of the transcript (this information can be found at the following website: ftp://ftp.ncbi.nih.gov/gene/DATA/). All selected Accession Numbers should be curated RefSeqs records (such as those beginning with NM_, NR_, NP_ accession prefixes). This list of transcripts was used to identify those miRNA that are predicted to regulate them, as follows:*

1. Access microRNA.org (http://www.microrna.com/) [9] (*see* **Note 2**).
2. From the section download, on the left hand side, go to August 2010 release downloads (*see* **Note 3**), and download Target

Site Predictions in "Human," with "Good mirSVR Score, conserved miRNA" (*see* **Note 4**).

3. Starting from this list, select transcripts of interest uniquely identified by their NCBI Accession Number (beginning with NM_) (*see* **Note 5**). We selected all the transcripts identified as important in CTLs responses in physiological or pathological conditions; these are included into the selected pathways described in Table 1.
4. For each transcript, select those miRNAs predicted to regulate their expression (Table 2). Identify each miRNA with their unique mirBASE accession number (MIMAT).
5. Once the list of the predicted miRNA has been generated, these can be used to choose primer sets from Exiqon's collection of validated sensitive LNA™ microRNA PCR primer sets to generate the custom PCR panel (*see* **Note 6**). The design tool is free of charge. Table 3 reports the list of the MIMAT Accession Numbers and miRNA names we generated to study CTLs and to create the PCR panel layout.
6. To design your miRNA PCR plate access to EXIQON web site (http://www.exiqon.com/pick-and-mix) and follow the guided procedure by selecting the "configure your plate" button. Select the plate format as 384 well and follow indications for all other steps (*see* **Note 7**). Include in your plate design control assays and reference assays (*see* **Note 8**). At the end of the procedure your plate is completed and you can proceed with the purchase. Each plate can be used to detect miRNA expression in one sample and contain in each well the selected dried microRNA LNA™ PCR primer sets.

3.2 Human Peripheral Blood Mononuclear Cell (PBMC) Separation, miRNA Extraction, and Quantification

The collection of human blood samples must be approved by your local ethical committee. All the procedures should be performed by well-instructed personnel able to work with potential infectious material.

1. To perform PBMC Isolation from human whole blood using Ficoll-Hypaque density gradient, dilute blood 1:2 with PBS 1× pH 7.4/1 mM EDTA and carefully overlay on 1/4 total volume of Ficoll-Hypaque (*see* **Note 9**)
2. Centrifuge tubes for 30 min at 460 × *g* at room temperature without brake, to avoid the mixtures of the phases.
3. Discard excess serum and collect the PBMC layer at the Ficoll-Hypaque interface in new tubes. Refill the tubes with PBS 1× pH 7.4/EDTA 1 mM and invert a few times to wash cells.
4. Centrifuge at 250 × *g* for 12 min at 4 °C and discard supernatant. Suspend the pellet in 30 ml PBS 1× pH 7.4/1 mM EDTA. Centrifuge again at 175 × *g* for 12 min at 4 °C and discard supernatant.

5. Suspend pellets in 10 ml PBS 1× pH 7.4/1 mM EDTA and unify in one tube. Use an aliquot for counting.
6. Centrifuge at 110×*g* for 12 min at 4 °C and discard supernatant.
7. PBMC can be directly used to isolate DNA-free RNA by the miRNeasy Mini Kit according to the manufacturer's instructions (*see* **Note 10**).
8. Quantify your RNA sample by a Spectrophotometer (*see* **Note 11**). Adjust RNA concentration to 5 ng/μl using nuclease-free water.

3.3 cDNA Generation and qRT-PCR Performance and Analysis

This protocol includes two parts: the first strand cDNA synthesis, obtained with a poly-T primer, after a poly-A tail is added to the mature miRNA templates, and the Real-time PCR amplification with SYBR Green. It is important to optimize the amount of starting RNA depending on miRNA expression levels and the possible presence of inhibitors.

1. Generate cDNA for each sample using the Universal cDNA Synthesis Kit II as described by the producer. Briefly, add into nuclease-free tubes 5× reaction buffer, enzyme mix, synthetic RNA Spike ins, template total RNA, and nuclease-free water to 20 μl total volume per sample (*see* **Note 12**).
2. Incubate the tubes for 60 min at 42 °C in a Thermocycler, then inactivate the enzyme for 5 min at 95 °C and immediately cool to 4 °C. The generated cDNA can be stored at 4 °C for short-time usage, or frozen for long-term storage.
3. To perform Real-time PCR, follow the instruction manual for Pick-&-Mix panels. Briefly, dilute the cDNA template in nuclease-free water to a final dilution 100×. Do not store the diluted cDNA. Mix the 2× PCR master mix with the 100× diluted cDNA, at 1:1 ratio and add 10 μl of the mix to each well of the Pick-&-Mix 384-well custom designed microRNA qPCR plate (*see* **Note 13**).
4. Perform Real-time PCR amplification and melting curve analysis to confirm specific amplification, according to the instruction manual using the described protocol for each instrument. On the 7900HT Fast Real-Time PCR System instrument (Life Technologies) we use the following cycle conditions: 10 min at 95 °C; 10 s at 95 °C followed by 60 s at 60 °C for 40 amplification cycles.
5. Data analysis can be performed by different softwares by the use of the comparative Ct method or $2^{-\Delta\Delta Ct}$ method [10] (*see* **Notes 14** and **15**). miRNAs relative expression (corrected to the reference miRNAs) can be reported as the relative fold change (increased or decreased) versus a control sample (healthy subject or unstimulated cells).

Table 1
List of the canonical pathways involved in CTLs differentiation and activity

Ingenuity canonical signaling pathways	CTLs-specific signaling
Apoptosis	Apoptosis signaling, apoptosis in toxicity pathway, calcium-induced T-lymphocytes apoptosis, cytotoxic T lymphocytes mediated apoptosis of target cells, Jak/Stat signaling, death receptor signaling, lymphotoxin beta receptor signaling, myc mediated apoptosis signaling, Nur77 signaling in T lymphocytes, PTEN signaling, SAPK/JNK signaling, LPS-stimulated MAPK signaling, april mediated signaling, tool-like receptor signaling, TWEAK signaling, TNFR1 signaling, TNFR2 signaling
Cancer	FAK signaling, role of BDCA1 in DNA damage response, Wnt/beta-catenin signaling
Cell cycle regulation	Cell cycle: G1/S checkpoint regulation, cell cycle: G2/M DNA damage checkpoint regulation, cell cycle control of chromosomal replication, cyclins and cell cycle regulation, DNA methylation and transcriptional repression signaling, cell cycle regulation by BTG family proteins
Cellular growth, proliferation, and development	Cdc42 signaling, TGFbeta signaling, mTOR signaling, antiproliferative role of TOB in T cell signaling
Cellular immune response	CD27 signaling in lymphocytes, CTLA4 signaling in cytotoxic T lymphocytes, role of cytokines in mediating communication between immune cells, granzyme A signaling, granzyme B signaling, interferon gamma signaling, IL2 signaling, primary immunodeficiency signaling, role of NFAT in regulation of immune response, PKCΘ signaling in T lymphocytes, T cell receptor signaling, CD28 signaling in T helper cells, CD40 signaling, CXCR4 signaling, iCOS iCOSL signaling in T helper, IL10 signaling, IL17 signaling, IL4 signaling, IL6 signaling, IL8 signaling, interferon signaling, natural killer cell signaling, NFkB signaling, OX40 signaling pathway, p38 MAPK signaling, signaling in T lymphocytes, IL15 signaling in T lymphocytes, dendritic cell maturation
Cellular stress and injury	HIF1alpha signaling
Cytokine signaling	Chemokine signaling
Humoral immune response	Antigen presentation pathway
Intracellular and second messenger signaling	Sphingosie-1-phosphate signaling

Table 2

miRNAs predicted to regulate selected transcripts involved in CTLs biogenesis and function Each transcript ID is associated to the corresponding gene symbol and indicated unambiguously by its Entrez Gene ID. miRNA names are indicated without the prefix *hsa-miR-*

Gene Symbol (Entrez Gene ID) Transcript ID	miRNAs
STAT2 (6773) NM_005419	143, 30c, 30d, 30e, 485-5p, 30a, 370, 30b, 24, 1297, 219-5p, 339-5p, 125a-3p, 330-5p, 488, 19b, 19a, 23a, 23b, 136, 98, 146b-5p, 26a, 10a, 653, let-7e, 10b, let-7b, let-7c, 31, let-7a, 26b, 222, 223, let-7i, 221, 494, 874, let-7g, 504
PTPRC (5788) NM_002838	599, 539, 30c, 410, 30d, 30e, 186, 30a, 27a, 27b, 30b, 25, 21, 367, 190, 362-3p, 363, 342-3p, 488, 150, 155, 137, 448, 590-3p, 33b, 190b, 33a, 92b, 92a, 381, 382, 543, 374b, 425, 653, 377, 205, 32, 340, 140-5p, 224, 590-5p, 876-5p, 300, 495, 329
EXOC7 (23265) NM_001145299	141, 129-5p, 152, 599, 200a, 491-5p, 370, 485-5p, 197, 148a, 148b, 339-5p, 19b, 19a
RPTOR (57521) NM_020761	9, 544, 495, 23a, 23b
NCK1 (4690) NM_006153	141, 431, 7, 186, 27a, 27b, 1, 148a, 190, 374a, 320d, 320c, 421, 129-5p, 490-3p, 613, 429, 425, 424, 140-5p, 224, 590-5p, 302b, 223, 497, 302a, 302c, 495, 494, 15a, 200b, 410, 200c, 200a, 520e, 542-3p, 24, 217, 219-5p, 376c, 15b, 448, 137, 590-3p, 320a, 33b, 320b, 33a, 190b, 381, 374b, 379, 206, 183, 340, 876-5p, 875-5p, 300
FAS (355) NM_152874	431, 361-5p, 539, 9, 27a, 27b, 1297, 335, 374a, 23a, 23b, 129-5p, 153, 425, 519d, 371-5p, 196b, 140-5p, 224, 196a, 495, 494, 181d, 599, 30c, 30d, 30e, 30a, 30b, 181a, 29a, 128, 29b, 181c, 29c, 181b, 146a, 22, 217, 376a, 376b, 363, 376c, 99b, 19b, 19a, 448, 137, 136, 98, 146b-5p, 106a, 92a, 17, 381, 544, 374b, 338-3p, 135a, 135b, let-7d, 183, let-7e, let-7b, let-7c, 216a, let-7a, 216b, 340, 505, 876-5p, 300, 26b, let-7i, 203, let-7f, let-7g
IL1F8 (27177) NM_014438	590-3p, 141, 154, 199a-5p, 92b, 200a, 92a, 544, 370, 199b-5p, 25, 142-3p, 204, 367, 486-5p, 32, 376c, 363, 211, 23a, 23b
IL17F (112744) NM_052872	590-3p, 155, 200b, 200c, 106b, 93, 106a, 17, 543, 429, 20a, 20b, 519d, 340, 374a
TCEB2 (6923) NM_207013	134
TLR1 (7096) NM_003263	590-3p, 421, 15a, 134, 599, 195, 224, 497, 542-3p, 15b, 16, 424
GIT2 (9815) NM_139201	181d, 127-3p, 200b, 200c, 186, 29a, 181a, 29b, 29c, 181c, 181b, 374a, 19b, 19a, 214, 448, 613, 543, 429, 374b, 197, 138, 205, 505, 224, 130a
PIK3R5 (23533) NM_014308	181d, 103, 539, 149, 181a, 1, 107, 24, 181c, 181b, 383, 335, 125a-3p, 374a, 330-5p, 210, 125a-5p, 136, 613, 374b, 138, 206, 378, let-7b, 182, 216a, 371-5p, 422a, 328, 125b, 326, 202, 873
MDC1 (9656) NM_014641	143, 185, 193b, 374a, 320d, 320c, 125a-5p, 193a-3p, 429, 520c-3p, 302b, 302a, 302d, 302c, 495, 302e, 124, 200b, 200c, 411, 20a, 20b, 365, 22, 212, 590-3p, 98, 320a, 320b, 132, 106b, 106a, 381, 17, 382, let-7d, let-7e, let-7b, let-7c, 216a, let-7a, 340, 125b, 506, 324-5p, 300, let-7i, let-7f, let-7g
CXCL10 (3627) NM_001565	200b, 200c, 139-5p, 7, 34a, 186, 142-3p, 217, 376c, 449b, 212, 449a, 590-3p, 448, 421, 153, 132, 429, 135a, 34c-5p, 135b, 206, 505, 208a, 208b, 499-5p, 221
MAST2 (23139) NM_015112	28-5p, 301a, 130b, 708, 130a, 454, 301b
IL6 (3569) NM_000600	144, 149, 1297, 190, 374a, 23a, 23b, 153, 429, 519d, 140-5p, 200b, 410, 451, 20a, 20b, 146a, 142-3p, 365, 217, 376a, 376b, 376c, 137, 448, 136, 98, 146b-5p, 26a, 190b, 106b, 106a, 93, 17, 381, 374b, 135a, 135b, let-7d, let-7e, let-7b, let-7c, let-7a, 340, 300, 26b, 202, let-7i, 203, let-7f, let-7g
TWSG1 (57045) NM_020648	141, 361-5p, 539, 139-5p, 9, 186, 27a, 27b, 148a, 148b, 335, 488, 155, 152, 224, 302b, 302d, 302c, 494, 124, 410, 200a, 20a, 1271, 20b, 142-3p, 217, 367, 218, 376a, 376b, 339-5p, 376c, 214, 590-3p, 137, 136, 96, 106b, 93, 106a, 381, 17, 382, 520d-3p, 338-3p, 135a, 135b, 216a, 373, 340, 505, 208a, 506, 300, 208b, 499-5p, 202, 520a-3p
TNFAIP6 (7130) NM_007115	181d, 141, 200c, 145, 200a, 128, 181a, 181c, 181b, 25, 384, 486-5p, 367, 376a, 376b, 194, 335, 363, 376c, 374a, 488, 212, 23a, 214, 23b, 448, 155, 590-3p, 137, 153, 129-5p, 134, 132, 92b, 92a, 381, 543, 374b, 32, 340, 876-5p, 300
CKS1B (1163) NM_001826	124, 361-5p, 181d, 101, 539, 485-5p, 20a, 181a, 29a, 29b, 181c, 29c, 20b, 181b, 383, 22, 194, 421, 106b, 93, 106a, 17, 382, 197, 135a, 135b, 519d, 371-5p, 224, 876-5p, 506, 494
BTG1 (694) NM_001731	361-5p, 145, 185, 186, 485-5p, 520b, 1297, 383, 190, 301a, 708, 320d, 374a, 320c, 488, 23a, 150, 23b, 301b, 155, 199a-5p, 153, 421, 424, 653, 28-5p, 520c-3p, 32, 371-5p, 224, 590-5p, 302b, 302a, 302d, 302c, 494, 302e, 410, 520e, 29a, 29b, 454, 29c, 25, 146a, 22, 21, 362-3p, 367, 376a, 376b, 363, 376c, 125a-3p, 19b, 19a, 590-3p, 320a, 320b, 146b-5p, 134, 26a, 190b, 106b, 92b, 92a, 543, 199b-5p, 520d-3p, 374b, 338-3p, 16, 183, 182, 373, 372, 130b, 505, 26b, 875-5p, 130a, 499-5p, 202, 203, 520a-3p
IL10 (3586) NM_000572	431, 141, 361-5p, 296-3p, 200a, 20a, 20b, 384, 21, 194, 125a-3p, 374a, 211, 590-3p, 421, 98, 132, 106b, 106a, 93, 381, 17, 543, 374b, let-7d, 653, let-7e, 204, let-7b, let-7c, let-7a, 140-5p, 590-5p, 496, 202, 203, let-7i, 495, 494, let-7f, let-7g
FAS (355) NM_152872	431, 361-5p, 539, 9, 27a, 27b, 335, 374a, 23a, 23b, 129-5p, 153, 425, 519d, 371-5p, 224, 196b, 140-5p, 196a, 495, 494, 181d, 599, 30c, 30d, 30e, 30a, 30b, 181a, 29a, 128, 29b, 29c, 181c, 181b, 146a, 22, 217, 376a, 376b, 99b, 19b, 19a, 448, 137, 136, 98, 146b-5p, 106a, 381, 544, 17, 374b, 338-3p, 135a, 135b, let-7d, let-7e, 183, let-7b, let-7c, 216a, let-7a, 216b, 340, 876-5p, 300, 203, let-7i, let-7f, let-7g
CARD11 (84433) NM_032415	590-3p, 155, 181d, 539, 149, 370, 374b, 338-3p, 181a, 181c, 181b, 362-3p, 339-5p, 374a, 494, 329
MMP9 (4318) NM_004994	154, 183, 204, 491-5p, 149, 211, 494
VDR (7421) NM_000376	433, 145, 520e, 485-5p, 520b, 21, 374a, 330-5p, 214, 448, 155, 136, 129-5p, 544, 520d-3p, 374b, 16, 10a, 10b, 520c-3p, 373, 372, 302b, 302a, 223, 326, 302d, 302c, 520a-3p, 494, 302e
GATA4 (2626) NM_002052	361-5p, 219-5p, 200b, 216b, 200c, 491-5p, 185, 485-5p, 429, 496
GSK3B (2932) NM_002093	144, 9, 185, 1297, 374a, 320d, 708, 488, 320c, 23a, 23b, 155, 199a-5p, 129-5p, 491-5p, 425, 28-5p, 32, 31, 224, 302a, 495, 124, 181d, 101, 410, 30c, 200b, 200c, 30e, 30b, 128, 29a, 29b, 542-3p, 29c, 24, 25, 146a, 217, 219-5p, 367, 376c, 363, 342-3p, 214, 590-3p, 137, 320a, 134, 33b, 320b, 146b-5p, 33a, 26a, 92b, 92a, 544, 543, 382, 199b-5p, 374b, 520d-3p, 135a, 16, 135b, 346, 377, 182, 373, 372, 506, 26b, 875-5p, 203, 874
TLR2 (7097) NM_003264	144, 101, 143, 410, 186, 542-3p, 146a, 22, 148a, 218, 148b, 376a, 376b, 376c, 320d, 374a, 320c, 214, 590-3p, 154, 320a, 320b, 146b-5p, 152, 544, 374b, 425, 340, 505, 328
HMOX1 (3162) NM_002133	200b, 200c, 485-5p, 429, 128, 338-3p, 135a, 135b, 22, 217, 377, 218, 505, 342-3p, 328, 873
TLR4 (7099) NM_138554	144, 145, 7, 485-5p, 1297, 384, 374a, 449b, 449a, 23a, 23b, 125a-5p, 421, 197, 425, 32, 31, 371-5p, 140-5p, 590-5p, 495, 329, 103, 181d, 410, 122, 34a, 181a, 107, 542-3p, 181c, 181b, 25, 146a, 365, 217, 21, 219-5p, 590-3p, 448, 137, 146b-5p, 26a, 543, 34c-5p, 10a, 206, 10b, 216b, 340, 130b, 125b, 26b, 203
CDKN2D (1032) NM_001800	362-3p, 340, 342-3p, 149, 125b, 543, 374a, 451, 374b, 329, 214
ANGPT2 (285) NM_001147	431, 141, 144, 539, 145, 7, 185, 186, 485-5p, 27a, 27b, 383, 301a, 374a, 320d, 320c, 301b, 125a-5p, 155, 421, 153, 129-5p, 133a, 133b, 429, 197, 653, 519d, 371-5p, 495, 124, 181d, 599, 410, 200c, 122, 200a, 128, 20a, 181a, 542-3p, 181c, 20b, 181b, 376a, 376b, 19b, 19a, 590-3p, 448, 320a, 320b, 106b, 93, 106a, 17, 543, 374b, 135a, 135b, 138, 183, 378, 205, 340, 505, 422a, 876-5p, 506, 875-5p, 203, 503
TANK (10010) NM_004180	144, 101, 30c, 410, 539, 145, 30d, 30e, 186, 30a, 27a, 27b, 30b, 128, 20a, 20b, 1297, 384, 190, 362-3p, 376a, 376b, 376c, 590-3p, 421, 129-5p, 26a, 190b, 106b, 93, 106a, 17, 382, 519d, 378, 346, 377, 216a, 340, 224, 422a, 26b, 496, 495, 203, 494, 329
BTG2 (7832) NM_006763	431, 144, 433, 539, 185, 149, 27a, 485-5p, 27b, 195, 330-5p, 125a-5p, 199a-5p, 424, 519d, 32, 328, 590-5p, 497, 103, 15a, 101, 410, 370, 128, 20a, 107, 25, 20b, 146a, 365, 21, 367, 218, 363, 339-5p, 125a-3p, 15b, 214, 146b-5p, 134, 92b, 106b, 92a, 106a, 93, 17, 199b-5p, 338-3p, 16, 340, 125b, 202
LYN (4067) NM_002350	539, 185, 384, 194, 301a, 320d, 320c, 301b, 154, 429, 371-5p, 222, 221, 495, 494, 599, 30c, 200b, 200c, 30d, 30e, 30a, 370, 30b, 454, 376a, 376b, 376c, 212, 320a, 98, 320b, 132, 544, let-7d, 378, let-7e, let-7b, 205, let-7c, let-7a, 372, 422a, 130b, 130a, 202, let-7i, let-7f, let-7g
TAB1 (10454) NM_153497	590-3p, 129-5p, 134, 152, 539, 371-5p, 340, 224, 491-5p, 374a, 374b, 130a

(continued)

Table 2 (continued)

Gene Symbol (Entrez Gene ID) Transcript ID	miRNAs
BCAR1 (9564) NM_014567	362-3p, 329
S1PR2 (9294) NM_004230	410, 34a, 485-5p, 451, 20a, 128, 454, 24, 20b, 339-5p, 301a, 19b, 488, 449b, 19a, 449a, 301b, 96, 106b, 106a, 93, 17, 133a, 133b, 34c-5p, 10a, 519d, 10b, 205, 130b, 130a
IGF1 (3479) NM_001111283	433, 599, 410, 186, 29a, 454, 29b, 1, 29c, 1297, 215, 142-3p, 22, 148a, 148b, 192, 194, 301a, 19b, 488, 19a, 23b, 301b, 590-3p, 137, 155, 129-5p, 152, 26a, 613, 299-3p, 758, 425, 206, 340, 130b, 222, 26b, 130a, 499-5p, 221, 495
CABIN1 (23523) NM_012295	376a, 18a, 376b, 93, 505
IGF1 (3479) NM_001111285	205, 599, 544, 214
FCER2 (2208) NM_002002	184, 22, 431, 122, 708, 330-5p, 326, 299-3p
NOS2 (4843) NM_000625	136, 15a, 26a, 539, 7, 149, 485-5p, 128, 16, 1297, 424, 28-5p, 195, 26b, 708, 497, 499-5p, 15b
TP53 (7157) NM_001126113	431, 296-3p, 143, 410, 539, 185, 186, 485-5p, 27a, 27b, 22, 218, 19b, 19a, 150, 125a-5p, 421, 98, 381, 491-5p, 338-3p, let-7d, 379, let-7e, let-7b, let-7c, let-7a, 340, 125b, 300, let-7i, let-7f, 504, let-7g
NBN (4683) NM_002485	141, 139-5p, 185, 149, 186, 1, 384, 301a, 374a, 301b, 429, 31, 371-5p, 495, 221, 494, 329, 181d, 200b, 410, 200c, 200a, 181a, 454, 181c, 181b, 217, 362-3p, 339-5p, 211, 212, 590-3p, 448, 136, 33b, 26a, 33a, 132, 106b, 543, 374b, 135a, 135b, 379, 206, 378, 204, 182, 205, 216a, 373, 372, 340, 130b, 26b, 130a, 499-5p, 874, 873
AIFM1 (9131) NM_004208	361-5p, 381, 186, 543, 653, 215, 383, 367, 192, 376c, 222, 300, 221
IL3 (3562) NM_000588	181d, 129-5p, 146b-5p, 15a, 143, 539, 613, 181a, 1, 181c, 16, 424, 181b, 206, 146a, 377, 195, 342-3p, 497, 223, 15b, 203, 214
TP53 (7157) NM_001126116	431, 143, 296-3p, 539, 410, 185, 186, 27a, 485-5p, 27b, 1297, 22, 218, 376a, 376b, 19b, 19a, 150, 125a-5p, 421, 98, 26a, 491-5p, 381, 338-3p, let-7d, 379, let-7e, let-7b, let-7c, let-7a, 340, 125b, 26b, 300, let-7i, let-7f, 504, let-7g
CDKN1B (1027) NM_004064	433, 539, 139-5p, 149, 520b, 148a, 148b, 190, 194, 374a, 488, 449b, 449a, 150, 23a, 23b, 155, 199a-5p, 154, 421, 152, 429, 758, 520c-3p, 140-5p, 196b, 222, 302b, 302a, 196a, 302d, 496, 302c, 221, 495, 494, 302e, 181d, 599, 200b, 200c, 122, 34a, 455-5p, 520e, 181a, 181c, 24, 181b, 1271, 142-3p, 218, 219-5p, 342-3p, 590-3p, 136, 98, 134, 96, 190b, 543, 199b-5p, 520d-3p, 374b, 34c-5p, let-7d, 379, let-7e, 182, 377, let-7b, let-7c, let-7a, 373, 372, 505, let-7i, 520a-3p, let-7f, let-7g
SH3BP2 (6452) NM_001145856	155, let-7d, 98, 185, let-7f, 494
DFFB (1677) NM_004402	124, 143, 200b, 145, 200c, 485-5p, 27b, 181a, 181c, 1297, 365, 22, 339-5p, 487b, 708, 214, 137, 448, 421, 26a, 429, 425, 138, 10a, 10b, 28-5p, 377, 371-5p, 340, 506, 26b, 203, 495, 494, 874, 504
SMAD2 (4087) NM_001003652	653, 486-5p
CDC45 (8318) NM_003504	184, 590-3p, 145, 371-5p, 488, 181a, 181c, 135a, 135b
TGFB1 (7040) NM_000660	142-3p, 139-5p, 185, 425, 214
IL6R (3570) NM_000565	124, 15a, 30c, 30d, 30e, 34a, 185, 149, 451, 30a, 30b, 146a, 195, 194, 320d, 320c, 449b, 449a, 212, 15b, 23a, 125a-5p, 23b, 320a, 320b, 146b-5p, 132, 490-3p, 491-5p, 16, 424, 138, 34c-5p, 653, 378, 371-5p, 216b, 140-5p, 224, 422a, 208a, 125b, 506, 208b, 497, 496, 499-5p, 495
SET (6418) NM_003011	539, 145, 9, 185, 186, 1, 1297, 335, 194, 23a, 23b, 125a-5p, 199a-5p, 613, 519d, 371-5p, 224, 590-5p, 496, 495, 494, 103, 101, 599, 30c, 30d, 30e, 411, 30a, 30b, 29a, 20a, 128, 29b, 107, 29c, 20b, 365, 21, 376a, 376b, 376c, 15b, 590-3p, 136, 26a, 106b, 106a, 93, 381, 17, 199b-5p, 338-3p, 184, 206, 125b, 300, 26b, 873
NFKBIB (4793) NM_002503	146a, 146b-5p, 296-3p
PABPC4 (8761) NM_001135653	141, 18a, 200a, 18b, 381, 520e, 520d-3p, 520b, 215, 520c-3p, 205, 218, 192, 373, 372, 708, 302b, 300, 330-5p, 302a, 326, 499-5p, 302d, 302c, 520a-3p, 302e
DGKZ (8525) NM_001105540	30c, 30d, 30e, 34a, 186, 543, 30a, 370, 30b, 34c-5p, 449b, 449a, 214
NRG1 (3084) NM_013962	186, 520b, 1297, 195, 23a, 23b, 758, 424, 519d, 520c-3p, 302b, 302a, 497, 302d, 302c, 494, 329, 302e, 181d, 15a, 411, 520e, 20a, 181a, 29a, 542-3p, 29b, 181c, 29c, 181b, 20b, 365, 362-3p, 342-3p, 15b, 137, 590-3p, 448, 26a, 106b, 106a, 93, 17, 543, 520d-3p, 374b, 16, 377, 373, 340, 372, 26b, 499-5p, 203, 520a-3p
LY96 (23643) NM_015364	136, 200b, 200c, 429
INPP5D (3635) NM_005541	124, 599, 34a, 186, 1, 1271, 362-3p, 335, 708, 210, 449b, 449a, 155, 153, 96, 18a, 613, 18b, 544, 299-3p, 138, 34c-5p, 653, 206, 28-5p, 377, 506, 329
PAK3 (5063) NM_001128168	103, 431, 433, 539, 122, 149, 20a, 107, 20b, 21, 488, 23a, 23b, 98, 129-5p, 106b, 106a, 93, 544, 17, 543, 519d, let-7d, let-7e, 378, let-7b, let-7c, let-7a, 422a, 590-5p, let-7i, 495, let-7f, 874, let-7g
TRAF5 (7188) NM_001033910	361-5p, 143, 9, 7, 190, 192, 374a, 488, 23a, 23b, 153, 18a, 18b, 425, 653, 495, 494, 296-3p, 410, 29a, 29b, 29c, 24, 215, 365, 218, 125a-3p, 214, 590-3p, 136, 320a, 320b, 190b, 544, 382, 374b, 338-3p, 135a, 138, 135b, let-7d, 378, let-7e, let-7b, let-7c, let-7a, 340, 422a, 202, let-7i, let-7f, let-7g
CD244 (51744) NM_016382	455-5p, 7, 185, 451, 542-3p, 1, 22, 217, 193b, 320d, 320c, 330-5p, 125a-5p, 320a, 320b, 613, 193a-3p, 338-3p, 135a, 206, 653, 876-5p, 125b, 326, 499-5p, 203, 495
CDH1 (999) NM_004360	143, 139-5p, 185, 485-5p, 148a, 148b, 374a, 330-5p, 23a, 23b, 199a-5p, 18a, 18b, 197, 425, 424, 653, 371-5p, 224, 497, 326, 495, 329, 599, 296-3p, 411, 24, 146a, 22, 362-3p, 219-5p, 339-5p, 342-3p, 590-3p, 98, 146b-5p, 544, 382, 199b-5p, 374b, 338-3p, 10a, let-7d, 10b, let-7e, let-7b, let-7c, let-7a, 340, 875-5p, 202, let-7i, let-7f, let-7g, 504
HIF1A (3091) NM_181054	361-5p, 144, 433, 143, 139-5p, 186, 520b, 1, 384, 148a, 148b, 194, 335, 301a, 708, 374a, 320d, 488, 320c, 301b, 155, 199a-5p, 153, 152, 18a, 18b, 613, 133a, 133b, 758, 653, 519d, 28-5p, 520c-3p, 371-5p, 302b, 222, 302a, 223, 302d, 302c, 221, 494, 302e, 103, 410, 411, 520e, 370, 20a, 542-3p, 107, 454, 24, 1271, 20b, 142-3p, 217, 376a, 376b, 376c, 19b, 210, 211, 19a, 212, 590-3p, 448, 320a, 33b, 320b, 96, 33a, 132, 106b, 106a, 93, 17, 543, 199b-5p, 374b, 520d-3p, 338-3p, 135a, 138, 135b, 10a, 206, 10b, 346, 204, 182, 373, 340, 372, 130b, 130a, 203, 520a-3p
CD40 (958) NM_001250	103, 15a, 145, 370, 107, 195, 374a, 330-5p, 15b, 590-3p, 448, 199a-5p, 153, 320a, 421, 320b, 381, 544, 199b-5p, 197, 135a, 424, 135b, 16, 10a, 10b, 371-5p, 340, 300, 497, 326
CD44 (960) NM_001001392	124, 181d, 144, 143, 410, 30c, 145, 185, 520e, 186, 485-5p, 520b, 181b, 142-3p, 194, 708, 330-5p, 211, 590-3p, 154, 152, 96, 26a, 132, 544, 520d-3p, 653, 28-5p, 204, 520c-3p, 216a, 216b, 373, 372, 340, 130b, 328, 506, 302b, 302a, 326, 302d, 202, 302c, 495, 520a-3p, 302e
NCR2 (9436) NM_004828	590-3p, 181d, 543, 181a, 494, 181c, 181b
PTPRH (5794) NM_002842	132, 9, 544, 491-5p, 133a, 133b, 222, 212
NUMA1 (4926) NM_006185	124, 7, 411, 520e, 520b, 454, 1297, 148a, 148b, 193b, 301a, 125a-3p, 301b, 214, 152, 26a, 193a-3p, 381, 543, 520d-3p, let-7d, 378, 520c-3p, 373, 422a, 328, 506, 300, 26b, 302b, 130a, 302a, 520a-3p, 873
CD58 (965) NM_001144822	141, 144, 152, 599, 122, 200a, 149, 142-3p, 183, 148a, 148b, 216a, 140-5p, 214, 504
TANK (10010) NM_133484	539
CEBPB (1051) NM_005194	539, 410, 139-5p, 20a, 20b, 191, 376a, 376b, 376c, 374a, 155, 154, 421, 33b, 33a, 106b, 93, 106a, 17, 381, 374b, 299-3p, 519d, 371-5p, 590-5p, 300, 495
BRCA1 (672) NM_007300	141, 200b, 200c, 7, 34a, 200a, 186, 485-5p, 1, 146a, 190, 218, 125a-3p, 320d, 320c, 449b, 15b, 212, 449a, 199a-5p, 153, 421, 320a, 320b, 146b-5p, 190b, 132, 613, 543, 429, 199b-5p, 34c-5p, 206, 205, 216b, 224, 494
PTGS2 (5743) NM_000963	141, 144, 539, 9, 1297, 148a, 148b, 192, 301a, 708, 374a, 488, 301b, 155, 152, 429, 758, 28-5p, 32, 196a, 494, 181d, 101, 200b, 410, 200c, 200a, 411, 181a, 128, 542-3p, 181c, 181b, 146a, 215, 362-3p, 367, 125a-3p, 212, 137, 448, 33b, 146b-5p, 33a, 26a, 132, 381, 543, 374b, 379, 183, 340, 130b, 26b, 300, 202, 203
MAPK8 (5599) NM_139049	377, 129-5p, 208a, 208b, 499-5p
TLR5 (7100) NM_003268	136, 154, 539, 34a, 185, 382, 34c-5p, let-7d, 218, 376a, 376b, 130b, 19b, 449b, 19a, 449a, let-7g

Gene Symbol (Entrez Gene ID) Transcript ID	miRNAs
RBBP8 (5932) NM_203292	20a, 454, 20b, 148a, 148b, 301a, 488, 19b, 19a, 301b, 590-3p, 136, 152, 18a, 106a, 18b, 17, 377, 205, 340, 130b, 222, 130a, 202, 221, 495
IL5 (3567) NM_000879	590-3p, 129-5p, 200b, 200c, 132, 613, 543, 186, 451, 429, 1, 206, 182, 194, 328, 495, 212, 203
TCEB1 (6921) NM_005648	144, 200b, 200c, 139-5p, 186, 1271, 21, 217, 194, 374a, 488, 19b, 19a, 212, 137, 590-3p, 448, 153, 96, 132, 429, 374b, 758, 653, 378, 182, 422a, 224, 590-5p, 223, 202
CDKN2A (1029) NM_000077	590-3p, 136, 365, 134, 410, 9, 340, 544, 186, 125b, 128, 125a-5p
CD14 (929) NM_001040021	296-3p, 340, 491-5p
TYK2 (7297) NM_003331	124, 506, 485-5p, 222, 221, 24
ROCK1 (6093) NM_005406	431, 144, 9, 139-5p, 27a, 27b, 148a, 148b, 190, 335, 194, 301a, 488, 449b, 449a, 301b, 199a-5p, 129-5p, 153, 421, 152, 429, 32, 371-5p, 196b, 224, 196a, 495, 221, 494, 124, 101, 599, 30c, 200b, 200c, 30d, 30e, 34a, 30a, 30b, 454, 25, 217, 367, 376a, 376b, 363, 376c, 448, 136, 98, 190b, 92b, 92a, 381, 199b-5p, 135a, 34c-5p, 135b, let-7d, let-7e, 183, let-7b, 182, let-7c, 216a, let-7a, 216b, 340, 130b, 506, 324-5p, 300, 130a, 202, let-7i, 203, let-7f, let-7g
FASLG (356) NM_000639	186, 149, 520b, 384, 192, 708, 519d, 28-5p, 520c-3p, 32, 590-5p, 328, 302b, 302a, 196a, 302d, 302c, 329, 302e, 520e, 20a, 24, 25, 20b, 215, 21, 367, 362-3p, 219-5p, 363, 590-3p, 136, 98, 106b, 92b, 93, 106a, 92a, 17, 543, 520d-3p, 10a, let-7d, let-7e, 10b, let-7b, let-7c, 216a, 216b, let-7a, 373, 372, 324-5p, 203, let-7i, let-7f, 520a-3p, let-7g
NRG1 (3084) NM_013956	431, 144, 145, 7, 27a, 27b, 384, 335, 301a, 374a, 488, 23a, 23b, 155, 18a, 18b, 429, 32, 222, 496, 221, 495, 124, 181d, 101, 200b, 410, 200c, 455-5p, 411, 128, 29a, 29b, 454, 29c, 25, 1271, 146a, 363, 125a-3p, 448, 590-3p, 137, 146b-5p, 96, 543, 382, 338-3p, 183, 340, 505, 506, 203
RAD51 (5888) NM_001164270	124, 9, 411, 186, 542-3p, 1271, 383, 148a, 148b, 219-5p, 193b, 194, 374a, 320d, 320c, 211, 421, 320a, 320b, 152, 96, 193a-3p, 544, 382, 197, 374b, 758, 653, 378, 204, 422a, 876-5p, 506, 222, 499-5p, 203, 221, 494
MTOR (2475) NM_004958	103, 144, 101, 100, 145, 139-5p, 7, 187, 370, 107, 1271, 190, 99b, 99a, 23a, 23b, 214, 421, 33b, 33a, 96, 190b, 381, 758, 135a, 135b, 183, let-7b, 182, let-7c, 371-5p, 224, 140-5p, 505, 300, 222, 496, let-7i, 221, 495, 503, let-7g
BCL9 (607) NM_004326	141, 15a, 101, 30c, 200b, 200c, 30d, 30e, 455-5p, 200a, 185, 186, 30a, 30b, 22, 217, 218, 362-3p, 195, 488, 211, 15b, 590-3p, 429, 338-3p, 425, 424, 16, 653, 10a, 204, 216a, 140-5p, 505, 324-5p, 497, 496, 503, 329, 494
DIABLO (56616) NM_019887	383, 148a, 191, 152, 148b, 376c, 487b, 324-5p, 499-5p, 203
CXCL5 (6374) NM_002994	181d, 141, 410, 200a, 149, 186, 27b, 181a, 1, 181c, 25, 181b, 384, 21, 367, 193b, 376a, 376b, 376c, 363, 342-3p, 708, 374a, 23a, 23b, 448, 590-3p, 421, 129-5p, 92b, 92a, 193a-3p, 613, 544, 543, 374b, 424, 206, 28-5p, 32, 876-5p, 203, 495, 494
RAG1 (5896) NM_000448	361-5p, 139-5p, 145, 186, 27a, 148a, 190, 148b, 193b, 301a, 150, 301b, 154, 421, 153, 152, 18a, 429, 32, 140-5p, 124, 181d, 200b, 410, 30c, 200c, 30d, 30e, 455-5p, 30a, 30b, 29a, 29b, 454, 29c, 25, 181b, 367, 362-3p, 363, 448, 134, 33b, 190b, 33a, 92b, 92a, 544, 381, 382, 338-3p, 182, 377, 505, 130b, 506, 208b, 300, 130a, 499-5p, 202, 203
TLR6 (10333) NM_006068	28-5p, 181d, 708, 181a, 494
GAS2 (2620) NM_005256	431, 539, 139-5p, 520b, 1, 195, 155, 154, 153, 129-5p, 613, 133a, 133b, 429, 425, 424, 653, 519d, 520c-3p, 222, 302b, 302a, 497, 302d, 302c, 221, 302e, 103, 15a, 200b, 200c, 520e, 20a, 128, 107, 20b, 486-5p, 376a, 376b, 339-5p, 376c, 342-3p, 15b, 448, 134, 190b, 106b, 106a, 93, 381, 17, 543, 520d-3p, 374b, 16, 206, 377, 375, 373, 372, 340, 300, 203, 520a-3p
PTPN6 (5777) NM_080549	186, 128
PTPN6 (5777) NM_080548	186, 485-5p, 128
KLRK1 (22914) NM_007360	137, 431, 433, 132, 9, 34a, 133a, 133b, 149, 138, 34c-5p, 218, 216b, 326, 330-5p, 449b, 212, 449a
TNFSF12 (8742) NM_003809	136, 421, 200b, 200c, 122, 186, 543, 429, 27a, 374b, 27b, 299-3p, 135a, 135b, 28-5p, 365, 204, 505, 374a, 708, 211, 874
ARNT (405) NM_001668	361-5p, 431, 9, 1, 383, 190, 193b, 195, 374a, 320d, 320c, 23a, 23b, 421, 129-5p, 18a, 193a-3p, 18b, 429, 758, 424, 653, 371-5p, 140-5p, 590-5p, 222, 223, 497, 495, 221, 103, 181d, 15a, 200b, 410, 200c, 455-5p, 370, 29a, 107, 29b, 29c, 181b, 21, 376c, 342-3p, 15b, 212, 590-3p, 98, 320a, 320b, 132, 381, 374b, 338-3p, 135a, 16, 135b, 206, let-7d, 10a, 10b, 378, let-7e, let-7b, 377, let-7c, 216a, let-7a, 340, 422a, 875-5p, 300, let-7i, let-7f, 504, let-7g
RB1 (5925) NM_000321	361-5p, 144, 143, 539, 145, 139-5p, 7, 1297, 192, 335, 194, 374a, 449b, 449a, 199a-5p, 129-5p, 490-3p, 519d, 590-5p, 450a, 223, 495, 494, 410, 34a, 128, 20a, 29b, 1271, 20b, 215, 142-3p, 376c, 342-3p, 212, 590-3p, 136, 26a, 96, 132, 106b, 106a, 93, 17, 382, 199b-5p, 374b, 34c-5p, 183, 378, 377, 216a, 216b, 340, 422a, 26b, 202, 499-5p, 203, let-7i, let-7g
ORC2L (4999) NM_006190	431, 143, 145, 186, 1, 374a, 320d, 320c, 488, 449b, 449a, 125a-5p, 301b, 129-5p, 153, 613, 197, 32, 140-5p, 495, 124, 200b, 30c, 30d, 200c, 30e, 122, 34a, 30a, 30b, 25, 218, 367, 363, 448, 137, 136, 320a, 33b, 320b, 33a, 92b, 92a, 381, 382, 374b, 34c-5p, 206, 183, 340, 506, 125b, 300, 875-5p, 130a, 203, 873
HMMR (3161) NM_001142556	361-5p, 200b, 200c, 9, 34a, 411, 1271, 142-3p, 21, 374a, 449b, 449a, 23a, 23b, 590-3p, 421, 96, 381, 543, 382, 429, 374b, 34c-5p, 379, 182, 31, 505, 590-5p, 300, 223, 202, 495, 503
EXOC2 (55770) NM_018303	103, 181d, 433, 143, 15a, 539, 145, 455-5p, 27a, 27b, 181a, 542-3p, 107, 181c, 181b, 384, 21, 195, 212, 15b, 214, 590-3p, 132, 543, 424, 16, 378, 422a, 497, 499-5p, 202, 203, 495, 504
DCLRE1C (64421) NM_001033855	181d, 431, 410, 149, 186, 520e, 187, 20a, 520b, 29b, 181c, 181b, 20b, 190, 125a-5p, 448, 154, 136, 129-5p, 18a, 106b, 106a, 18b, 93, 17, 520d-3p, 425, 519d, 520c-3p, 373, 372, 140-5p, 125b, 302b, 302a, 302d, 221, 302c, 520a-3p, 302e
TFE3 (7030) NM_006521	361-5p, 136, 320a, 320b, 200b, 200c, 145, 122, 133a, 491-5p, 133b, 186, 429, 485-5p, 24, 653, 184, 383, 205, 31, 335, 320d, 320c, 203
WASL (8976) NM_003941	144, 9, 520b, 1, 301a, 23a, 301b, 23b, 129-5p, 152, 613, 758, 519d, 302b, 302a, 302d, 302c, 302e, 124, 599, 128, 454, 142-3p, 19b, 19a, 448, 590-3p, 137, 136, 134, 26a, 92b, 92a, 374b, 506, 26b, 433, 539, 139-5p, 186, 27b, 148a, 190, 148b, 195, 374a, 488, 424, 520c-3p, 32, 196b, 196a, 223, 497, 496, 329, 494, 181d, 15a, 520e, 20a, 181a, 181c, 20b, 25, 181b, 218, 362-3p, 367, 363, 342-3p, 211, 15b, 98, 33b, 33a, 106b, 106a, 93, 17, 544, 543, 382, 520d-3p, 299-3p, 16, 379, 206, let-7d, let-7e, let-7b, 182, 204, let-7c, 216a, let-7a, 216b, 373, 372, 130b, 130a, 202, let-7i, 203, let-7f, 520a-3p, let-7g
HOXB9 (3219) NM_024017	129-5p, 539, 139-5p, 122, 7, 128, 542-3p, 206, 346, 28-5p, 21, 375, 328, 222, 708, 551a, 495, 551b, 23a, 494, 23b
GH1 (2688) NM_000515	590-3p, 138
DDR1 (780) NM_013994	142-3p, 199a-5p, 599, 195, 185, 125a-3p, 125b, 199b-5p, 542-3p, 494, 125a-5p, 16
MDM2 (4193) NM_006879	181d, 141, 145, 200a, 185, 29a, 181a, 29b, 29c, 181c, 181b, 25, 384, 383, 367, 193b, 363, 194, 23a, 23b, 590-3p, 92b, 92a, 193a-3p, 374b, 338-3p, 758, 379, 377, 373, 140-5p, 222, 302b, 223, 302a, 302d, 496, 221, 495, 302c, 504
NRG1 (3084) NM_004495	103, 141, 30d, 122, 30e, 200a, 30a, 107, 21, 362-3p, 376c, 342-3p, 125a-3p, 448, 421, 153, 544, 338-3p, 183, 346, 377, 182, 216b, 876-5p, 590-5p, 223, 495, 329
FAM175A (84142) NM_139076	141, 144, 143, 145, 185, 186, 520b, 384, 190, 193b, 335, 194, 320d, 320c, 488, 23a, 23b, 193a-3p, 429, 425, 653, 520c-3p, 371-5p, 140-5p, 302b, 302a, 302d, 302c, 302e, 296-3p, 599, 200b, 200c, 200a, 520e, 142-3p, 219-5p, 125a-3p, 211, 448, 590-3p, 320a, 320b, 381, 520d-3p, 338-3p, 204, 205, 216b, 373, 372, 300, 875-5p, 520a-3p, 504
CCR7 (1236) NM_001838	21, 218, 339-5p, 335, 320d, 320c, 330-5p, 125a-5p, 214, 199a-5p, 320a, 98, 320b, 199b-5p, let-7d, let-7e, 378, let-7b, 204, let-7c, let-7a, 422a, 125b, 590-5p, let-7i, let-7f, let-7g
CRK (1398) NM_005206	361-5p, 141, 145, 186, 27a, 27b, 520b, 191, 193b, 192, 194, 449b, 449a, 23a, 23b, 490-3p, 193a-3p, 133a, 133b, 653, 519d, 520c-3p, 31, 328, 302b, 302a, 302d, 302c, 329, 302e, 200a, 34a, 520e, 181a, 20a, 181c, 20b, 142-3p, 215, 362-3p, 212, 136, 132, 106b, 93, 106a, 381, 17, 520d-3p, 34c-5p, 183, 373, 372, 208a, 300, 208b, 499-5p, 203, 520a-3p, 874

(continued)

Table 2 (continued)

Gene Symbol (Entrez Gene ID) Transcript ID	miRNAs
WAS (7454) NM_000377	146a, 129-5p, 146b-5p, 185, 491-5p, 214
DDIT4 (54541) NM_019058	181d, 433, 101, 30c, 200b, 30d, 139-5p, 200c, 30e, 7, 30a, 30b, 128, 181a, 181c, 1297, 25, 181b, 383, 22, 217, 367, 363, 212, 448, 137, 153, 26a, 132, 92b, 92a, 133a, 133b, 429, 183, 32, 26b, 496, 495, 494, 504
FYN (2534) NM_153047	141, 200b, 539, 410, 200c, 200a, 7, 186, 1271, 376c, 125a-3p, 374a, 23a, 23b, 590-3p, 155, 448, 137, 129-5p, 33b, 96, 33a, 429, 374b, 653, 183, 182, 876-5p, 494
GADD45A (1647) NM_001924	181d, 599, 145, 9, 411, 181a, 454, 181e, 181b, 146a, 148a, 217, 148b, 376c, 301a, 374a, 19b, 19a, 301b, 590-3p, 129-5p, 421, 152, 146b-5p, 381, 374b, 135a, 135b, 216a, 375, 130b, 876-5p, 300, 130a, 202, 496, 499-5p
UNG (7374) NM_080911	448, 199a-5p, 141, 101, 539, 18a, 18b, 34a, 544, 199b-5p, 374b, 454, 34c-5p, 22, 377, 204, 31, 335, 506, 374a, 496, 211, 449b, 495, 449a, 150
PTPRC (5788) NM_080923	103, 15a, 433, 410, 411, 107, 191, 219-5p, 195, 376c, 374a, 15b, 590-3p, 199a-5p, 98, 33b, 33a, 381, 544, 199b-5p, 374b, 338-3p, 425, 424, 16, 653, 184, let-7d, let-7e, let-7b, 205, let-7c, 216a, let-7a, 340, 505, 196b, 208a, 300, 208b, 196a, 497, 223, 499-5p, let-7i, let-7f, 873, let-7g
TNFRSF17 (608) NM_001192	320a, 320b, 96, 539, 106b, 106a, 93, 17, 27a, 27b, 20a, 425, 20b, 519d, 21, 320d, 320c, 150, 873
EDN1 (1906) NM_001955	141, 144, 539, 1, 384, 383, 194, 301a, 301b, 154, 613, 653, 224, 495, 494, 599, 101, 30c, 410, 30d, 122, 30e, 455-5p, 200a, 30a, 30b, 454, 376a, 376b, 376c, 212, 214, 590-3p, 448, 98, 134, 33b, 33a, 132, 382, 299-3p, 135a, 135b, 206, 379, let-7d, let-7e, 378, let-7b, let-7c, let-7a, 216b, 340, 422a, 130b, 876-5p, 130a, 203, let-7i, let-7f, let-7g, 873
MYD88 (4615) NM_002468	433, 30c, 200b, 200c, 30d, 122, 30e, 455-5p, 185, 187, 30a, 370, 30b, 24, 365, 218, 376a, 376b, 330-5p, 23a, 23b, 98, 152, 491-5p, 429, 135a, 135b, 138, let-7d, let-7e, let-7b, let-7c, let-7a, 340, 326, 202, let-7i, 203, let-7f, let-7g
DFFA (1676) NM_213566	129-5p, 421, 320a, 320b, 132, 185, 149, 27a, 485-5p, 27b, 299-3p, 138, 182, 190, 339-5p, 505, 196b, 208a, 590-5p, 208b, 320d, 320c, 196a, 212, 873
IL4 (3565) NM_000589	590-3p, 320a, 320b, 433, 410, 200b, 200c, 186, 429, 376a, 376b, 340, 320d, 320c
IL25 (64806) NM_172314	181d, 15a, 30c, 30d, 30e, 149, 370, 30a, 30b, 20a, 181a, 181c, 181b, 20b, 195, 449b, 449a, 15b, 214, 106b, 106a, 93, 17, 16, 424, 519d, 216a, 216b, 340, 140-5p, 328, 497, 495
NFKBIA (4792) NM_020529	181d, 101, 30e, 34a, 30a, 181b, 374a, 19b, 449b, 211, 19a, 449a, 590-3p, 129-5p, 133a, 381, 133b, 374b, 34c-5p, 653, 204, 196b, 208a, 300, 208b, 196a, 499-5p, 495
BRCC3 (79184) NM_024332	361-5p, 144, 143, 410, 145, 27a, 27b, 29a, 29b, 29c, 142-3p, 383, 21, 217, 218, 330-5p, 211, 23a, 125a-5p, 23b, 590-3p, 136, 421, 653, 204, 377, 340, 590-5p, 125b, 875-5p, 222, 326, 221, 203, 494
IL17RA (23765) NM_014339	103, 365, 183, 377, 205, 373, 149, 708, 19b, 19a, 107, 24
SMAD6 (4091) NR_027654	144, 410, 186, 20a, 24, 20b, 1297, 25, 367, 363, 374a, 488, 330-5p, 125a-5p, 155, 136, 98, 134, 26a, 92b, 106b, 92a, 93, 106a, 17, 381, 374b, 519d, let-7d, let-7e, let-7b, let-7c, 32, let-7a, 340, 505, 125b, 300, 26b, 326, let-7i, 874, 503, let-7f, let-7g
RPL11 (6135) NM_000975	137, 185
UBE2V1 (7335) NM_001032288	181d, 144, 101, 15a, 296-3p, 200b, 139-5p, 200c, 145, 455-5p, 185, 370, 27a, 485-5p, 27b, 29a, 1, 29b, 29c, 362-3p, 218, 190, 195, 19b, 19a, 15b, 18b, 429, 135a, 135b, 138, 424, 16, 206, let-7b, let-7c, let-7a, 140-5p, 506, 497, 499-5p, 494, 329
CD86 (942) NM_175862	141, 181d, 144, 101, 410, 200a, 7, 24, 181b, 146a, 486-5p, 218, 376c, 150, 590-3p, 98, 129-5p, 146b-5p, 18a, 18b, 133a, 133b, 429, 338-3p, 135a, 135b, let-7d, 379, let-7e, 182, let-7b, let-7c, let-7a, 373, 196b, 196a, 223, 202, 496, let-7i, let-7f, 504, let-7g, 873
ATR (545) NM_001184	448, 590-3p, 361-5p, 146b-5p, 410, 539, 613, 185, 374b, 1, 146a, 206, 383, 374a
CDKN1A (1026) NM_000389	101, 186, 485-5p, 370, 20a, 454, 20b, 22, 365, 335, 301a, 708, 212, 301b, 98, 132, 106b, 93, 106a, 491-5p, 17, 519d, let-7d, 379, let-7e, 28-5p, 378, let-7b, let-7c, 205, let-7a, 224, 422a, 130b, 130a, 499-5p, let-7i, let-7f, let-7g, 873
ICAM1 (3383) NM_000201	141, 431, 129-5p, 296-3p, 9, 200a, 411, 490-3p, 491-5p, 338-3p, 299-3p, 454, 138, 383, 182, 21, 486-5p, 216b, 301a, 130b, 223, 130a, 203, 495, 301b
MAP3K2 (10746) NM_006609	144, 539, 139-5p, 9, 7, 186, 485-5p, 520b, 1297, 190, 195, 335, 708, 374a, 320d, 330-5p, 320c, 449b, 449a, 150, 23a, 23b, 129-5p, 758, 424, 519d, 653, 28-5p, 520c-3p, 302b, 450a, 302a, 326, 497, 302d, 302c, 495, 302e, 15a, 30c, 410, 30d, 122, 30e, 520e, 30a, 30b, 20a, 454, 24, 20b, 1271, 218, 342-3p, 19b, 15b, 137, 590-3p, 136, 320a, 320b, 33b, 33a, 190b, 26a, 106b, 106a, 93, 17, 544, 374b, 520d-3p, 299-3p, 16, 379, 182, 377, 373, 372, 340, 875-5p, 26b, 520a-3p
LAT (27040) NM_001014988	146a, 146b-5p, 193b, 216b, 18a, 18b, 363, 193a-3p, 342-3p, 876-5p
STAT6 (6778) NM_003153	361-5p, 103, 144, 101, 599, 139-5p, 411, 107, 142-3p, 486-5p, 219-5p, 125a-3p, 210, 150, 590-3p, 154, 153, 18a, 106b, 18b, 106a, 93, 17, 491-5p, 135a, 135b, 377, 216a, 590-5p, 496
PSMB6 (5694) NM_002798	487b, 758
IFNGR2 (3460) NM_005534	361-5p, 15a, 200b, 200c, 145, 9, 381, 429, 142-3p, 300, 497, 496, 495, 15b
TAPBP (6892) NM_172208	136, 296-3p, 139-5p, 544, 491-5p, 149, 485-5p, 370, 197, 299-3p, 542-3p, 24, 379, 28-5p, 383, 21, 371-5p, 125a-3p, 590-5p, 496, 494, 873
AZI2 (64343) NM_001134433	653, 21, 296-3p, 190, 410, 190b, 132, 411, 590-5p, 496, 212
GNAQ (2776) NM_002072	141, 144, 30c, 30d, 30e, 200a, 411, 185, 451, 30a, 30b, 29b, 142-3p, 218, 342-3p, 320d, 374a, 19b, 320c, 19a, 590-3p, 448, 320a, 320b, 490-3p, 544, 374b, 425, 135a, 135b, 183, 377, 182, 205, 371-5p, 224, 590-5p, 202, 496, 495
RAB11FIP2 (22841) NM_014904	141, 431, 361-5p, 144, 433, 539, 186, 384, 195, 194, 374a, 320d, 320c, 449b, 449a, 23a, 23b, 155, 199a-5p, 153, 18a, 18b, 429, 424, 32, 196b, 224, 590-5p, 497, 196a, 495, 494, 181d, 103, 15a, 200b, 410, 30d, 200c, 34a, 200a, 128, 181a, 29b, 107, 29c, 181c, 181b, 142-3p, 21, 367, 376b, 363, 376c, 19b, 19a, 15b, 448, 590-3p, 136, 320a, 320b, 190b, 381, 382, 374b, 135a, 16, 34c-5p, 340, 506, 300, 875-5p, 202, 504
NODAL (4838) NM_018055	320a, 146b-5p, 143, 320b, 92b, 92a, 193a-3p, 197, 135a, 135b, 146a, 346, 377, 219-5p, 218, 205, 193b, 505, 320d, 320c, 495, 874, 873
TNFAIP3 (7128) NM_006290	141, 186, 335, 301a, 374a, 330-5p, 23a, 23b, 301b, 125a-5p, 154, 421, 18a, 18b, 429, 758, 425, 519d, 653, 326, 495, 494, 329, 103, 200b, 200c, 200a, 455-5p, 20a, 29a, 128, 107, 454, 29b, 29c, 20b, 146a, 362-3p, 19b, 19a, 211, 448, 98, 146b-5p, 106b, 93, 106a, 17, 544, 374b, 135a, 135b, let-7d, let-7e, let-7b, 204, let-7c, let-7a, 340, 130b, 505, 125b, 130a, 203, let-7i, let-7f, let-7g, 873
GAST (2520) NM_000805	383
PITX2 (5308) NM_000325	141, 144, 139-5p, 145, 186, 520b, 1, 190, 487b, 320d, 374a, 708, 320c, 488, 23a, 150, 23b, 155, 199a-5p, 613, 758, 653, 28-5p, 520c-3p, 140-5p, 590-5p, 302b, 302a, 302d, 494, 599, 410, 30c, 200b, 30e, 200a, 451, 30a, 30b, 128, 142-3p, 217, 21, 363, 376c, 342-3p, 211, 137, 590-3p, 320a, 320b, 190b, 381, 199b-5p, 374b, 206, 377, 204, 340, 505, 324-5p, 875-5p, 300, 203
CDC42BPA (8476) NM_003607	361-5p, 186, 320d, 320c, 449b, 449a, 154, 193a-3p, 758, 653, 181d, 410, 30c, 30d, 30e, 34a, 30a, 30b, 29a, 181a, 542-3p, 29b, 181c, 29c, 181b, 218, 339-5p, 125a-3p, 19b, 19a, 590-3p, 98, 320a, 320b, 33b, 33a, 544, 381, 382, 135a, 34c-5p, 135b, 378, let-7b, 182, let-7c, 205, 216b, 372, 422a, 876-5p, 300, let-7i, let-7g
CCL2 (6347) NM_002982	124, 421, 101, 33b, 33a, 9, 122, 613, 186, 543, 374b, 1, 206, 379, 22, 377, 373, 505, 506, 374a, 19b, 19a, 495, 494, 23a, 23b
DAXX (1616) NM_001141970	146a, 137, 144, 146b-5p, 101, 340, 186, 543, 494
MYLK (4638) NM_053025	143, 539, 139-5p, 7, 520b, 1, 193b, 192, 195, 335, 374a, 320d, 320c, 488, 449b, 449a, 155, 154, 129-5p, 18a, 18b, 193a-3p, 613, 429, 424, 653, 519d, 520c-3p, 32, 590-5p, 302b, 302a, 497, 496, 302d, 302c, 495, 302e, 15a, 200b, 200c, 34a, 520e, 20a, 25, 20b, 215, 142-3p, 146a, 365, 367, 376c, 363, 211, 15b, 590-3p, 320a, 320b, 146b-5p, 190b, 92b, 106b, 106a, 92a, 93, 17, 520d-3p, 374b, 16, 34c-5p, 206, 182, 204, 373, 372, 340, 130b, 208a, 208b, 130a, 499-5p, 203, 520a-3p, 503

Gene Symbol (Entrez Gene ID) Transcript ID	miRNAs
FCGR2B (2213) NM_004001	103, 433, 30c, 30d, 30e, 186, 30a, 30b, 128, 107, 1, 191, 376a, 376b, 339-5p, 194, 342-3p, 125a-3p, 374a, 212, 590-3p, 154, 98, 132, 18a, 18b, 613, 543, 520d-3p, 374b, 138, 206, let-7c, 340, 140-5p, 302b, 302a, 203, let-7f, 494, let-7g
FANCG (2189) NM_004629	590-3p, 421, 216a, 539, 18a, 18b, 203, 23a, 23b
EGFR (1956) NM_005228	141, 103, 539, 455-5p, 200a, 7, 520e, 27a, 370, 27b, 520b, 107, 365, 342-3p, 155, 129-5p, 134, 133a, 491-5p, 133b, 520d-3p, 299-3p, 520c-3p, 373, 372, 875-5p, 302b, 450a, 302a, 302d, 203, 302c, 874, 520a-3p, 302e
HDAC9 (9734) NM_178425	361-5p, 7, 485-5p, 27a, 27b, 1297, 383, 320d, 320c, 488, 155, 199a-5p, 129-5p, 490-3p, 425, 424, 519d, 32, 302b, 223, 302a, 495, 494, 124, 181d, 30c, 30d, 30e, 455-5p, 30a, 30b, 181a, 128, 29a, 20a, 29b, 181c, 29c, 1271, 25, 20b, 181b, 365, 217, 486-5p, 367, 376c, 363, 342-3p, 211, 320a, 320b, 96, 26a, 92b, 106b, 93, 106a, 92a, 17, 199b-5p, 338-3p, 377, 204, 205, 373, 372, 208a, 506, 208b, 26b, 499-5p, 874, 873
EXOC1 (55763) NM_001024924	144, 433, 101, 539, 139-5p, 542-3p, 215, 367, 192, 335, 374a, 320d, 330-5p, 320c, 23a, 23b, 214, 155, 590-3p, 129-5p, 320a, 33b, 320b, 33a, 543, 374b, 205, 32, 371-5p, 224, 505, 326, 496, 499-5p
RAF1 (5894) NM_002880	15a, 410, 7, 185, 149, 485-5p, 542-3p, 217, 148a, 362-3p, 195, 125a-3p, 19b, 488, 19a, 15b, 125a-5p, 590-3p, 134, 18a, 18b, 491-5p, 199b-5p, 16, 424, 216a, 125b, 497, 495, 874, 329
NAA10 (8260) NM_003491	152
MAP3K3 (4215) NM_002401	9, 1, 190, 194, 708, 374a, 449b, 449a, 23a, 150, 23b, 133a, 133b, 424, 519d, 28-5p, 302a, 497, 326, 181d, 103, 410, 30d, 34a, 30a, 20a, 181a, 107, 24, 181c, 20b, 181b, 1271, 217, 211, 15b, 212, 33b, 96, 33a, 132, 106b, 93, 106a, 544, 17, 374b, 135a, 34c-5p, 135b, 206, 204, 505
IFNG (3458) NM_000619	181d, 101, 200b, 410, 200c, 411, 149, 27a, 27b, 181a, 29a, 29b, 24, 181c, 29c, 181b, 25, 1297, 362-3p, 367, 363, 374a, 23a, 125a-5p, 23b, 155, 448, 137, 590-3p, 136, 421, 26a, 92b, 93, 92a, 382, 429, 374b, 758, 653, 377, 32, 340, 505, 125b, 26b, 495, 329
EXOC5 (10640) NM_006544	141, 144, 539, 145, 27a, 27b, 1297, 148a, 148b, 195, 194, 301a, 374a, 488, 301b, 154, 129-5p, 152, 424, 28-5p, 32, 371-5p, 224, 196b, 497, 196a, 181d, 15a, 101, 100, 410, 411, 200a, 181a, 454, 181c, 24, 181b, 25, 146a, 217, 367, 376a, 376b, 363, 99b, 19b, 19a, 15b, 590-3p, 146b-5p, 26a, 92b, 92a, 374b, 338-3p, 16, 10a, 10b, 378, 182, 216a, 216b, 340, 130b, 505, 422a, 26b, 875-5p, 130a, 504
CKS2 (1164) NM_001827	124, 421, 144, 152, 134, 33a, 26a, 139-5p, 30d, 7, 30a, 181c, 1297, 148a, 21, 148b, 32, 371-5p, 363, 506, 590-5p, 26b, 495, 494
BCL2L10 (10017) NM_020396	141, 377, 193b, 18a, 200a, 7, 18b, 193a-3p, 342-3p, 27a, 27b, 197
PAK4 (10298) NM_001014832	181d, 433, 224, 506, 485-5p, 181a, 24, 181c, 425, 181b
LMNA (4000) NM_170707	124, 129-5p, 539, 9, 185, 34c-5p, 138, let-7d, 10a, 142-3p, 10b, 28-5p, let-7e, let-7b, let-7c, 205, 371-5p, let-7a, 506, 708, 449b, 449a
TNFRSF13B (23495) NM_012452	378, 22, 148a, 367, 32, 92b, 92a, 363, 422a, 25, 214
TNFRSF9 (3604) NM_001561	9, 186, 29a, 542-3p, 29b, 29c, 486-5p, 339-5p, 374a, 320d, 320c, 590-3p, 448, 137, 320a, 33b, 320b, 33a, 490-3p, 382, 374b, 10a, 10b, 378, 371-5p, 340, 422a, 876-5p, 328, 203, 495, 504
ARG2 (384) NM_001172	124, 103, 144, 101, 9, 181a, 128, 520b, 107, 542-3p, 181b, 148a, 148b, 376c, 374a, 155, 448, 137, 154, 98, 152, 26a, 18b, 543, 374b, 379, let-7d, 10a, let-7e, 10b, let-7b, let-7c, 520c-3p, let-7a, 506, let-7i, 494, let-7f, let-7g
NFKB2 (4791) NM_001077494	491-5p
BCL2A1 (597) NM_001114735	137, 181d, 182, 144, 421, 122, 376c, 411, 185, 505, 381, 382, 300, 181c
CCR3 (1232) NM_178329	181d, 599, 296-3p, 410, 200b, 200c, 18a, 18b, 133a, 544, 543, 133b, 149, 429, 181a, 181c, 181b, 138, 340, 335, 125a-3p, 214
LAIR1 (3903) NM_002287	141, 145, 34a, 200a, 24, 25, 384, 22, 367, 363, 125a-3p, 708, 320d, 210, 320c, 330-5p, 449b, 212, 449a, 23a, 23b, 214, 590-3p, 129-5p, 320a, 134, 320b, 132, 92b, 92a, 758, 424, 34c-5p, 138, 28-5p, 32, 876-5p, 326, 202

Gene Symbol (Entrez Gene ID) Transcript ID	miRNAs
MAP2K4 (6416) NM_003010	127-3p, 141, 431, 144, 433, 539, 139-5p, 9, 185, 186, 149, 27a, 27b, 194, 335, 487b, 374a, 199a-5p, 421, 129-5p, 18a, 490-3p, 18b, 429, 653, 519d, 32, 371-5p, 31, 224, 221, 124, 181d, 200b, 200c, 200a, 181a, 128, 29a, 29b, 542-3p, 181c, 29c, 181b, 25, 22, 367, 363, 125a-3p, 211, 136, 92b, 92a, 544, 381, 382, 199b-5p, 374b, 135a, 135b, 204, 375, 340, 505, 506, 300, 203, 503, 874
KLRD1 (3824) NM_002262	141, 144, 186, 149, 485-5p, 187, 190, 301a, 488, 449b, 449a, 301b, 491-5p, 425, 519d, 32, 140-5p, 590-5p, 223, 494, 410, 411, 34a, 200a, 20a, 454, 25, 20b, 365, 367, 363, 590-3p, 106b, 92b, 93, 106a, 92a, 381, 17, 543, 299-3p, 34c-5p, let-7e, 183, 130b, 300, 130a, 203, let-7f, 873
NGF (4803) NM_002506	141, 320a, 98, 320b, 200a, 186, 429, 374b, let-7d, let-7e, 217, let-7b, let-7c, let-7a, 340, 125a-3p, 320d, 374a, 320c, let-7i, let-7f, let-7g
IL22 (50616) NM_020525	101, 433, 410, 186, 20a, 1, 454, 20b, 1297, 21, 219-5p, 335, 374a, 448, 26a, 106b, 93, 106a, 613, 17, 429, 374b, 206, 519d, 340, 130b, 590-5p, 875-5p, 26b, 130a, 203, 494
VASP (7408) NM_003370	124, 103, 200b, 200c, 20a, 542-3p, 107, 1, 20b, 1297, 22, 376a, 376b, 211, 150, 26a, 106b, 93, 613, 106a, 17, 544, 338-3p, 206, 519d, 204, 506, 26b, 324-5p
PTPN22 (26191) NM_012411	200b, 200c, 429
TTRAP (51567) NM_016614	143, 7, 186, 1, 21, 148a, 148b, 486-5p, 23b, 590-3p, 33b, 152, 33a, 613, 491-5p, 544, 135a, 135b, 206, 653, 183, 375, 216a, 216b, 590-5p, 499-5p, 495, 203
CASP8 (841) NM_033358	590-3p, 217, 371-5p, 335, 544, 543
TRAF2 (7186) NM_021138	183, 134, 342-3p, 222, 330-5p, 302a
CSTB (1476) NM_000100	590-3p, 124, 143, 539, 7, 186, 149, 27b, 379, 21, 377, 590-5p, 876-5p, 506, 488, 203
CLIP1 (6249) NM_002956	141, 144, 433, 143, 145, 7, 149, 186, 384, 148a, 148b, 193b, 487b, 301a, 320d, 320c, 150, 301b, 154, 199a-5p, 152, 18a, 193a-3p, 18b, 429, 758, 653, 196b, 302b, 196a, 495, 494, 124, 103, 181d, 599, 101, 410, 200b, 200c, 411, 200a, 451, 181a, 454, 107, 181c, 181b, 376c, 125a-3p, 19b, 19a, 211, 212, 590-3p, 448, 320a, 320b, 132, 381, 543, 199b-5p, 138, 183, let-7e, 204, 205, 130b, 506, 300, 130a, 202, let-7i, 203, let-7g
SMURF2 (64750) NM_022739	144, 539, 9, 27a, 485-5p, 27b, 1297, 195, 335, 708, 488, 155, 18a, 18b, 429, 758, 424, 28-5p, 32, 196b, 590-5p, 326, 497, 196a, 496, 494, 103, 126, 296-3p, 15a, 200b, 200c, 122, 128, 107, 146a, 21, 15b, 590-3p, 137, 98, 134, 26a, 33a, 381, 382, 338-3p, 135a, 16, 135b, let-7d, 379, let-7e, let-7h, let-7c, let-7a, 216b, 340, 300, 26b, let-7i, 203, 503, let-7f, let-7g
IRF8 (3394) NM_002163	433, 186, 1, 190, 194, 335, 301a, 330-5p, 23a, 150, 301b, 23b, 155, 153, 613, 429, 425, 519d, 326, 496, 495, 329, 181d, 103, 200b, 410, 200c, 200a, 455-5p, 181a, 20a, 542-3p, 107, 454, 181c, 20b, 181b, 365, 362-3p, 218, 376c, 19b, 19a, 212, 448, 190b, 106b, 93, 106a, 381, 17, 338-3p, 135a, 135b, 206, 346, 182, 340, 130b, 506, 300, 324-5p, 130a, 202, 203, 504
SUV39H1 (6839) NM_003173	181d, 296-3p, 149, 520e, 27a, 27b, 520b, 454, 181b, 486-5p, 376c, 301a, 125a-3p, 19b, 330-5p, 19a, 125a-5p, 301b, 153, 491-5p, 520d-3p, 653, 346, 520c-3p, 373, 372, 130b, 196b, 328, 125b, 302b, 130a, 326, 196a, 302a, 302d, 302c, 520a-3p, 302e
CNOT7 (29883) NM_054026	124, 539, 200b, 145, 200c, 34a, 185, 29a, 29b, 29c, 383, 374a, 449b, 449a, 155, 154, 129-5p, 134, 96, 490-3p, 429, 374b, 34c-5p, 340, 196b, 506, 222, 196a, 499-5p, 221
AICDA (57379) NM_020661	181d, 361-5p, 143, 296-3p, 410, 200b, 539, 9, 200c, 185, 186, 27a, 27b, 29a, 181a, 29b, 29c, 181c, 181b, 21, 190, 376a, 376b, 376c, 335, 708, 150, 155, 590-3p, 136, 129-5p, 190b, 543, 429, 135a, 135b, 10a, 28-5p, 10b, 377, 205, 340, 875-5p

(continued)

Table 2
(continued)

Gene Symbol (Entrez Gene ID) Transcript ID	miRNAs
MAP3K1 (4214) NM_005921	144, 143, 9, 7, 520b, 1, 193b, 23a, 23b, 129-5p, 193a-3p, 613, 758, 519d, 371-5p, 302b, 302a, 302d, 302c, 302e, 124, 101, 599, 30c, 200b, 30d, 200c, 30e, 30a, 451, 30b, 219-5p, 486-5p, 19b, 19a, 590-3p, 137, 136, 134, 26a, 92b, 92a, 10a, 10b, 505, 506, 875-5p, 26b, 433, 139-5p, 186, 1297, 191, 192, 194, 335, 488, 421, 18a, 18b, 429, 197, 520c-3p, 31, 196b, 590-5p, 196a, 221, 495, 494, 410, 411, 520e, 20a, 29b, 29c, 20b, 25, 215, 21, 367, 339-5p, 342-3p, 98, 33b, 33a, 106b, 106a, 93, 544, 17, 382, 543, 520d-3p, 338-3p, let-7d, 206, 379, let-7e, 377, let-7b, let-7c, 216a, let-7a, 373, 372, 340, 876-5p, 499-5p, 202, 203, let-7i, 874, 520a-3p, let-7f, let-7g
MDM2 (4193) NM_006881	590-3p, 141, 145, 193a-3p, 200a, 185, 374b, 338-3p, 29a, 29b, 758, 181c, 29c, 379, 384, 383, 377, 193b, 194, 140-5p, 223, 496, 495, 23a, 23b
CD80 (941) NM_005191	103, 141, 15a, 539, 30c, 200b, 200c, 145, 30d, 30e, 200a, 186, 149, 30a, 30b, 29a, 107, 29b, 29c, 146a, 22, 195, 211, 15b, 137, 98, 146b-5p, 544, 381, 133a, 133b, 429, 424, 16, let-7d, let-7e, 204, let-7b, let-7c, let-7a, 497, let-7i, let-7f, 494, let-7g
CD300A (11314) NM_007261	448, 204, 96, 149, 211, 542-3p, 150, 1271
CBL (867) NM_005188	141, 200a, 425
IL6R (3570) NM_181359	431, 185, 149, 195, 194, 320d, 320c, 449b, 449a, 23a, 23b, 125a-5p, 490-3p, 491-5p, 424, 653, 371-5p, 224, 140-5p, 497, 496, 495, 124, 15a, 30c, 30d, 30e, 34a, 451, 30a, 30b, 146a, 15b, 212, 137, 320a, 320b, 146b-5p, 132, 16, 34c-5p, 378, 216b, 422a, 125b, 506, 208b, 499-5p, 202
TNFRSF1A (7132) NM_001065	590-3p, 142-3p, 181d, 218, 194, 335, 29a, 29b, 24, 29c, 181b, 138
CIITA (4261) NM_000246	33b, 152, 296-3p, 146b-5p, 33a, 374b, 146a, 10a, 142-3p, 10b, 22, 148a, 148b, 371-5p, 194, 339-5p, 374a, 330-5p, 874, 873
MED14 (9282) NM_004229	144, 143, 139-5p, 145, 185, 186, 149, 27a, 27b, 1, 384, 193b, 192, 23a, 23b, 129-5p, 421, 18a, 490-3p, 613, 193a-3p, 18b, 491-5p, 133a, 133b, 653, 496, 494, 329, 124, 181d, 101, 410, 30c, 30d, 30e, 30a, 30b, 128, 181b, 1271, 215, 362-3p, 376c, 448, 137, 590-3p, 136, 96, 381, 543, 135b, 10a, 206, 10b, 182, 340, 876-5p, 300, 202, 203, 504
CD247 (919) NM_198053	181d, 199a-5p, 144, 320a, 320b, 101, 410, 96, 132, 411, 199b-5p, 181a, 181b, 22, 486-5p, 376c, 222, 196a, 330-5p, 326, 19b, 488, 19a, 212, 874, 214
EXOC4 (60412) NM_001037126	182, 219-5p, 96, 9, 224, 876-5p, 23a, 1271, 873, 138, 23b
SFN (2810) NM_006142	383, 431, 362-3p, 130b, 329
CDC6 (990) NM_001254	186, 520e, 485-5p, 520b, 1, 1297, 218, 376a, 376b, 339-5p, 342-3p, 19a, 23a, 23b, 155, 137, 199a-5p, 26a, 132, 613, 490-3p, 199b-5p, 520d-3p, 135a, 135b, 206, 10a, 10b, 520c-3p, 31, 373, 208b, 26b, 302d, 499-5p, 495
CDK7 (1022) NM_001799	103, 361-5p, 144, 100, 139-5p, 107, 25, 383, 367, 363, 335, 99b, 374a, 99a, 23a, 23b, 448, 590-3p, 136, 199a-5p, 33b, 33a, 92b, 92a, 199b-5p, 374b, 338-3p, 222, 496, 221, 495
CD27 (939) NM_001242	124, 140-5p, 506, 299-3p, 214
MAPK14 (1432) NM_139013	182, 9, 133a, 133b
MAPK14 (1432) NM_139014	124, 433, 539, 27a, 27b, 128, 22, 376b, 194, 335, 374a, 320d, 320c, 19b, 19a, 23a, 125a-5p, 23b, 320a, 421, 320b, 33b, 33a, 381, 133a, 382, 133b, 374b, 135a, 346, 377, 216b, 340, 224, 506, 125b, 876-5p, 302b, 300, 302a
SH2D2A (9047) NM_001161444	145
MAPK14 (1432) NM_139012	124, 433, 539, 27a, 27b, 128, 22, 376b, 194, 335, 374a, 19b, 19a, 23a, 23b, 125a-5p, 421, 33b, 33a, 381, 133a, 382, 133b, 374b, 135a, 346, 377, 216b, 340, 224, 876-5p, 125b, 506, 300, 302b, 302a
PDIA3 (2923) NM_005313	144, 200b, 539, 200c, 9, 34a, 185, 186, 454, 25, 148a, 486-5p, 148b, 367, 219-5p, 363, 194, 301a, 488, 449b, 212, 449a, 150, 125a-5p, 301b, 590-3p, 152, 134, 132, 133a, 381, 133b, 429, 32, 130b, 590-5p, 125b, 300, 130a, 494, 873
SIN3A (25942) NM_015477	431, 141, 144, 9, 7, 185, 27a, 27b, 1, 193b, 320d, 374a, 320c, 488, 150, 125a-5p, 193a-3p, 491-5p, 429, 496, 101, 200b, 200c, 200a, 370, 24, 1271, 376c, 339-5p, 210, 211, 214, 448, 136, 320a, 320b, 96, 199b-5p, 374b, 138, 206, 10a, 379, 183, 346, 10b, 204, 216a, 125b, 876-5p, 499-5p, 874, 504
BIRC2 (329) NM_001166	421, 143, 539, 145, 197, 29a, 29b, 135a, 29c, 135b, 146a, 148a, 204, 211, 495, 203
TIRAP (114609) NM_001039661	361-5p, 199a-5p, 599, 134, 152, 433, 410, 145, 7, 199b-5p, 370, 374b, 135a, 142-3p, 183, 217, 148a, 148b, 125a-3p, 374a, 875-5p, 326, 330-5p, 495, 23a, 23b
BAX (581) NM_138763	365
IRF4 (3662) NM_002460	433, 186, 27a, 27b, 1297, 148a, 148b, 195, 301a, 320d, 320c, 150, 125a-5p, 421, 129-5p, 152, 491-5p, 429, 424, 653, 371-5p, 224, 497, 495, 103, 15a, 30c, 200b, 30d, 200c, 30e, 30a, 30b, 128, 454, 107, 1271, 181b, 339-5p, 376c, 211, 15b, 590-3p, 320a, 320b, 96, 26a, 16, 204, 216a, 505, 130b, 125b, 26b, 130a, 203, 873
NOX1 (27035) NM_007052	590-3p, 141, 129-5p, 134, 26a, 30c, 30d, 139-5p, 30e, 490-3p, 200a, 93, 186, 30a, 30b, 542-3p, 1297, 371-5p, 372, 224, 222, 26b, 302d
IL4R (3566) NM_001008699	217, 190, 190b, 491-5p, 876-5p
LILRB1 (10859) NM_001081637	519d, 384, 217, 143, 145, 106b, 122, 93, 106a, 17, 185, 20a, 150, 20b
PLCG2 (5336) NM_002661	410, 340, 491-5p, 382, 186, 488
RBBP4 (5928) NM_005610	206, 383, 377, 218, 599, 539, 613, 381, 140-5p, 186, 300, 499-5p, 1, 24
EGR1 (1958) NM_001964	143, 9, 186, 27a, 27b, 1297, 191, 192, 335, 23a, 150, 23b, 129-5p, 429, 197, 32, 371-5p, 31, 224, 223, 124, 181d, 101, 200b, 410, 200c, 411, 181a, 181c, 25, 181b, 215, 217, 367, 363, 19b, 211, 19a, 212, 590-3p, 26a, 132, 92b, 92a, 381, 543, 34c-5p, 135b, let-7d, 206, 183, 204, 377, 340, 506, 300, 26b, 203, let-7g
JAK1 (3716) NM_002227	9, 139-5p, 186, 520b, 148a, 148b, 301a, 708, 23a, 301b, 23b, 421, 152, 490-3p, 519d, 28-5p, 520c-3p, 302b, 302a, 302d, 302c, 302e, 30c, 30d, 30e, 455-5p, 520e, 30a, 30b, 20a, 454, 20b, 181b, 125a-3p, 214, 448, 106b, 106a, 93, 17, 520d-3p, 10a, 10b, 373, 372, 340, 499-5p, 203, 520a-3p
MLH1 (4292) NM_000249	361-5p, 152, 520e, 520d-3p, 374b, 128, 520b, 148a, 148b, 520c-3p, 362-3p, 31, 373, 372, 340, 374a, 302b, 302a, 302d, 302c, 520a-3p, 329, 302e
IGLL1 (3543) NM_020070	296-3p, 138
RASGRP1 (10125) NM_005739	431, 144, 433, 539, 9, 485-5p, 383, 148a, 190, 148b, 195, 194, 320d, 374a, 320c, 152, 429, 758, 196b, 328, 590-5p, 222, 223, 196a, 221, 494, 200b, 200c, 370, 146a, 21, 486-5p, 376a, 376b, 590-3p, 320a, 98, 134, 146b-5p, 320b, 190b, 381, 544, 382, 374b, let-7d, let-7e, 378, 182, 377, let-7b, 205, let-7c, let-7a, 422a, 506, 875-5p, let-7i, let-7f, let-7g, 504, 873
MAP4K1 (11184) NM_007181	143, 187
MAPKAPK2 (9261) NM_004759	124, 296-3p, 433, 15a, 539, 9, 7, 24, 362-3p, 195, 335, 15b, 137, 136, 320a, 320b, 544, 135a, 16, 135b, 424, 183, 31, 224, 506, 875-5p, 497, 496, 495, 329, 873
CXCL12 (6387) NM_199168	141, 431, 144, 185, 186, 149, 383, 148a, 148b, 301a, 320d, 708, 320c, 23a, 23b, 301b, 153, 152, 28-5p, 31, 221, 329, 494, 181d, 101, 410, 200a, 455-5p, 370, 29a, 181a, 454, 29b, 29c, 181c, 181b, 365, 22, 362-3p, 219-5p, 448, 137, 590-3p, 320a, 33b, 320b, 33a, 381, 543, 199b-5p, 135a, 135b, 138, 375, 340, 130b, 300, 130a, 203
ORC4L (5000) NM_181742	141, 181d, 433, 200b, 539, 410, 139-5p, 9, 200a, 186, 520e, 370, 520b, 542-3p, 1, 181b, 215, 190, 192, 376c, 374a, 212, 590-3p, 190b, 132, 490-3p, 613, 381, 374b, 520d-3p, 520c-3p, 216a, 31, 373, 372, 224, 302b, 300, 302a, 302d, 203, 302c, 520a-3p, 504, 302e
GH1 (2688) NM_022562	590-3p, 138

Gene Symbol (Entrez Gene ID) Transcript ID	miRNAs
AZI2 (64343) NM_022461	141, 144, 433, 539, 9, 186, 1, 383, 374a, 150, 23a, 23b, 125a-5p, 153, 129-5p, 421, 613, 653, 371-5p, 196b, 302b, 222, 302a, 196a, 496, 495, 221, 302c, 494, 329, 124, 181d, 103, 101, 30c, 30d, 30e, 200a, 30a, 30b, 20a, 181a, 107, 1271, 181b, 362-3p, 376c, 448, 590-3p, 96, 106a, 17, 374b, 520d-3p, 338-3p, 206, 377, 216a, 216b, 373, 340, 505, 876-5p, 125b, 506, 499-5p, 203
PAG1 (55824) NM_018440	519d, 144, 106b, 93, 106a, 544, 17, 20a, 202, 135a, 20b
BAK1 (578) NM_001188	410, 145, 185, 520e, 27a, 451, 27b, 29a, 29b, 29c, 1297, 25, 384, 367, 363, 125a-3p, 330-5p, 125a-5p, 26a, 92b, 92a, 32, 373, 125b, 302b, 26b, 326, 302a, 302d, 495, 302c, 520a-3p, 302e
CDC42SE1 (56882) NM_020239	141, 145, 185, 186, 1, 383, 125a-5p, 129-5p, 613, 429, 197, 519d, 31, 371-5p, 124, 103, 200b, 30c, 30d, 200c, 30e, 122, 200a, 370, 30a, 30b, 20a, 29a, 107, 29b, 29c, 20b, 146a, 22, 125a-3p, 214, 590-3p, 98, 146b-5p, 106b, 106a, 93, 17, 206, 10a, 10b, 378, 216a, 372, 422a, 125b, 202, 499-5p, 203, let-7f, 504, 873
AIFM1 (9131) NM_001130847	141, 361-5p, 145, 520b, 125a-5p, 199a-5p, 425, 653, 520c-3p, 32, 371-5p, 302b, 222, 223, 302a, 302d, 302c, 221, 302e, 103, 200a, 520e, 107, 24, 25, 22, 367, 363, 98, 33b, 33a, 92b, 92a, 381, 543, 520d-3p, let-7d, let-7e, let-7b, let-7c, let-7a, 373, 372, 125b, 300, 202, let-7i, 874, 520a-3p, let-7f, let-7g
STAT1 (6772) NM_139266	590-3p, 361-5p, 181d, 421, 129-5p, 30c, 9, 30d, 30e, 381, 30a, 30b, 181a, 181c, 135a, 135b, 181b, 340, 300, 875-5p, 488
BAG4 (9530) NM_004874	433, 145, 9, 1, 1297, 384, 190, 194, 301a, 320d, 320c, 488, 301b, 421, 613, 133a, 133b, 429, 758, 653, 140-5p, 224, 497, 181d, 30c, 200b, 30d, 200c, 30e, 122, 30a, 370, 30b, 20a, 181a, 542-3p, 181c, 20b, 1271, 181b, 217, 19b, 211, 19a, 137, 590-3p, 136, 320a, 320b, 26a, 96, 190b, 106b, 543, 199b-5p, 206, 182, 375, 340, 130b, 26b, 130a
MAP3K11 (4296) NM_002419	520e, 485-5p, 370, 520b, 20a, 542-3p, 20b, 142-3p, 125a-3p, 150, 125a-5p, 214, 199a-5p, 134, 106b, 106a, 93, 17, 491-5p, 199b-5p, 520d-3p, 299-3p, 424, 34c-5p, 138, 519d, 520c-3p, 373, 372, 196b, 125b, 302b, 302a, 499-5p, 302d, 302c, 520a-3p, 302e
NCR1 (9437) NM_004829	199a-5p, 186, 199b-5p
BLNK (29760) NM_013314	653, 590-3p, 181d, 433, 539, 132, 106b, 181c, 135a, 181b, 20b
IL10RA (3587) NM_001558	124, 181d, 431, 15a, 143, 539, 455-5p, 185, 370, 181a, 181c, 181b, 486-5p, 193b, 195, 320d, 330-5p, 320c, 15b, 23a, 125a-5p, 421, 320a, 320b, 544, 520d-3p, 197, 299-3p, 135a, 135b, 424, 16, 378, 377, 373, 422a, 506, 125b, 875-5p, 497, 450a, 326, 499-5p, 495, 520a-3p
POU2F1 (5451) NM_002697	199a-5p, 204, 490-3p, 140-5p, 199b-5p, 223, 128, 211, 23a, 23b
SMAD4 (4089) NM_005359	144, 599, 410, 411, 34a, 27a, 27b, 20a, 454, 1297, 20b, 146a, 219-5p, 376c, 301a, 125a-3p, 19b, 449b, 19a, 449a, 301b, 590-3p, 153, 146b-5p, 26a, 106b, 106a, 613, 93, 17, 34c-5p, 519d, 205, 216b, 224, 140-5p, 130b, 208a, 590-5p, 208b, 26b, 130a, 495, 221
HMGA1 (3159) NM_145901	361-5p, 15a, 185, 520e, 542-3p, 1297, 142-3p, 217, 195, 15b, 98, 134, 26a, 133a, 133b, 197, 520d-3p, 138, 16, 424, let-7d, let-7e, let-7b, 520c-3p, let-7c, let-7a, 31, 373, 196b, 26b, 497, 196a, let-7i, let-7f, let-7g
MBD2 (8932) NM_003927	144, 433, 539, 139-5p, 7, 186, 520b, 1297, 384, 383, 190, 320d, 374a, 320c, 155, 199a-5p, 129-5p, 421, 491-5p, 520c-3p, 32, 371-5p, 140-5p, 224, 590-5p, 302b, 222, 302a, 302d, 302c, 221, 494, 302e, 124, 410, 30c, 30d, 30e, 520e, 30a, 30b, 128, 25, 22, 218, 367, 363, 125a-3p, 590-3p, 320a, 320b, 33b, 26a, 190b, 33a, 92b, 92a, 543, 199b-5p, 374b, 520d-3p, 138, 378, 375, 373, 340, 372, 422a, 506, 26b, 874, 520a-3p
BCL10 (8915) NM_003921	143, 145, 186, 187, 485-5p, 520b, 384, 320d, 374a, 320c, 488, 155, 129-5p, 18b, 133a, 133b, 653, 519d, 520c-3p, 32, 224, 302b, 302a, 302d, 302c, 495, 494, 329, 302e, 30c, 30d, 30e, 520e, 30a, 370, 30b, 20a, 128, 20b, 217, 219-5p, 362-3p, 342-3p, 212, 590-3p, 136, 320a, 33b, 320b, 33a, 132, 106b, 106a, 93, 17, 374b, 520d-3p, 183, 377, 182, 216a, 375, 373, 340, 372, 875-5p, 203, 520a-3p, 873
DNMT3B (1789) NM_006892	539, 145, 335, 23a, 23b, 18a, 18b, 491-5p, 429, 425, 519d, 653, 590-5p, 222, 496, 494, 124, 30c, 200b, 30d, 200c, 30e, 370, 30a, 30b, 20a, 29a, 29b, 29c, 24, 20b, 21, 339-5p, 15b, 590-3p, 106b, 93, 106a, 17, 299-3p, 379, let-7d, let-7b, let-7c, 375, let-7a, 505, 506, 203, let-7f, 874, let-7g
TNIP1 (10318) NM_006058	30c, 30d, 30e, 520e, 149, 30a, 520d-3p, 30b, 425, 424, 182, 486-5p, 373, 302b, 19b, 302a, 19a, 302d, 302c, 214
IL4R (3566) NM_000418	205, 339-5p, 125a-3p, 338-3p, 425
NLRC5 (84166) NM_032206	141, 431, 100, 34a, 200a, 7, 542-3p, 384, 21, 148a, 148b, 190, 486-5p, 99b, 449b, 449a, 99a, 125a-5p, 214, 137, 448, 152, 33b, 190b, 33a, 425, 34c-5p, 377, 340, 125b, 590-5p
SH2D2A (9047) NM_003975	103, 421, 599, 15a, 381, 107, 24, 16, 424, 195, 300, 497, 495, 15b, 150
ARNT (405) NM_178426	361-5p, 431, 9, 7, 187, 485-5p, 1, 383, 190, 193b, 195, 320d, 374a, 320c, 23a, 23b, 129-5p, 421, 18a, 18b, 193a-3p, 429, 758, 424, 653, 371-5p, 140-5p, 590-5p, 222, 223, 497, 221, 495, 494, 181d, 103, 15a, 410, 200b, 200c, 455-5p, 370, 29a, 107, 29b, 454, 29c, 181b, 21, 376c, 342-3p, 212, 15b, 590-3p, 320a, 98, 320b, 132, 381, 374b, 338-3p, 16, 10a, 206, let-7d, 378, 10b, 183, let-7e, let-7b, 377, let-7c, 216a, let-7a, 340, 422a, 300, 875-5p, 130a, let-7i, let-7f, 504, let-7g
APEX1 (328) NM_080649	384, 539, 149, 299-3p, 135a, 135b
IL13 (3596) NM_002188	431, 101, 149, 520e, 520b, 362-3p, 339-5p, 125a-3p, 19b, 150, 125a-5p, 155, 590-3p, 199a-5p, 98, 381, 199b-5p, 520d-3p, 135a, 135b, let-7d, 346, let-7e, let-7b, 377, let-7c, 520c-3p, 216a, let-7a, 373, 372, 125b, 208a, 302b, 208b, 300, 302a, 302d, 499-5p, let-7i, 302c, let-7f, 329, 520a-3p, let-7g, 504
TEK (7010) NM_000459	144, 433, 139-5p, 27a, 187, 27b, 148a, 148b, 301a, 488, 23a, 150, 301b, 23b, 199a-5p, 153, 421, 152, 18a, 18b, 425, 32, 31, 224, 181d, 101, 200c, 455-5p, 181a, 454, 181c, 25, 181b, 217, 367, 486-5p, 376c, 363, 125a-3p, 19b, 19a, 214, 448, 137, 33a, 92b, 92a, 381, 199b-5p, 378, 340, 130b, 422a, 300, 130a
EP300 (2033) NM_001429	431, 433, 539, 139-5p, 186, 1, 1297, 148a, 191, 148b, 190, 195, 194, 374a, 449b, 449a, 150, 155, 154, 421, 129-5p, 152, 18a, 18b, 613, 429, 653, 519d, 32, 224, 196b, 222, 326, 196a, 495, 221, 494, 124, 296-3p, 101, 30c, 410, 200b, 30d, 200c, 30e, 34a, 30a, 30b, 29a, 128, 20a, 29b, 24, 29c, 25, 20b, 1271, 22, 367, 363, 339-5p, 376c, 342-3p, 211, 212, 137, 448, 590-3p, 190b, 96, 26a, 132, 106b, 92b, 92a, 106a, 93, 17, 543, 374b, 138, 34c-5p, 10a, 206, 10b, 182, 204, 377, 340, 505, 506, 26b, 499-5p
ARID4D (51742) NM_016374	141, 127-3p, 144, 9, 145, 149, 520b, 1, 193b, 301a, 301b, 129-5p, 152, 613, 193a-3p, 519d, 302b, 302a, 302d, 302c, 302e, 124, 599, 101, 200b, 30c, 200c, 30d, 30e, 30a, 451, 30b, 128, 454, 486-5p, 376a, 376b, 19b, 19a, 137, 590-3p, 136, 132, 374b, 34c-5p, 505, 506, 300, 139-5p, 186, 148a, 148b, 194, 374a, 449b, 449a, 421, 18a, 18b, 429, 653, 520c-3p, 224, 328, 495, 221, 494, 181d, 410, 455-5p, 34a, 520e, 370, 20a, 181a, 24, 181c, 20b, 181b, 218, 342-3p, 125a-3p, 212, 33b, 33a, 106b, 93, 106a, 544, 381, 17, 543, 382, 520d-3p, 206, 183, 182, 377, 205, 373, 372, 340, 130b, 876-5p, 130a, 520a-3p
IRF9 (10379) NM_006084	590-3p, 199a-5p, 106b, 93, 106a, 17, 520e, 199b-5p, 520d-3p, 20a, 520b, 20b, 519d, 384, 520c-3p, 371-5p, 373, 340, 372, 302b, 302a, 302d, 302c, 520a-3p, 302e
MAP2K6 (5608) NM_002758	181d, 143, 30c, 30d, 30e, 185, 186, 451, 30a, 30b, 181a, 181c, 181b, 142-3p, 190, 376c, 374a, 211, 448, 137, 590-3p, 136, 153, 129-5p, 190b, 18a, 18b, 374b, 425, 653, 183, 378, 204, 216a, 371-5p, 216b, 340, 422a, 495, 494
VCAM1 (7412) NM_001078	181d, 30c, 539, 30d, 145, 30e, 122, 186, 30a, 187, 30b, 181a, 181c, 181b, 384, 21, 219-5p, 190, 376c, 708, 374a, 488, 211, 212, 590-3p, 448, 33b, 33a, 190b, 132, 18a, 490-3p, 18b, 381, 382, 543, 374b, 758, 425, 183, 346, 204, 590-5p, 300, 202, 495, 203, 494
DUSP8 (1850) NM_004420	448, 137, 33b, 33a, 200b, 145, 200c, 106b, 106a, 93, 491-5p, 17, 429, 374b, 20a, 24, 20b, 519d, 21, 590-5p, 374a, 488, 873
SRC (6714) NM_198291	137, 141, 144, 153, 599, 613, 455-5p, 34a, 200a, 491-5p, 485-5p, 1, 34c-5p, 206, 184, 31, 488, 19b, 19a, 449b, 203, 449a
CSF3 (1440) NM_000759	141, 143, 15a, 26a, 200a, 485-5p, 374b, 542-3p, 16, 28-5p, 377, 195, 339-5p, 876-5p, 328, 708, 374a
IL23A (51561) NM_016584	181d, 421, 410, 381, 181a, 181b, 653, 204, 340, 505, 208a, 300, 208b, 223, 499-5p, 211
MAPKAP1 (79109) NM_001006617	103, 539, 410, 30c, 7, 485-5p, 27a, 27b, 30b, 520b, 107, 383, 191, 362-3p, 486-5p, 19b, 19a, 301b, 590-3p, 137, 153, 129-5p, 98, let-7b, 182, 520c-3p, 340, 208a, 875-5p, 26b, 208b, 499-5p, 203, let-7i, 329, 494

(continued)

Table 2
(continued)

Gene Symbol (Entrez Gene ID) Transcript ID	miRNAs
MAPKAP1 (79109) NM_001006618	141, 127-3p, 181d, 30c, 30d, 30e, 200a, 30a, 30b, 181a, 542-3p, 181c, 181b, 365, 19b, 19a, 212, 590-3p, 421, 33b, 33a, 132, 491-5p, 223, 329
FOXH1 (8928) NM_003923	134, 296-3p, 18a, 18b, 339-5p, 125a-3p, 485-5p, 150, 138
CD44 (960) NM_000610	124, 181d, 144, 143, 410, 30c, 145, 185, 520e, 186, 485-5p, 520b, 181b, 194, 708, 330-5p, 211, 590-3p, 154, 152, 26a, 96, 132, 520d-3p, 653, 28-5p, 204, 520c-3p, 216a, 216b, 373, 340, 372, 130b, 506, 328, 302b, 326, 302a, 202, 302d, 495, 302c, 520a-3p, 302e
SMAD7 (4092) NM_005904	485-5p, 520b, 1297, 148a, 148b, 195, 301a, 374a, 23a, 301b, 23b, 152, 424, 519d, 520c-3p, 32, 590-5p, 302b, 302a, 497, 302d, 495, 302c, 494, 302e, 181d, 15a, 599, 410, 122, 520e, 181a, 20a, 454, 181c, 181b, 20b, 1271, 25, 21, 367, 363, 212, 15b, 590-3p, 33b, 26a, 96, 33a, 132, 106b, 92b, 92a, 93, 106a, 381, 17, 543, 382, 374b, 520d-3p, 16, 182, 205, 216a, 375, 216b, 373, 372, 340, 130b, 876-5p, 26b, 300, 130a, 203, 503, 520a-3p
IL21 (59067) NM_021803	496
PKMYT1 (9088) NM_004203	519d, 106b, 93, 106a, 17, 185, 20a, 150, 20b
NR5A2 (2494) NM_205860	433, 139-5p, 9, 186, 27a, 27b, 1, 335, 374a, 488, 23a, 155, 153, 491-5p, 429, 31, 224, 326, 196a, 450a, 496, 494, 200b, 30c, 410, 200c, 30d, 30e, 30a, 451, 30b, 146a, 217, 219-5p, 376c, 590-3p, 136, 33b, 26a, 33a, 381, 374b, 34c-5p, 10a, 10b, 182, 216a, 373, 300, 499-5p, 520a-3p, 873
NME1 (4830) NM_198175	146a, 346, 141, 146b-5p, 486-5p, 335, 200a
ITK (3702) NM_005546	7, 185, 186, 149, 485-5p, 190, 195, 194, 301a, 320d, 708, 374a, 320c, 330-5p, 449b, 449a, 301b, 155, 199a-5p, 613, 758, 424, 28-5p, 371-5p, 140-5p, 497, 302d, 103, 15a, 30c, 30d, 30e, 34a, 30a, 30b, 454, 107, 125a-3p, 15b, 590-3p, 448, 320a, 98, 320b, 134, 190b, 543, 199b-5p, 520d-3p, 374b, 135a, 135b, 16, 34c-5p, 138, let-7d, 206, let-7e, let-7b, 182, let-7c, 216a, let-7a, 130b, 130a, let-7i, let-7f, let-7g
IL24 (11009) NM_006850	361-5p, 200b, 200c, 30e, 186, 30a, 29a, 1, 29b, 29c, 22, 342-3p, 125a-3p, 214, 154, 613, 381, 382, 429, 425, 34c-5p, 206, 346, 377, 205, 216b, 324-5p, 300, 203
ATF1 (466) NM_005171	144, 143, 9, 145, 27a, 27b, 383, 190, 192, 374a, 449b, 449a, 153, 129-5p, 421, 371-5p, 224, 495, 494, 181d, 101, 410, 30c, 30d, 30e, 34a, 30a, 30b, 181a, 181c, 1271, 181b, 215, 217, 19b, 211, 19a, 590-3p, 448, 136, 96, 381, 543, 374b, 138, 34c-5p, 182, 216b, 340, 505, 300, 203
BAD (572) NM_032989	127-3p, 153, 129-5p, 7
CDKN2B (1030) NM_004936	144, 433, 100, 200b, 200c, 451, 1, 25, 217, 148a, 190, 148b, 125a-3p, 708, 23a, 125a-5p, 23b, 137, 152, 93, 92a, 429, 138, 28-5p, 346, 182, 216b, 340, 196b, 505, 130b, 125b, 876-5p, 222, 130a, 196a, 203, 221, 495, 504
GRAP2 (9402) NM_004810	181d, 144, 296-3p, 143, 181a, 454, 1, 542-3p, 181c, 181b, 301a, 708, 211, 449b, 449a, 301b, 136, 613, 382, 543, 138, 34c-5p, 206, 204, 205, 373, 505, 223, 302a, 130a, 494
RUNX2 (860) NM_001024630	361-5p, 141, 143, 433, 139-5p, 9, 520b, 148a, 148b, 335, 301a, 320d, 374a, 488, 320c, 23a, 301b, 23b, 155, 154, 152, 490-3p, 520c-3p, 371-5p, 224, 302b, 222, 302a, 302d, 221, 495, 302c, 302e, 103, 30c, 30d, 122, 30e, 411, 520e, 30a, 30b, 20a, 181a, 29a, 107, 29b, 454, 24, 29c, 25, 146a, 365, 217, 486-5p, 218, 367, 376a, 376b, 363, 376c, 125a-3p, 19b, 211, 19a, 590-3p, 320a, 146b-5p, 33b, 320b, 134, 190b, 33a, 543, 374b, 520d-3p, 338-3p, 183, 377, 182, 204, 205, 373, 372, 340, 130b, 505, 876-5p, 324-5p, 130a, 499-5p, 203, 520a-3p, 873
SYK (6850) NM_003177	145, 27a, 27b, 128, 20a, 1271, 20b, 384, 148a, 219-5p, 148b, 488, 15b, 590-3p, 421, 152, 96, 106b, 106a, 93, 17, 382, 197, 135a, 135b, 519d, 377, 371-5p, 196a, 203, 495
TAB1 (10454) NM_006116	134, 491-5p, 299-3p, 29a, 181a, 29b, 758, 425, 29c, 135a, 181b, 135b, 10a, 10b, 504
FANCF (2188) NM_022725	539, 520e, 485-5p, 520b, 1297, 383, 218, 342-3p, 320d, 320c, 488, 210, 590-3p, 137, 448, 155, 320a, 320b, 26a, 190b, 490-3p, 544, 543, 520d-3p, 135a, 135b, 184, 519d, 378, 205, 520c-3p, 373, 340, 224, 876-5p, 26b, 495, 221, 520a-3p
IRS1 (3667) NM_005544	361-5p, 141, 144, 143, 539, 145, 7, 186, 27a, 27b, 384, 148a, 148b, 195, 335, 487b, 421, 152, 490-3p, 429, 424, 653, 371-5p, 222, 223, 497, 495, 221, 181d, 15a, 200b, 410, 30c, 30d, 200c, 30e, 200a, 30a, 30b, 128, 181a, 181c, 181b, 1271, 15b, 590-3p, 33b, 26a, 96, 33a, 544, 543, 338-3p, 16, 183, 182, 340, 505, 875-5p, 203
SIVA1 (10572) NM_006427	124, 154, 340, 301a, 130b, 506, 19b, 130a, 19a, 551b, 454, 301b
CD40LG (959) NM_000074	127-3p, 296-3p, 143, 410, 139-5p, 122, 185, 186, 24, 146a, 374a, 210, 330-5p, 212, 136, 146b-5p, 132, 381, 544, 429, 374b, 182, 31, 876-5p, 300, 326, 202
SP1 (6667) NM_138473	141, 361-5p, 539, 7, 149, 520b, 384, 383, 192, 374a, 150, 23a, 23b, 155, 199a-5p, 491-5p, 28-5p, 520c-3p, 590-5p, 302b, 302a, 223, 496, 302d, 495, 302c, 296-3p, 410, 200a, 520e, 128, 24, 215, 21, 376c, 211, 136, 134, 199b-5p, 374b, 520d-3p, 135a, 34c-5p, 135b, 10a, 377, 204, 373, 505, 875-5p, 499-5p, 203, 520a-3p
HNF4A (3172) NM_178850	377, 362-3p, 134, 342-3p, 485-5p, 138
ORC5L (5001) NM_002553	361-5p, 9, 411, 185, 186, 370, 27a, 27b, 128, 146a, 383, 218, 219-5p, 193b, 363, 374a, 212, 590-3p, 448, 199a-5p, 129-5p, 421, 146b-5p, 132, 193a-3p, 382, 199b-5p, 374b, 135a, 135b, 10a, 10b, 182, 371-5p, 31, 216b, 876-5p, 450a
RFX5 (5993) NM_000449	144, 145, 411, 186, 128, 454, 301a, 374a, 708, 19b, 19a, 15b, 301b, 448, 98, 134, 520d-3p, 374b, 135a, 135b, 16, let-7d, 519d, 378, 28-5p, let-7e, let-7b, 205, let-7c, 520c-3p, 216b, let-7a, 373, 372, 130b, 876-5p, 302b, 302a, 130a, 497, 302d, let-7i, 203, let-7f, 520a-3p, let-7g
INSR (3643) NM_000208	361-5p, 185, 186, 520b, 383, 195, 301a, 154, 18a, 18b, 424, 519d, 520c-3p, 497, 495, 302e, 181d, 15a, 520e, 20a, 181b, 20b, 25, 218, 342-3p, 15b, 214, 590-3p, 136, 98, 134, 106b, 106a, 93, 544, 17, 382, 520d-3p, 16, 379, let-7d, let-7e, let-7b, 182, let-7c, 216a, let-7a, 372, 505, 130b, let-7i, 520a-3p, 503, let-7f, let-7g
RBX1 (9978) NM_014248	96, 139-5p, 7, 27a, 27b, 128, 135a, 425, 1271, 135b, 378, 377, 194, 376c, 224, 422a, 222, 495, 221, 494, 214
CASP6 (839) NM_001226	124, 599, 186, 20a, 542-3p, 20b, 21, 301a, 125a-3p, 150, 301b, 125a-5p, 155, 129-5p, 106b, 93, 106a, 381, 17, 519d, 371-5p, 373, 340, 876-5p, 125b, 506, 590-5p, 300
MX1 (4599) NM_002462	141, 204, 205, 539, 200a, 223, 197, 211
ARHGAP26 (23092) NM_015071	144, 30c, 30d, 106b, 30e, 34a, 106a, 93, 17, 186, 30a, 30b, 20a, 20b, 34c-5p, 519d, 183, 204, 377, 219-5p, 216a, 449b, 211, 499-5p, 449a
COPS5 (10987) NM_006837	361-5p, 144, 200b, 200c, 520b, 20a, 29a, 29b, 29c, 20b, 383, 21, 335, 708, 106b, 106a, 93, 17, 429, 519d, 28-5p, 520c-3p, 371-5p, 373, 302b, 302c
SAP30 (8819) NM_003864	361-5p, 144, 101, 30c, 539, 30d, 30e, 186, 30a, 30b, 383, 21, 320d, 320c, 212, 590-3p, 199a-5p, 320a, 320b, 132, 543, 199b-5p, 216b, 590-5p, 222, 221, 495, 494, 873
BCL2L11 (10018) NM_207002	590-3p, 185
CXCL11 (6373) NM_005409	127-3p, 144, 139-5p, 9, 7, 27a, 27b, 1, 384, 190, 488, 449b, 449a, 155, 154, 421, 18a, 613, 133a, 133b, 197, 224, 196b, 590-5p, 222, 196a, 496, 495, 221, 101, 30c, 30d, 30e, 411, 34a, 455-5p, 30a, 30b, 128, 25, 21, 367, 219-5p, 376a, 376b, 376c, 590-3p, 137, 190b, 92b, 92a, 543, 138, 34c-5p, 206, 379, 505, 208a, 499-5p
CCR1 (1230) NM_001295	143, 200b, 539, 200c, 411, 34a, 186, 128, 24, 383, 320d, 708, 320c, 330-5p, 449b, 449a, 23a, 150, 214, 23b, 590-3p, 320a, 129-5p, 320b, 429, 197, 135a, 34c-5p, 206, 378, 28-5p, 373, 372, 340, 422a, 326, 223, 450a, 302a, 221, 203, 495
GJA1 (2697) NM_000165	141, 144, 139-5p, 9, 185, 186, 1, 193b, 301a, 374a, 23a, 301b, 23b, 125a-5p, 421, 193a-3p, 613, 429, 758, 519d, 653, 520c-3p, 371-5p, 495, 124, 101, 30c, 200c, 30d, 30e, 455-5p, 200a, 30a, 30b, 20a, 454, 20b, 142-3p, 217, 219-5p, 218, 19b, 19a, 214, 590-3p, 137, 106b, 106a, 93, 17, 381, 382, 374b, 135a, 135b, 206, 340, 372, 130b, 505, 506, 125b, 300, 130a, 499-5p, 873

Gene Symbol (Entrez Gene ID) Transcript ID	miRNAs
TAP2 (6891) NM_000544	433, 185, 186, 384, 195, 320d, 320c, 23a, 125a-5p, 23b, 613, 429, 424, 520c-3p, 31, 371-5p, 590-5p, 450a, 497, 223, 302d, 124, 181d, 599, 15a, 296-3p, 200b, 200c, 370, 181a, 128, 181c, 24, 181b, 1271, 142-3p, 217, 21, 486-5p, 376c, 15b, 448, 137, 590-3p, 136, 320a, 320b, 96, 381, 520d-3p, 135a, 16, 135b, 184, let-7d, 346, let-7e, let-7b, let-7c, 216a, let-7a, 340, 125b, 506, 300, let-7f, 520a-3p, 873
TRAF3IP2 (10758) NM_147686	590-3p, 30c, 30d, 106b, 30e, 106a, 411, 491-5p, 17, 149, 543, 30a, 30b, 20a, 193b, 195
CD28 (940) NM_006139	141, 144, 101, 15a, 145, 34a, 200a, 27a, 27b, 1, 215, 146a, 384, 383, 219-5p, 192, 195, 449b, 211, 15b, 449a, 212, 23a, 23b, 590-3p, 137, 136, 146b-5p, 132, 613, 544, 424, 34c-5p, 16, 206, 183, 204, 216a, 371-5p, 31, 216b, 340, 224, 497, 499-5p, 221, 503, 494
SFRP1 (6422) NM_003012	144, 101, 149, 27a, 27b, 542-3p, 29b, 1, 181c, 1297, 191, 486-5p, 195, 335, 488, 23a, 23b, 26a, 613, 93, 382, 425, 184, 206, 378, 216a, 31, 422a, 328, 26b, 203, 873
TRAF4 (9618) NM_004295	433, 520e, 370, 29a, 520b, 20a, 29b, 29c, 20b, 194, 339-5p, 330-5p, 15b, 106b, 93, 106a, 17, 520d-3p, 424, 519d, 346, 520c-3p, 205, 373, 372, 328, 302b, 302a, 326, 302d, 302c, 494, 520a-3p, 302e
TBK1 (29110) NM_013254	144, 539, 186, 27a, 27b, 191, 192, 195, 301a, 374a, 23a, 23b, 301b, 155, 429, 425, 424, 653, 520c-3p, 371-5p, 590-5p, 497, 124, 200b, 410, 200c, 454, 215, 365, 21, 362-3p, 218, 19b, 19a, 15b, 212, 214, 448, 590-3p, 134, 132, 92a, 381, 374b, 135a, 135b, 340, 505, 130b, 506, 300, 130a, 203, 503
GAB2 (9846) NM_080491	590-3p, 124, 181d, 421, 134, 132, 9, 520e, 543, 186, 485-5p, 520d-3p, 181a, 454, 29b, 181c, 29c, 181b, 384, 218, 373, 505, 506, 212
VCL (7414) NM_014000	141, 9, 383, 195, 320d, 488, 320c, 449b, 449a, 23a, 23b, 199a-5p, 153, 152, 613, 491-5p, 424, 32, 371-5p, 590-5p, 497, 495, 124, 181d, 103, 15a, 30c, 410, 30d, 30e, 455-5p, 34a, 200a, 30a, 30b, 128, 181a, 107, 181c, 24, 181b, 25, 1271, 21, 367, 376a, 376b, 376c, 363, 342-3p, 15b, 214, 137, 448, 320a, 98, 320b, 33b, 96, 33a, 92b, 92a, 382, 199b-5p, 338-3p, 299-3p, 16, 34c-5p, let-7d, 346, let-7e, 378, let-7b, 182, let-7c, let-7a, 340, 422a, 506, let-7i, let-7f, let-7g
MSH6 (2956) NM_000179	383, 320a, 320b, 340, 505, 224, 186, 320d, 320c, 223
CCND1 (595) NM_053056	186, 520b, 193b, 195, 374a, 449b, 449a, 23a, 23b, 193a-3p, 490-3p, 424, 519d, 520c-3p, 224, 302b, 497, 450a, 302a, 302d, 495, 302c, 494, 302e, 15a, 410, 34a, 520e, 20a, 20b, 1271, 142-3p, 218, 19b, 19a, 15b, 96, 132, 106b, 93, 106a, 17, 374b, 520d-3p, 338-3p, 34c-5p, 16, 373, 372, 340, 202, 203, 503, 520a-3p
PAK1 (5058) NM_001128620	141, 145, 7, 186, 485-5p, 1297, 195, 374a, 320d, 320c, 199a-5p, 491-5p, 758, 371-5p, 196b, 222, 196a, 302d, 221, 494, 200a, 411, 455-5p, 20a, 542-3p, 20b, 1271, 218, 219-5p, 342-3p, 19a, 98, 320a, 320b, 26a, 96, 106b, 106a, 17, 199b-5p, 374b, 299-3p, 16, let-7d, let-7e, 377, let-7b, let-7c, 375, 216a, let-7a, 26b, 203, let-7i, let-7f, let-7g
BID (637) NM_197966	124, 181d, 144, 101, 30c, 30d, 30e, 520e, 30a, 485-5p, 370, 30b, 181a, 128, 520b, 20a, 181c, 20b, 1297, 181b, 142-3p, 148a, 219-5p, 212, 137, 199a-5p, 154, 26a, 132, 106b, 93, 106a, 17, 543, 199b-5p, 520d-3p, 299-3p, 519d, 520c-3p, 216b, 371-5p, 373, 140-5p, 224, 506, 26b, 302a, 495, 520a-3p
ICOSLG (23308) NM_015259	155, 129-5p, 488, 24
BARD1 (580) NM_000465	101, 543, 374a, 19b, 374b, 19a, 203
SPHK1 (8877) NM_182965	206, 124, 613, 506, 875-5p, 485-5p, 708, 495, 1
UBE2N (7334) NM_003348	144, 7, 185, 186, 27a, 27b, 384, 383, 193b, 708, 330-5p, 488, 155, 153, 193a-3p, 429, 197, 425, 653, 28-5p, 31, 222, 326, 495, 221, 494, 124, 101, 200b, 200c, 411, 128, 486-5p, 219-5p, 376c, 590-3p, 136, 33b, 33a, 338-3p, 205, 216a, 125b, 208a, 506, 208b, 499-5p, 203, 873
CCNH (902) NM_001239	384, 590-3p, 190, 190b, 539, 340, 488, 23a, 23b
S1PR5 (53637) NM_030760	590-3p, 361-5p, 136, 152, 7, 186, 27b, 24, 10a, 384, 10b, 148a, 377, 148b, 342-3p, 224, 450a, 203, 23a, 23b
NRG1 (3084) NM_001160008	181d, 103, 204, 143, 335, 324-5p, 485-5p, 211, 181a, 338-3p, 107, 181c, 181b
CSK (1445) NM_001127190	30c, 30d, 30e, 186, 485-5p, 30a, 30b, 454, 365, 148a, 191, 362-3p, 148b, 487b, 301a, 374a, 488, 301b, 152, 374b, 184, 346, 216a, 371-5p, 216b, 130b, 130a, 329, 494
MYL2 (4633) NM_000432	539, 876-5p
TNFRSF21 (27242) NM_014452	361-5p, 144, 539, 9, 520b, 148a, 190, 148b, 193b, 301a, 320d, 374a, 320c, 301b, 199a-5p, 152, 490-3p, 193a-3p, 197, 519d, 520c-3p, 371-5p, 224, 302b, 302a, 302d, 495, 302c, 329, 302e, 124, 101, 410, 520e, 20a, 454, 542-3p, 20b, 217, 362-3p, 125a-3p, 590-3p, 320a, 33b, 320b, 33a, 106b, 93, 106a, 17, 381, 199b-5p, 520d-3p, 374b, 135a, 135b, 183, 373, 340, 372, 130b, 422a, 506, 876-5p, 300, 130a, 520a-3p
TAP2 (6891) NM_018833	433, 200b, 200c, 139-5p, 371-5p, 339-5p, 429
NRG1 (3084) NM_001160004	431, 144, 145, 7, 149, 485-5p, 27a, 27b, 384, 335, 301a, 374a, 708, 330-5p, 488, 23a, 23b, 155, 18a, 18b, 429, 28-5p, 222, 326, 496, 495, 221, 124, 181d, 101, 599, 410, 200b, 200c, 34a, 411, 455-5p, 615-3p, 370, 29a, 128, 29b, 454, 29c, 1271, 146a, 125a-3p, 214, 448, 137, 146b-5p, 96, 543, 382, 183, 216a, 340, 505, 876-5p, 506, 203
FANCE (2178) NM_021922	421, 26a, 485-5p, 29a, 338-3p, 29b, 29c, 34c-5p, 1297, 138, 10a, 10b, 365, 216a, 371-5p, 335, 194, 342-3p, 224, 26b, 330-5p, 326, 874, 873
CD1A (909) NM_001763	590-3p, 448, 361-5p, 421, 33b, 146b-5p, 33a, 146a, 28-5p, 383, 21, 217, 31, 590-5p, 708, 19a, 495, 873, 214
RAG2 (5897) NM_000536	296-3p, 599, 410, 539, 30c, 30d, 30e, 186, 30a, 30b, 25, 146a, 383, 367, 193b, 363, 374a, 488, 590-3p, 154, 146b-5p, 33b, 33a, 92b, 193a-3p, 92a, 374b, 299-3p, 653, 182, 32, 340, 328, 875-5p, 496, 495
BAX (581) NR_027882	181d, 433, 132, 145, 133a, 543, 133b, 29a, 181a, 29b, 29c, 181b, 138, 22, 346, 365, 339-5p, 125a-3p, 449b, 449a, 212
CD8A (925) NM_171827	590-3p, 144, 190b, 7, 197, 758, 138, 346, 28-5p, 190, 376a, 376b, 340, 140-5p, 125b, 488, 326, 330-5p, 150, 873, 125a-5p
MAP3K4 (4216) NM_005922	144, 101, 15a, 139-5p, 186, 451, 27a, 27b, 128, 384, 142-3p, 22, 148a, 148b, 195, 212, 15b, 214, 590-3p, 152, 132, 424, 16, 653, 183, 497, 495, 504
RFXANK (8625) NM_003721	22, 544, 125b, 223, 125a-5p
IFNB1 (3456) NM_002176	653, 101, 433, 875-5p, 374b, 29a, 29b, 29c
CANX (821) NM_001024649	431, 141, 144, 139-5p, 186, 520b, 148a, 148b, 195, 194, 301a, 320d, 320c, 488, 150, 301b, 153, 152, 425, 520c-3p, 495, 494, 103, 15a, 122, 200a, 520e, 370, 29a, 128, 29b, 454, 107, 29c, 146a, 365, 217, 486-5p, 590-3p, 320a, 320b, 93, 381, 338-3p, 16, 205, 372, 505, 130b, 324-5p, 300, 130a, 504
TOB1 (10140) NM_005749	141, 144, 139-5p, 7, 186, 27a, 27b, 1, 1297, 191, 190, 194, 487b, 301a, 320d, 374a, 320c, 301b, 129-5p, 421, 613, 429, 197, 32, 371-5p, 590-5p, 223, 450a, 496, 495, 302c, 494, 124, 200b, 410, 200c, 200a, 451, 454, 1271, 25, 21, 486-5p, 367, 218, 363, 125a-3p, 19b, 19a, 212, 590-3p, 137, 320a, 320b, 190b, 26a, 96, 132, 92b, 92a, 381, 374b, 206, 10a, 10b, 182, 340, 130b, 208a, 506, 208b, 26b, 300, 130a, 499-5p
NLK (51701) NM_016231	141, 144, 150, 23a, 23b, 155, 199a-5p, 154, 129-5p, 152, 28-5p, 371-5p, 140-5p, 101, 296-3p, 30c, 200b, 30d, 200c, 30e, 30a, 451, 30b, 142-3p, 219-5p, 376a, 376b, 376c, 19b, 19a, 590-3p, 26a, 132, 92b, 92a, 199b-5p, 135a, 135b, 10a, 208a, 300, 26b, 208b, 433, 139-5p, 186, 27a, 27b, 1297, 384, 148a, 190, 148b, 194, 335, 487b, 708, 374a, 330-5p, 421, 429, 197, 653, 32, 590-5p, 222, 326, 221, 495, 494, 329, 181d, 410, 455-5p, 181a, 29a, 542-3p, 29b, 29c, 24, 181c, 25, 181b, 146a, 21, 217, 367, 362-3p, 363, 342-3p, 125a-3p, 212, 98, 33b, 146b-5p, 190b, 33a, 381, 543, 382, let-7d, let-7e, 377, let-7b, 205, let-7c, 216a, let-7a, 340, 499-5p, let-7i, 203, let-7f, let-7g
CXCR4 (7852) NM_003467	101, 410, 9, 139-5p, 185, 186, 520e, 520b, 1, 486-5p, 487b, 211, 590-3p, 613, 381, 133a, 133b, 520d-3p, 338-3p, 206, 204, 520c-3p, 373, 372, 340, 224, 302b, 300, 302a, 223, 302d, 302c, 495, 494, 520a-3p, 302e
DKK1 (22943) NM_012242	433, 520b, 1, 148a, 148b, 335, 374a, 488, 449b, 449a, 155, 152, 613, 653, 520c-3p, 32, 196b, 302b, 223, 302a, 196a, 496, 302d, 302c, 302e, 181d, 103, 410, 34a, 520e, 181a, 107, 25, 146a, 217, 367, 376a, 376b, 363, 590-3p, 137, 136, 146b-5p, 33b, 33a, 92b, 92a, 543, 520d-3p, 374b, 34c-5p, 206, 373, 372, 202, 203, 520a-3p

(continued)

Table 2 (continued)

Gene Symbol (Entrez Gene ID) Transcript ID	miRNAs
CUL2 (8453) NM_003591	103, 144, 15a, 599, 539, 30c, 30d, 30e, 30a, 30b, 107, 21, 362-3p, 195, 342-3p, 374a, 211, 15b, 23a, 214, 23b, 590-3p, 154, 381, 374b, 424, 16, 371-5p, 340, 590-5p, 300, 223, 497, 203, 329, 503, 873
STK11 (6794) NM_000455	519d, 106b, 93, 106a, 17, 186, 330-5p, 326, 20a, 150, 20b
IFNAR2 (3455) NM_207585	124, 539, 30c, 30d, 30e, 149, 186, 30a, 485-5p, 30b, 128, 20a, 20b, 218, 339-5p, 153, 134, 106b, 18a, 18b, 93, 106a, 491-5p, 17, 10a, 519d, 379, let-7d, let-7e, 10b, 377, let-7b, let-7c, let-7a, 506, 203, 551b, let-7i, let-7f, 494, let-7g
IGF1 (3479) NM_000618	599, 433, 410, 186, 29a, 1, 454, 29b, 29c, 1297, 215, 142-3p, 22, 148a, 148b, 192, 194, 301a, 19b, 488, 19a, 301b, 23b, 155, 137, 590-3p, 129-5p, 152, 26a, 613, 299-3p, 758, 425, 206, 340, 130b, 26b, 222, 130a, 499-5p, 495, 221
MSH2 (4436) NM_000251	590-3p, 137, 136, 433, 296-3p, 410, 132, 382, 374b, 183, 21, 205, 371-5p, 340, 590-5p, 212, 495
CR2 (1380) NM_001877	149, 520b, 148a, 148b, 301a, 320d, 320c, 488, 449b, 449a, 23a, 23b, 301b, 152, 520c-3p, 371-5p, 302b, 302a, 302d, 496, 302c, 494, 329, 302e, 200b, 34a, 520e, 30b, 454, 362-3p, 19b, 19a, 448, 590-3p, 320a, 320b, 146b-5p, 381, 520d-3p, 34c-5p, 205, 216b, 373, 340, 372, 130b, 300, 130a, 203, 520a-3p
PRKCQ (5588) NM_006257	410, 200b, 145, 200c, 122, 34a, 411, 455-5p, 186, 1297, 25, 215, 362-3p, 367, 193b, 192, 363, 125a-3p, 449b, 449a, 136, 134, 26a, 92b, 92a, 193a-3p, 381, 382, 429, 34c-5p, 653, 183, 377, 32, 31, 224, 876-5p, 26b, 300, 875-5p, 203, 329, 873
BRIP1 (83990) NM_032043	590-3p, 361-5p, 421, 33b, 101, 33a, 92b, 18a, 18b, 7, 490-3p, 92a, 186, 543, 370, 425, 25, 138, 10a, 10b, 367, 32, 363, 499-5p
SRF (6722) NM_003131	200b, 200c, 7, 186, 542-3p, 22, 365, 148a, 486-5p, 335, 342-3p, 320d, 320c, 488, 23a, 23b, 590-3p, 154, 320a, 320b, 491-5p, 429, 653, 184, let-7e, 377, let-7b, let-7c, 216a, let-7a, 371-5p, 224, 300, 324-5p, 496, 503, 874
SIGLEC7 (27036) NM_014385	216a, 371-5p, 615-3p
IRAK3 (11213) NM_007199	124, 653, 361-5p, 320a, 421, 320b, 539, 335, 224, 506, 320d, 199b-5p, 320c, 494
IFIT1 (3434) NM_001548	106b, 613, 186, 543, 374b, 520d-3p, 20a, 29a, 128, 1, 29b, 29c, 20b, 384, 653, 206, 362-3p, 373, 372, 374a, 302a, 488, 302d, 203, 329
FADD (8772) NM_003824	361-5p, 129-5p, 320a, 153, 320b, 134, 185, 382, 370, 128, 138, 206, 28-5p, 182, 505, 342-3p, 708, 320d, 320c, 503
RPS6KA1 (6195) NM_001006665	139-5p, 520b, 193b, 708, 320d, 320c, 330-5p, 125a-5p, 421, 193a-3p, 519d, 28-5p, 520c-3p, 140-5p, 302b, 302a, 326, 302d, 302c, 302e, 124, 520e, 20a, 128, 20b, 339-5p, 342-3p, 212, 214, 320a, 320b, 132, 106b, 93, 106a, 17, 520d-3p, 138, 135b, 10a, 378, 10b, 183, 373, 372, 422a, 125b, 506, 520a-3p, 504
ULK1 (8408) NM_003565	410, 520e, 20a, 520b, 128, 454, 1297, 20b, 22, 210, 150, 26a, 106b, 93, 106a, 17, 520d-3p, 519d, 377, 520c-3p, 373, 372, 130b, 302b, 26b, 130a, 302a, 302d, 302c, 520a-3p, 302e
FRAT1 (10023) NM_005479	144, 15a, 539, 122, 485-5p, 1297, 383, 367, 190, 195, 15b, 23a, 23b, 136, 190b, 26a, 199b-5p, 16, 424, 183, 205, 31, 328, 876-5p, 26b, 223, 497
CDC42 (998) NM_001791	141, 361-5p, 433, 539, 9, 185, 186, 27a, 27b, 1, 190, 301a, 488, 301b, 199a-5p, 129-5p, 153, 421, 18a, 613, 18b, 429, 32, 31, 224, 496, 495, 494, 329, 101, 296-3p, 200b, 30c, 30d, 200c, 30e, 200a, 30a, 30b, 29a, 454, 29b, 29c, 25, 367, 363, 342-3p, 19b, 19a, 212, 448, 137, 590-3p, 33a, 190b, 132, 92b, 92a, 381, 543, 299-3p, 206, 377, 205, 130b, 505, 300, 130a, 499-5p
WIF1 (11197) NM_007191	141, 361-5p, 144, 539, 139-5p, 7, 27a, 27b, 192, 195, 335, 194, 374a, 708, 320d, 320c, 488, 330-5p, 150, 199a-5p, 154, 129-5p, 421, 490-3p, 429, 758, 424, 653, 28-5p, 222, 497, 302a, 326, 496, 221, 495, 329, 494, 181d, 103, 101, 15a, 599, 200b, 410, 200c, 200a, 29a, 181a, 128, 29b, 107, 24, 29c, 181c, 181b, 215, 365, 22, 362-3p, 342-3p, 211, 212, 15b, 137, 590-3p, 320a, 320b, 33b, 33a, 132, 381, 543, 199b-5p, 520d-3p, 374b, 16, 346, 204, 216b, 373, 340, 208a, 300, 875-5p, 208b, 203, 503
MAPK13 (5603) NM_002754	421, 134, 26a, 200b, 200c, 34a, 185, 544, 429, 454, 34c-5p, 383, 377, 324-5p, 488, 496, 449b, 449a, 150
RAD51 (5888) NM_002875	124, 411, 186, 370, 542-3p, 1271, 383, 148a, 148b, 219-5p, 193b, 194, 374a, 320d, 320c, 211, 421, 320a, 320b, 152, 96, 193a-3p, 544, 382, 374b, 197, 758, 653, 378, 204, 422a, 506, 876-5p, 222, 499-5p, 203, 221, 494
KAT2B (8850) NM_003884	361-5p, 433, 539, 185, 520b, 191, 148a, 148b, 374a, 23a, 301b, 23b, 155, 199a-5p, 129-5p, 152, 429, 519d, 520c-3p, 32, 140-5p, 590-5p, 302b, 302a, 302d, 302c, 495, 494, 302e, 181d, 101, 599, 200b, 410, 200c, 34a, 411, 520e, 181a, 20a, 542-3p, 181c, 181b, 20b, 25, 142-3p, 217, 367, 376a, 376b, 376c, 363, 342-3p, 125a-3p, 448, 590-3p, 137, 33b, 33a, 92b, 106b, 92a, 93, 106a, 17, 382, 543, 199b-5p, 520d-3p, 374b, 299-3p, 377, 205, 216a, 216b, 373, 372, 340, 130b, 876-5p, 499-5p, 520a-3p, 873, 504
HMGN1 (3150) NM_004965	145, 1, 454, 181a, 1297, 217, 335, 301a, 330-5p, 301b, 448, 590-3p, 136, 199a-5p, 421, 33b, 26a, 33a, 613, 381, 199b-5p, 338-3p, 206, 140-5p, 26b, 300, 326, 494
TRAT1 (50852) NM_016388	361-5p, 181d, 410, 200b, 539, 9, 200c, 370, 181a, 128, 29b, 181c, 181b, 384, 383, 194, 488, 330-5p, 212, 590-3p, 155, 129-5p, 421, 98, 33b, 33a, 132, 429, 520d-3p, 653, let-7d, let-7c, let-7a, 224, 875-5p, 326, 202, 496, 203, let-7f, 494
TNS1 (7145) NM_022648	141, 181d, 139-5p, 200a, 185, 520e, 520b, 181a, 20a, 181c, 20b, 181b, 487b, 374a, 320d, 320c, 590-3p, 137, 421, 320a, 33b, 320b, 33a, 106b, 93, 106a, 491-5p, 17, 374b, 520d-3p, 519d, 182, 520c-3p, 31, 373, 372, 340, 876-5p, 302b, 302a, 302d, 302c, 520a-3p, 302e
PLCB2 (5330) NM_004573	141, 98, 200a, 185, 425, let-7d, let-7e, let-7b, let-7c, let-7a, 875-5p, let-7i, 874, let-7f, 214, let-7g
BIRC6 (57448) NM_016252	9, 149, 520b, 1, 301a, 301b, 155, 153, 129-5p, 152, 613, 519d, 28-5p, 140-5p, 302b, 302a, 302d, 302c, 302e, 124, 599, 30c, 100, 200b, 30d, 200c, 30e, 122, 30a, 30b, 454, 486-5p, 376a, 376b, 376c, 19b, 19a, 99a, 590-3p, 136, 134, 135a, 34c-5p, 135b, 506, 300, 186, 384, 148a, 148b, 190, 194, 708, 449b, 449a, 429, 653, 520c-3p, 196b, 223, 196a, 496, 495, 494, 181d, 410, 455-5p, 34a, 411, 520e, 181a, 29a, 29b, 181c, 29c, 1271, 181b, 365, 217, 362-3p, 218, 342-3p, 211, 98, 33b, 33a, 96, 190b, 106b, 106a, 544, 17, 381, 382, 543, 520d-3p, 206, let-7d, 183, let-7e, 204, let-7b, 182, let-7c, let-7a, 373, 372, 130b, 130a, let-7i, 203, 520a-3p, let-7f, let-7g
CCL11 (6356) NM_002986	136, 33b, 134, 410, 33a, 200b, 200c, 543, 186, 429, 374b, 542-3p, 384, 32, 224, 876-5p, 374a
YWHAH (7533) NM_003405	361-5p, 431, 433, 1297, 195, 708, 320d, 320c, 488, 129-5p, 421, 424, 28-5p, 32, 31, 224, 497, 495, 494, 103, 15a, 30c, 30d, 30e, 30a, 30b, 107, 29b, 25, 365, 367, 363, 212, 15b, 590-3p, 136, 320a, 320b, 33b, 26a, 33a, 132, 92b, 92a, 381, 543, 382, 338-3p, 16, 182, 340, 300, 26b, 503
IL12B (3593) NM_002187	141, 361-5p, 144, 101, 143, 599, 30c, 30d, 30e, 200a, 186, 30a, 30b, 383, 217, 219-5p, 376b, 376c, 194, 320d, 374a, 320c, 212, 23a, 23b, 590-3p, 154, 129-5p, 320a, 421, 320b, 33b, 33a, 132, 93, 544, 382, 543, 183, 205, 328, 223, 495, 494, 873
S1PR4 (8698) NM_003775	377, 491-5p, 324-5p
ILK (3611) NM_004517	379, 34a, 370, 374a, 374b, 128, 542-3p, 758
GZMB (3002) NM_004131	378, 199a-5p, 422a, 328, 199b-5p, 202
NFATC2 (4773) NM_173091	431, 383, 143, 488, 135a, 135b
MBD3 (53615) NM_003926	218
VEGFA (7422) NM_001033756	361-5p, 141, 144, 1, 23a, 150, 23b, 155, 199a-5p, 153, 129-5p, 613, 519d, 140-5p, 302b, 302a, 302c, 302e, 103, 126, 101, 30c, 200b, 30d, 200c, 30e, 200a, 451, 30a, 30b, 107, 486-5p, 376c, 448, 590-3p, 136, 134, 26a, 199b-5p, 374b, 138, 505, 300, 503, 539, 185, 186, 383, 148a, 191, 148b, 190, 195, 374a, 449b, 449a, 429, 424, 653, 31, 497, 495, 494, 329, 15a, 410, 520e, 20a, 29a, 29b, 29c, 20b, 362-3p, 339-5p, 342-3p, 125a-3p, 15b, 190b, 106b, 93, 106a, 381, 17, 382, 543, 299-3p, 16, 206, 377, 205, 216a, 373, 340, 372, 876-5p, 202, 499-5p, 203, 520a-3p
ROCK2 (9475) NM_004850	144, 139-5p, 27a, 485-5p, 27b, 520b, 190, 301a, 374a, 301b, 155, 153, 152, 429, 653, 519d, 520c-3p, 31, 302b, 302a, 302d, 495, 302c, 302e, 124, 101, 410, 200b, 200c, 520e, 20a, 454, 20b, 142-3p, 376a, 376b, 590-3p, 448, 33b, 33a, 106b, 106a, 93, 381, 544, 17, 520d-3p, 135a, 138, 135b, 378, 373, 372, 340, 130b, 506, 300, 130a, 520a-3p
CTLA4 (1493) NM_005214	124, 143, 200b, 539, 145, 34a, 149, 370, 181a, 542-3p, 1297, 384, 190, 218, 488, 449b, 449a, 155, 590-3p, 33b, 33a, 190b, 429, 197, 34c-5p, 378, 205, 371-5p, 505, 422a, 506, 26b, 324-5p, 496, 203, 495, 494

Gene Symbol (Entrez Gene ID)	Transcript ID	miRNAs
ECSIT (51295)	NR_024551	142-3p, 143, 371-5p
IL13RA1 (3597)	NM_001560	141, 431, 361-5p, 539, 30c, 30d, 30e, 200a, 185, 30a, 370, 27a, 27b, 30b, 128, 215, 22, 190, 192, 335, 342-3p, 708, 488, 211, 590-3p, 129-5p, 190b, 382, 758, 135a, 135b, 28-5p, 182, 204, 216a, 31, 495
PTPN1 (5770)	NM_002827	410, 485-5p, 1, 215, 146a, 22, 362-3p, 192, 374a, 211, 214, 590-3p, 137, 199a-5p, 33b, 146b-5p, 33a, 613, 199b-5p, 374b, 135a, 135b, 206, 204, 205, 216a, 31, 224, 222, 221, 203, 329
BLM (641)	NM_000057	590-3p, 143, 33b, 146b-5p, 33a, 410, 186, 27a, 27b, 338-3p, 146a, 21, 224, 208a, 208b, 495
TYROBP (7305)	NM_198125	590-3p, 183, 433, 218, 205, 185, 496, 202
TNFSF13 (8741)	NM_172087	155, 590-3p, 383, 339-5p, 185, 222, 211, 221
RUVBL2 (10856)	NM_006666	27a, 27b, 128
MAP2K5 (5607)	NM_145160	199a-5p, 365, 103, 199b-5p, 107
TNFSF13 (8741)	NM_172088	590-3p, 155, 383, 185, 222, 221
EIF2AK2 (5610)	NM_001135651	361-5p, 431, 143, 186, 485-5p, 1, 25, 217, 190, 367, 339-5p, 363, 449b, 449a, 448, 129-5p, 190b, 92b, 613, 92a, 544, 543, 34c-5p, 10a, let-7d, 379, 10b, let-7e, let-7b, let-7c, 32, let-7a, 340, let-7i, 494, let-7f, 873, let-7g
MCRS1 (10445)	NM_001012300	378, 296-3p, 490-3p, 186
AXIN1 (8312)	NM_003502	124, 137, 141, 26a, 539, 132, 200a, 381, 128, 1297, 377, 31, 506, 26b, 300, 488, 212
MARK2 (2011)	NM_001039469	129-5p, 152, 143, 539, 9, 122, 193a-3p, 185, 491-5p, 543, 485-5p, 374b, 138, 146a, 365, 183, 182, 362-3p, 193b, 224, 125a-3p, 374a, 326, 330-5p, 329
TNFSF13 (8741)	NM_003808	590-3p, 155, 383, 339-5p, 185, 222, 211, 221
CDK2 (1017)	NM_001798	124, 141, 200b, 539, 410, 200c, 200a, 186, 29a, 29b, 542-3p, 29c, 339-5p, 335, 708, 214, 155, 18a, 18b, 490-3p, 544, 381, 429, 182, 375, 340, 140-5p, 506, 222, 300, 203, 495
IQGAP1 (8826)	NM_003870	141, 361-5p, 433, 539, 9, 185, 186, 485-5p, 195, 335, 708, 374a, 155, 421, 133a, 133b, 429, 425, 424, 519d, 28-5p, 497, 495, 124, 103, 296-3p, 15a, 200b, 200c, 122, 200a, 455-5p, 20a, 107, 24, 20b, 146a, 15b, 212, 137, 590-3p, 146b-5p, 132, 106b, 106a, 93, 544, 17, 543, 374b, 299-3p, 16, 379, 205, 216a, 340, 208a, 506, 208b, 499-5p, 203
IFITM1 (8519)	NM_003641	19b, 19a, 425
CHEK1 (1111)	NM_001274	103, 15a, 30c, 539, 30d, 30e, 7, 186, 30a, 30b, 107, 362-3p, 190, 195, 320d, 320c, 330-5p, 15b, 421, 320a, 129-5p, 320b, 190b, 197, 16, 424, 377, 505, 326, 497, 495, 329, 503, 873
TLR10 (81793)	NM_001017388	590-3p, 190, 219-5p, 433, 26a, 190b, 340, 374a, 374b
CRP (1401)	NM_000567	448, 137, 199a-5p, 15a, 143, 145, 7, 133a, 491-5p, 186, 133b, 199b-5p, 338-3p, 424, 16, 183, 365, 219-5p, 218, 195, 497, 15b, 150
FANCC (2176)	NM_000136	103, 361-5p, 149, 186, 107, 24, 146a, 486-5p, 219-5p, 125a-3p, 488, 19b, 19a, 15b, 98, 146b-5p, 152, 338-3p, 424, let-7d, 10a, let-7e, 183, 10b, let-7b, let-7c, 32, let-7a, 140-5p, 875-5p, 499-5p, let-7i, let-7f, let-7g
DFFA (1676)	NM_004401	127-3p, 154, 129-5p, 106b, 18a, 18b, 106a, 34a, 93, 17, 485-5p, 20a, 20b, 34c-5p, 138, 519d, 190, 196b, 590-5p, 196a, 449b, 449a
SHB (6461)	NM_003028	320a, 15a, 320b, 613, 1, 206, 28-5p, 362-3p, 195, 376c, 342-3p, 708, 320d, 320c, 488, 499-5p, 495, 329, 23a, 874, 23b
CXCR1 (3577)	NM_000634	141, 200a, 34a, 149, 135a, 24, 135b, 34c-5p, 16, 346, 205, 362-3p, 31, 195, 125a-3p, 876-5p, 708, 449b, 449a, 329, 873, 214
CRKL (1399)	NM_005207	124, 181d, 296-3p, 200b, 145, 200c, 200a, 186, 128, 29a, 181a, 29b, 29c, 181c, 1271, 181b, 365, 217, 191, 21, 376c, 125a-3p, 320d, 320c, 211, 137, 590-3p, 320a, 320b, 96, 18b, 429, 299-3p, 204, 216a, 140-5p, 224, 506, 590-5p, 222, 496, 221, 495, 873
IL7R (3575)	NM_002185	204, 211, 758, 874

Gene Symbol (Entrez Gene ID)	Transcript ID	miRNAs
ADA (100)	NM_000022	28-5p, 183, 96, 125a-3p, 708, 29a, 202, 338-3p, 29b, 135a, 29c
ARHGEF6 (9459)	NM_004840	361-5p, 139-5p, 185, 27a, 27b, 384, 193b, 320d, 488, 320c, 449b, 449a, 23a, 125a-5p, 23b, 193a-3p, 490-3p, 429, 425, 653, 371-5p, 450a, 496, 495, 329, 124, 200b, 30c, 30d, 200c, 30e, 30a, 30b, 128, 217, 362-3p, 219-5p, 211, 448, 590-3p, 136, 320a, 134, 320b, 33a, 544, 135a, 135b, 16, 204, 340, 506, 125b, 874, 873
VEGFA (7422)	NM_001025366	141, 361-5p, 144, 1, 23a, 150, 23b, 155, 199a-5p, 153, 613, 519d, 140-5p, 302b, 302a, 302c, 302e, 103, 126, 101, 200b, 30c, 30d, 200c, 30e, 200a, 451, 30a, 30b, 107, 486-5p, 376c, 590-3p, 448, 136, 134, 26a, 199b-5p, 374b, 138, 505, 300, 503, 539, 185, 186, 383, 148a, 191, 190, 148b, 195, 374a, 449b, 449a, 125a-5p, 429, 424, 653, 31, 497, 495, 329, 494, 15a, 410, 520e, 20a, 29a, 29b, 29c, 20b, 362-3p, 339-5p, 342-3p, 125a-3p, 15b, 190b, 106b, 93, 106a, 17, 381, 543, 382, 299-3p, 16, 206, 377, 205, 216a, 373, 340, 372, 125b, 876-5p, 202, 499-5p, 203, 520a-3p
ECSIT (51295)	NM_001142464	143
VEGFA (7422)	NM_001025369	141, 361-5p, 144, 539, 185, 186, 1, 383, 191, 148a, 190, 148b, 195, 374a, 449b, 449a, 150, 23a, 23b, 155, 199a-5p, 153, 613, 429, 424, 653, 519d, 31, 140-5p, 302b, 497, 302a, 495, 302c, 494, 329, 103, 126, 101, 15a, 30c, 200b, 410, 200c, 30d, 30e, 200a, 520e, 451, 30a, 30b, 29a, 20a, 29b, 107, 29c, 20b, 486-5p, 362-3p, 339-5p, 376c, 342-3p, 125a-3p, 15b, 448, 590-3p, 136, 134, 26a, 190b, 106b, 93, 106a, 17, 381, 543, 382, 199b-5p, 374b, 299-3p, 16, 138, 206, 377, 205, 216a, 373, 340, 372, 505, 876-5p, 300, 202, 499-5p, 203, 520a-3p, 503
SPTAN1 (6709)	NM_001130438	184, 101, 134, 185, 29a, 128, 758, 29b, 29c
MADD (8567)	NM_003682	181d, 103, 15a, 491-5p, 185, 543, 299-3p, 181a, 107, 542-3p, 181c, 424, 181b, 16, 377, 486-5p, 195, 340, 342-3p, 19b, 497, 19a, 15b, 23a, 23b
ORAI1 (84876)	NM_032790	519d, 377, 106b, 93, 106a, 130b, 17, 130a, 20a, 454, 425, 20b
DBF4 (10926)	NM_006716	30c, 30d, 145, 30e, 411, 186, 30a, 30b, 29a, 454, 29b, 542-3p, 29c, 25, 367, 486-5p, 363, 342-3p, 301a, 320d, 320c, 301b, 155, 590-3p, 199a-5p, 320a, 33b, 320b, 33a, 92b, 92a, 381, 199b-5p, 135a, 135b, 205, 32, 340, 300, 130a, 203
ATRIP (84126)	NM_130384	383, 370, 326, 330-5p, 197, 138
S1PR1 (1901)	NM_001400	127-3p, 144, 145, 186, 148a, 148b, 301a, 320d, 708, 320c, 301b, 155, 154, 152, 429, 519d, 653, 28-5p, 520c-3p, 32, 224, 196b, 590-5p, 302b, 223, 190a, 302c, 495, 101d, 101, 200b, 200c, 30e, 455-5p, 370, 181a, 20a, 454, 181c, 24, 25, 181b, 20b, 367, 218, 363, 19b, 19a, 590-3p, 320a, 33b, 320b, 33a, 106b, 92b, 92a, 106a, 93, 17, 543, 382, 378, 377, 373, 340, 130b, 422a, 324-5p, 130a, 203, 873
PTPN11 (5781)	NM_002834	124, 103, 143, 539, 455-5p, 185, 186, 107, 454, 181c, 1271, 21, 376a, 376b, 374a, 23a, 23b, 590-3p, 448, 129-5p, 96, 491-5p, 374b, 338-3p, 758, 138, 378, 182, 31, 216b, 224, 196b, 422a, 505, 590-5p, 506, 196a, 499-5p, 873
ICOS (29851)	NM_012092	539, 145, 149, 186, 27a, 27b, 190, 193b, 195, 320d, 374a, 320c, 153, 193a-3p, 758, 424, 224, 196b, 497, 450a, 196a, 103, 15a, 30b, 29a, 29b, 107, 29c, 376c, 19b, 19a, 15b, 590-3p, 98, 320a, 320b, 520d-3p, 374b, 338-3p, 16, 138, 379, let-7d, let-7e, let-7b, let-7c, let-7a, 216b, 203, let-7i, 520a-3p, 874, let-7f, let-7g
EIF4EBP1 (1978)	NM_004095	34a, 125b, 328, 370, 202, 874, 125a-5p, 138
CDKN2C (1031)	NM_078626	181d, 185, 20a, 181a, 542-3p, 181c, 181b, 20b, 146a, 22, 218, 488, 590-3p, 154, 129-5p, 146b-5p, 106b, 93, 106a, 544, 17, 425, 519d, 182, 340, 495
FAS (355)	NM_000043	431, 361-5p, 539, 9, 149, 27a, 27b, 335, 374a, 23a, 23b, 129-5p, 153, 425, 519d, 371-5p, 196b, 196a, 495, 494, 181d, 410, 30c, 30d, 30e, 30a, 30b, 128, 181a, 29a, 29b, 29c, 181c, 181b, 22, 217, 376a, 376b, 99b, 19b, 19a, 448, 137, 136, 98, 146b-5p, 106a, 544, 381, 17, 374b, 338-3p, let-7d, 183, let-7e, let-7b, let-7c, let-7a, 216b, 340, 300, 203, let-7i, let-7f, let-7g
SKI (6497)	NM_003036	141, 200a, 20a, 20b, 25, 21, 367, 363, 125a-3p, 374a, 137, 155, 448, 129-5p, 33b, 33a, 92b, 106b, 93, 92a, 106a, 544, 17, 374b, 338-3p, 758, 424, 519d, 10a, 32, 208a, 590-5p, 208b, 203

(continued)

Table 2 (continued)

Gene Symbol (Entrez Gene ID) Transcript ID	miRNAs
TNFRSF13C (115650) NM_052945	142-3p, 124, 218, 544, 506, 873
IL1F8 (27177) NM_173178	103, 15a, 152, 18a, 106b, 93, 106a, 18b, 17, 186, 20a, 107, 424, 20b, 16, 519d, 183, 182, 195, 497, 15b
FAS (355) NR_028035	361-5p, 431, 9, 27a, 27b, 1297, 194, 335, 374a, 23a, 23b, 425, 519d, 196b, 140-5p, 196a, 181d, 599, 181a, 29a, 29b, 29c, 181c, 181b, 25, 142-3p, 22, 217, 218, 376a, 376b, 376c, 99b, 19b, 19a, 212, 137, 448, 136, 98, 146b-5p, 33b, 33a, 132, 106a, 381, 17, 544, 374b, 338-3p, 138, let-7d, 183, let-7e, 182, let-7b, let-7c, let-7a, 216b, 505, 876-5p, 300, 26b, let-7i, let-7f, let-7g
FAS (355) NR_028034	431, 361-5p, 9, 27a, 27b, 1297, 194, 335, 374a, 23a, 23b, 425, 519d, 196b, 140-5p, 196a, 181d, 599, 181a, 29a, 29b, 29c, 181c, 181b, 25, 142-3p, 22, 217, 218, 376a, 376b, 376c, 99b, 19b, 19a, 212, 448, 137, 136, 98, 33b, 146b-5p, 33a, 132, 106a, 17, 544, 381, 374b, 338-3p, 138, let-7d, let-7e, 183, let-7b, let-7c, 216b, let-7a, 505, 876-5p, 26b, 300, let-7i, let-7f, let-7g
CHUK (1147) NM_001278	144, 1297, 148a, 148b, 190, 195, 335, 194, 301a, 23a, 23b, 301b, 152, 429, 197, 425, 424, 519d, 590-5p, 223, 497, 196a, 329, 494, 15a, 296-3p, 410, 200b, 411, 451, 20a, 454, 20b, 21, 219-5p, 362-3p, 376a, 376b, 376c, 339-5p, 342-3p, 15b, 448, 590-3p, 98, 190b, 26a, 106b, 106a, 93, 17, 382, 16, 379, let-7d, let-7e, let-7b, 377, let-7c, let-7a, 340, 130b, 876-5p, 208a, 26b, 208b, 130a, 499-5p, 203, let-7i, let-7f, let-7g
FAS (355) NR_028036	361-5p, 431, 9, 27a, 27b, 1297, 194, 335, 374a, 23a, 23b, 425, 140-5p, 196b, 196a, 181d, 599, 29a, 181a, 29b, 181c, 29c, 25, 181b, 142-3p, 22, 217, 218, 376a, 376b, 376c, 99b, 19b, 19a, 212, 448, 137, 136, 98, 146b-5p, 33b, 33a, 132, 381, 544, 374b, 338-3p, 138, let-7d, 183, let-7e, 182, 377, let-7b, let-7c, 205, let-7a, 216b, 505, 876-5p, 26b, 300, let-7i, let-7f, let-7g
IFI35 (3430) NM_005533	34a, 185, 125a-3p, 449b, 449a, 34c-5p
BAX (581) NM_004324	124, 98, 34a, 27a, 27b, 128, 34c-5p, let-7d, let-7e, let-7b, let-7c, let-7a, 506, 449b, 449a, let-7f, 214
CASP7 (840) NM_033340	361-5p, 539, 186, 27a, 27b, 194, 335, 301a, 320d, 320c, 23a, 23b, 301b, 129-5p, 18a, 18b, 197, 519d, 653, 371-5p, 224, 495, 451, 20a, 29a, 29b, 454, 29c, 20b, 146a, 486-5p, 376c, 19b, 19a, 212, 137, 136, 320a, 320b, 146b-5p, 132, 106b, 93, 106a, 544, 17, 543, 138, 10b, 378, 130b, 422a, 130a
SHARPIN (81858) NM_030974	206, 134, 328, 149
IGLL1 (3543) NM_152855	199a-5p, 362-3p, 433, 544, 543, 199b-5p, 449b, 449a, 329, 24, 34c-5p, 138
PRF1 (5551) NM_005041	136, 204, 134, 145, 132, 422a, 328, 370, 450a, 326, 330-5p, 211, 212, 24
CD79A (973) NM_001783	103, 378, 7, 328, 708, 485-5p, 488, 107
CASP7 (840) NM_033338	361-5p, 539, 186, 451, 27a, 27b, 20a, 29a, 29b, 454, 29c, 20b, 146a, 486-5p, 335, 194, 376c, 301a, 320d, 320c, 19b, 19a, 212, 23a, 23b, 301b, 136, 129-5p, 320a, 146b-5p, 320b, 132, 106b, 18a, 18b, 106a, 93, 17, 544, 543, 197, 138, 519d, 653, 10b, 371-5p, 130b, 224, 130a, 495
LTBR (4055) NM_002342	33a, 455-5p, 133a, 133b, 485-5p, 29a, 299-3p, 29b, 425, 29c, 204, 328, 211, 874, 150
IL18 (3606) NM_001562	590-3p, 377, 129-5p, 143, 411, 505, 197, 23a, 504, 23b
PSMB8 (5696) NM_148919	22, 410, 339-5p, 125b, 451, 24, 125a-5p
BRCA2 (675) NM_000059	145, 200c, 1, 1297, 146a, 142-3p, 21, 148a, 148b, 19b, 488, 211, 19a, 590-3p, 129-5p, 146b-5p, 152, 26a, 544, 429, 425, 206, 653, 182, 204, 140-5p, 26b, 496, 203
FAS (355) NR_028033	431, 361-5p, 9, 27a, 27b, 1297, 194, 335, 374a, 23a, 23b, 425, 519d, 140-5p, 196b, 196a, 181d, 599, 181a, 29a, 29b, 29c, 181c, 25, 181b, 142-3p, 22, 217, 218, 376a, 376b, 376c, 99b, 19b, 19a, 212, 137, 448, 136, 98, 146b-5p, 33b, 33a, 132, 106a, 17, 544, 381, 374b, 338-3p, 138, let-7d, let-7e, 183, 377, let-7b, 205, let-7c, 216b, let-7a, 505, 876-5p, 300, 26b, let-7i, let-7f, let-7g

Gene Symbol (Entrez Gene ID) Transcript ID	miRNAs
ATF2 (1386) NM_001880	15a, 186, 451, 20a, 128, 454, 1297, 20b, 217, 195, 301a, 374a, 211, 15b, 23a, 23b, 301b, 590-3p, 26a, 106b, 106a, 93, 381, 544, 17, 374b, 338-3p, 16, 519d, 204, 216a, 340, 130b, 224, 222, 300, 26b, 130a, 496, 221, 203
ORC6L (23594) NM_014321	448, 590-3p, 127-3p, 136, 132, 613, 543, 485-5p, 1, 206, 486-5p, 125a-3p, 212
ORC5L (5001) NM_181747	137, 320a, 433, 320b, 539, 410, 186, 374b, 138, 590-5p, 320d, 374a, 223, 320c, 150
NFKBID (84807) NM_139239	184, 296-3p, 185, 491-5p, 27a, 27b
TNFSF14 (8740) NM_003807	199a-5p, 106b, 93, 411, 106a, 17, 199b-5p, 20a, 20b, 519d, 125a-3p, 125b, 214, 125a-5p, 504
MBD2 (8932) NM_015832	200b, 30c, 30d, 200c, 30e, 381, 543, 27a, 429, 30a, 374b, 30b, 27b, 29a, 29b, 29c, 183, 182, 340, 224, 374a, 300, 19b, 19a, 495, 494
CD3E (916) NM_000733	15a, 122, 34a, 485-5p, 24, 34c-5p, 424, 16, 184, 31, 195, 505, 497, 449b, 449a, 15b
CD70 (970) NM_001252	129-5p, 15a, 195, 497, 15b, 503, 424, 16
IL1B (3553) NM_000576	144, 132, 185, 149, 485-5p, 299-3p, 184, 21, 204, 340, 328, 590-5p, 488, 330-5p, 326, 211, 212, 495
OAS1 (4938) NM_002534	448, 378, 182, 144, 134, 15a, 31, 422a, 186, 758, 16
MCL1 (4170) NM_182763	361-5p, 144, 139-5p, 186, 27a, 520b, 1297, 383, 193b, 192, 374a, 320d, 488, 320c, 125a-5p, 153, 193a-3p, 133a, 133b, 197, 519d, 520c-3p, 32, 224, 302b, 302a, 302d, 496, 495, 302c, 302e, 101, 410, 520e, 20a, 128, 29a, 29b, 29c, 25, 20b, 215, 217, 367, 376c, 363, 448, 320a, 320b, 33a, 26a, 106b, 92b, 93, 92a, 106a, 17, 381, 382, 520d-3p, 374b, 373, 372, 130b, 125b, 26b, 300, 130a, 520a-3p, 873
RELB (5971) NM_006509	28-5p, 204, 7, 34a, 491-5p, 485-5p, 708, 299-3p, 449b, 211, 449a, 34c-5p
SMURF1 (57154) NM_181349	431, 15a, 200b, 539, 145, 9, 200c, 30e, 370, 384, 486-5p, 376a, 376b, 195, 376c, 19b, 19a, 15b, 125a-5p, 448, 153, 152, 33a, 106b, 93, 490-3p, 429, 197, 425, 16, 424, 10a, 519d, 378, 10b, 340, 422a, 196b, 140-5p, 125b, 497, 196a, 221, 504
STAT3 (6774) NM_213662	181d, 410, 485-5p, 370, 29a, 181a, 20a, 29b, 454, 29c, 181c, 20b, 181b, 21, 301a, 342-3p, 125a-3p, 320d, 320c, 211, 301b, 125a-5p, 129-5p, 320a, 320b, 106b, 93, 106a, 544, 17, 519d, 204, 372, 130b, 590-5p, 125b, 130a, 499-5p, 495, 329, 874
IRF1 (3659) NM_002198	139-5p, 485-5p, 520b, 383, 190, 193b, 195, 335, 301a, 374a, 488, 23a, 301b, 23b, 129-5p, 193a-3p, 424, 519d, 520c-3p, 32, 31, 302b, 302a, 497, 302d, 302c, 302e, 124, 103, 181d, 15a, 520e, 20a, 454, 107, 24, 181b, 20b, 25, 367, 218, 363, 342-3p, 125a-3p, 15b, 590-3p, 134, 190b, 92b, 106b, 93, 92a, 106a, 17, 544, 374b, 520d-3p, 16, 183, 377, 216b, 373, 340, 372, 130b, 506, 300, 130a, 520a-3p
JUN (3725) NM_002228	141, 144, 101, 30c, 200b, 139-5p, 9, 200c, 30d, 30e, 200a, 186, 30a, 30b, 29a, 542-3p, 29b, 1, 29c, 24, 383, 190, 590-3p, 190b, 429, 758, 182, 377, 216b, 340, 203, 495, 494, 873
RXRA (6256) NM_002957	219-5p, 194, 342-3p, 876-5p
IFIT3 (3437) NM_001031683	137, 361-5p, 431, 143, 146b-5p, 200b, 539, 200c, 429, 374b, 299-3p, 29b, 29c, 146a, 32, 371-5p, 339-5p, 376c, 422a, 99b, 876-5p, 374a, 496, 203, 873
IL15RA (3601) NM_002189	448, 590-3p, 199a-5p, 96, 410, 411, 381, 149, 199b-5p, 370, 374b, 138, 1271, 184, 653, 183, 28-5p, 339-5p, 342-3p, 374a, 708, 300, 125a-5p
TICAM2 (353376) NM_021649	361-5p, 181d, 599, 539, 200b, 200c, 186, 181a, 181c, 181b, 384, 383, 376a, 376b, 335, 342-3p, 211, 23a, 23b, 590-3p, 129-5p, 491-5p, 381, 544, 543, 429, 183, 378, 204, 377, 182, 32, 340, 422a, 590-5p, 300, 223, 499-5p, 494
RPL5 (6125) NM_000969	376a, 376b
CCL4 (6351) NM_002984	590-3p, 33b, 410, 33a, 9, 122, 544, 542-3p, 425, 24, 183, 346, 217, 340, 125a-3p, 203, 873
MAP3K13 (9175) NM_004721	144, 101, 539, 139-5p, 185, 27a, 27b, 20a, 1, 25, 20b, 148a, 219-5p, 148b, 339-5p, 590-3p, 136, 129-5p, 152, 106b, 93, 613, 106a, 17, 653, 206, 519d, 377, 205, 216a, 371-5p, 216b, 31, 450a, 495, 203
NCR3 (259197) NM_147130	296-3p, 330-5p, 326
PSMB5 (5693) NM_001144932	142-3p, 155, 127-3p, 18b, 376c, 455-5p, 381, 300, 25

Gene Symbol (Entrez Gene ID) Transcript ID	miRNAs
ELK1 (2002) NM_005229	136, 143, 539, 9, 185, 491-5p, 382, 135a, 135b, 219-5p, 342-3p, 125b, 125a-3p, 326, 488, 330-5p, 495, 150, 125a-5p, 873
BTK (695) NM_000061	124, 590-3p, 21, 362-3p, 411, 876-5p, 506, 590-5p, 425, 329
RHOA (387) NM_001664	361-5p, 144, 539, 9, 185, 186, 485-5p, 27a, 27b, 383, 191, 194, 320d, 320c, 330-5p, 154, 129-5p, 490-3p, 429, 425, 519d, 31, 140-5p, 222, 326, 221, 495, 494, 101, 200b, 200c, 128, 20a, 542-3p, 1271, 20b, 146a, 217, 218, 376a, 376b, 125a-3p, 590-3p, 98, 320a, 320b, 146b-5p, 96, 190b, 93, 381, 135a, 135b, 379, 183, let-7c, let-7a, 340, 300, let-7i, let-7f, 504, let-7g
MAPK1 (5594) NM_138957	155, 590-3p, 28-5p, 190, 190b, 186, 708
IL26 (55801) NM_018402	181d, 141, 30c, 539, 9, 30d, 30e, 200a, 455-5p, 186, 30a, 30b, 454, 542-3p, 181b, 301a, 19b, 19a, 301b, 590-3p, 154, 544, 382, 758, 135a, 425, 135b, 371-5p, 340, 130b, 130a, 494
CTNNB1 (1499) NM_001904	181d, 101, 410, 539, 9, 185, 370, 217, 335, 301a, 320d, 488, 320c, 19b, 19a, 212, 150, 23a, 23b, 301b, 214, 448, 590-3p, 129-5p, 320a, 33b, 320b, 33a, 132, 106b, 93, 106a, 381, 17, 543, 382, 377, 182, 340, 130b, 140-5p, 300, 222, 130a, 496, 221
MYT1 (4661) NM_004535	144, 186, 485-5p, 27a, 27b, 520b, 301a, 374a, 449b, 449a, 23a, 301b, 23b, 125a-5p, 129-5p, 429, 519d, 28-5p, 520c-3p, 302b, 223, 302a, 302d, 495, 302c, 329, 302e, 200b, 410, 200c, 122, 34a, 520e, 20a, 454, 20b, 362-3p, 590-3p, 136, 106b, 93, 106a, 17, 520d-3p, 34c-5p, 373, 340, 372, 130b, 125b, 130a, 520a-3p, 873
CCRN4L (25819) NM_012118	10a, 10b, 339-5p, 130b, 301a, 543, 485-5p, 130a, 499-5p, 203, 454, 494, 301b
EPO (2056) NM_000799	320a, 33b, 320b, 122, 106a, 17, 338-3p, 20b, 378, 362-3p, 224, 125b, 125a-3p, 328, 320d, 320c, 330-5p, 326, 329, 125a-5p
RPRM (56475) NM_019845	33b, 539, 33a, 613, 338-3p, 1, 138, 206, 375, 371-5p, 335, 224, 495, 203, 494, 150, 214
SH2D1A (4068) NM_002351	431, 361-5p, 144, 410, 30e, 20a, 20b, 1271, 146a, 215, 192, 376a, 376b, 374a, 708, 211, 448, 155, 199a-5p, 146b-5p, 33a, 96, 18a, 18b, 106a, 381, 17, 199b-5p, 374b, 135a, 425, 135b, 28-5p, 204, 182, 205, 31, 340, 140-5p, 876-5p, 208a, 208b, 300, 450a, 496, 499-5p, 495
MPO (4353) NM_000250	146a, 183, 148a, 377, 146b-5p, 152, 148b, 193b, 193a-3p, 381, 300, 29b
ENDOG (2021) NM_004435	362-3p, 197, 329
FKBP1A (2280) NM_054014	141, 181d, 96, 34a, 200a, 543, 186, 181a, 181c, 1271, 181b, 34c-5p, 183, 22, 182, 376a, 376b, 340, 376c, 488, 449b, 449a
NCOA1 (8648) NM_147223	361-5p, 144, 7, 149, 301a, 23a, 301b, 23b, 129-5p, 152, 519d, 371-5p, 140-5p, 128, 454, 219-5p, 486-5p, 376c, 19b, 19a, 590-3p, 137, 448, 132, 92b, 92a, 374b, 135a, 34c-5p, 135b, 138, 300, 875-5p, 539, 186, 27a, 27b, 383, 148a, 148b, 190, 335, 374a, 330-5p, 449b, 449a, 421, 18a, 18b, 424, 32, 223, 496, 495, 329, 181d, 410, 34a, 181a, 20a, 181c, 24, 25, 181b, 20b, 146a, 22, 362-3p, 367, 363, 342-3p, 212, 98, 146b-5p, 190b, 106b, 93, 106a, 381, 544, 17, 543, let-7d, let-7e, 182, 377, let-7b, 205, let-7c, 216a, 216b, let-7a, 130b, 130a, 203, let-7i, let-7f, let-7g
NR4A1 (3164) NM_173157	124, 361-5p, 15a, 410, 187, 485-5p, 542-3p, 384, 383, 195, 125a-3p, 374a, 15b, 23a, 23b, 214, 544, 374b, 424, 16, let-7e, 371-5p, 340, 224, 506, 497, 873
IL15 (3600) NM_000585	141, 144, 139-5p, 186, 148a, 148b, 195, 194, 301a, 374a, 23a, 23b, 301b, 155, 421, 129-5p, 152, 424, 32, 497, 103, 15a, 101, 200a, 542-3p, 107, 454, 25, 367, 376a, 376b, 363, 19b, 19a, 15b, 212, 214, 137, 590-3p, 98, 92b, 92a, 544, 543, 374b, 338-3p, 16, let-7d, let-7e, 346, let-7b, let-7c, 205, let-7a, 340, 130b, 505, 130a, 202, let-7i, 203, let-7f, let-7g
PA2G4 (5036) NM_006191	127-3p, 15a, 143, 599, 433, 7, 185, 376a, 376b, 195, 19b, 19a, 15b, 150, 590-3p, 491-5p, 758, 424, 138, 16, let-7d, let-7b, let-7c, 216b, let-7a, 208a, 208b, 223, 497, let-7i, let-7f
CDKN2B (1030) NM_078487	144, 433, 100, 200b, 200c, 451, 1, 25, 217, 148a, 486-5p, 190, 148b, 125a-3p, 708, 23a, 125a-5p, 23b, 137, 152, 92a, 93, 429, 138, 28-5p, 346, 182, 216b, 340, 505, 196b, 130b, 125b, 876-5p, 222, 196a, 130a, 203, 495, 221

Gene Symbol (Entrez Gene ID) Transcript ID	miRNAs
EIF4E (1977) NM_001130678	141, 361-5p, 144, 433, 539, 9, 139-5p, 7, 186, 520b, 1, 1297, 148a, 148b, 192, 195, 374a, 320d, 320c, 23a, 150, 23b, 153, 152, 613, 429, 424, 519d, 520c-3p, 32, 224, 302b, 302a, 497, 223, 496, 302d, 302c, 495, 494, 302e, 103, 181d, 296-3p, 15a, 599, 200b, 200c, 200a, 520e, 20a, 29a, 107, 29b, 20b, 215, 367, 486-5p, 376c, 19a, 15b, 590-3p, 448, 320a, 320b, 26a, 106b, 106a, 544, 17, 381, 382, 374b, 520d-3p, 338-3p, 16, 206, 10a, 377, 373, 372, 340, 130b, 26b, 300, 130a, 499-5p, 203, 503, 520a-3p, 873
PARD6A (50855) NM_016948	125a-3p
TAB2 (23118) NM_015093	141, 143, 539, 7, 186, 1297, 192, 374a, 320d, 320c, 488, 449b, 449a, 23a, 23b, 155, 153, 429, 32, 590-5p, 223, 495, 124, 103, 181d, 599, 30c, 200b, 410, 200c, 200a, 34a, 455-5p, 29a, 181a, 107, 29b, 29c, 181c, 181b, 25, 215, 142-3p, 217, 21, 218, 367, 219-5p, 376a, 376b, 363, 376c, 214, 590-3p, 448, 98, 320a, 33b, 320b, 26a, 33a, 92b, 92a, 381, 374b, 34c-5p, let-7d, 183, let-7e, 377, let-7b, let-7c, 216a, let-7a, 340, 506, 300, 26b, 202, let-7i, let-7f, let-7g
RASA1 (5921) NM_002890	141, 361-5p, 144, 539, 145, 186, 1, 384, 335, 301a, 374a, 320d, 330-5p, 320c, 488, 301b, 153, 421, 613, 425, 653, 31, 371-5p, 196b, 196a, 223, 326, 496, 495, 494, 30c, 30d, 30e, 200a, 30a, 30b, 454, 24, 1271, 146a, 21, 218, 376a, 376b, 342-3p, 19b, 19a, 211, 212, 590-3p, 320a, 146b-5p, 320b, 33b, 96, 33a, 132, 381, 382, 374b, 338-3p, 206, 182, 377, 204, 375, 130b, 505, 300, 130a, 873
PAK1 (5058) NM_002576	141, 145, 7, 186, 485-5p, 1297, 195, 374a, 320d, 320c, 199a-5p, 491-5p, 758, 371-5p, 196b, 222, 196a, 302d, 221, 494, 200a, 455-5p, 411, 20a, 542-3p, 1271, 20b, 218, 342-3p, 19a, 98, 320a, 320b, 26a, 96, 106b, 106a, 17, 199b-5p, 374b, 299-3p, 16, let-7d, let-7e, 377, let-7b, let-7c, 216a, let-7a, 26b, let-7i, 203, let-7f, let-7g
MYC (4609) NM_002467	599, 296-3p, 539, 145, 34a, 149, 186, 24, 376c, 374a, 449b, 449a, 590-3p, 98, 33b, 613, 381, 374b, 135a, 34c-5p, 135b, let-7d, 183, let-7e, 182, let-7b, let-7c, 31, let-7a, 300, 223, let-7i, 494, let-7f, let-7g
TGIF1 (7050) NM_170695	144, 433, 139-5p, 7, 186, 27a, 27b, 1, 194, 301a, 320d, 374a, 320c, 23a, 23b, 301b, 155, 129-5p, 613, 429, 32, 495, 494, 124, 101, 410, 200b, 200c, 455-5p, 128, 454, 25, 146a, 367, 363, 342-3p, 19b, 19a, 211, 212, 320a, 134, 146b-5p, 320b, 132, 92b, 92a, 543, 374b, 299-3p, 206, 204, 216a, 216b, 340, 130b, 506, 130a, 873
GZMA (3001) NM_006144	124, 590-3p, 132, 224, 19b, 488, 19a, 758, 212
RUNX3 (864) NM_004350	145, 139-5p, 27a, 27b, 20a, 542-3p, 454, 20b, 194, 301a, 374a, 210, 19b, 330-5p, 19a, 214, 301b, 137, 129-5p, 106b, 106a, 93, 17, 544, 382, 374b, 424, 519d, 371-5p, 130b, 130a, 326, 495
DIAPH3 (81624) NM_001042517	539, 9, 145, 186, 1297, 383, 148a, 190, 148b, 301a, 374a, 125a-5p, 301b, 199a-5p, 152, 758, 32, 31, 224, 494, 124, 410, 181a, 454, 181c, 181b, 25, 365, 367, 219-5p, 363, 376c, 19b, 19a, 590-3p, 98, 26a, 190b, 92b, 92a, 382, 199b-5p, 374b, 135a, 135b, let-7d, let-7e, 183, 182, let-7b, let-7c, let-7a, 340, 130b, 506, 26b, 130a, 202, 499-5p, let-7i, let-7f, let-7g
CDC42 (998) NM_044472	103, 361-5p, 599, 15a, 539, 139-5p, 186, 107, 25, 383, 367, 376a, 195, 376b, 363, 194, 335, 211, 15b, 214, 590-3p, 137, 136, 153, 33b, 33a, 92b, 18a, 18b, 92a, 338-3p, 424, 16, 184, 204, 32, 340, 505, 224, 497, 499-5p, 495, 873
PKMYT1 (9088) NM_182687	519d, 371-5p, 106b, 93, 106a, 185, 17, 125a-3p, 20a, 150, 24, 20b
HNRNPK (3190) NM_002140	431, 144, 539, 186, 1, 1297, 384, 374a, 708, 421, 153, 129-5p, 613, 429, 653, 28-5p, 590-5p, 222, 495, 221, 103, 30c, 200b, 200c, 30d, 30e, 370, 30a, 30b, 29a, 29b, 107, 29c, 21, 376c, 339-5p, 342-3p, 590-3p, 448, 26a, 93, 544, 374b, 338-3p, 135a, 135b, 206, 10a, 10b, 377, 205, 26b, 203, 873
GSC (145258) NM_173849	431, 204, 93, 34a, 211
ZFYVE9 (9372) NM_004799	145, 7, 520b, 148a, 148b, 192, 194, 301a, 320d, 320c, 150, 301b, 153, 152, 519d, 520c-3p, 590-5p, 302b, 302a, 302d, 495, 302c, 302e, 520e, 20a, 454, 20b, 215, 22, 21, 486-5p, 376a, 376b, 376c, 19b, 19a, 320a, 320b, 106b, 106a, 93, 17, 520d-3p, 373, 372, 130b, 130a, 203, 520a-3p, 873

(continued)

Table 2 (continued)

Gene Symbol (Entrez Gene ID) Transcript ID	miRNAs
TNF (7124) NM_000594	361-5p, 185, 149, 520b, 383, 148a, 191, 148b, 335, 301a, 320d, 374a, 320c, 150, 301b, 152, 519d, 520c-3p, 140-5p, 222, 302b, 302a, 302d, 221, 302c, 495, 494, 302e, 124, 103, 181d, 599, 520e, 20a, 181a, 107, 542-3p, 454, 181c, 24, 1271, 181b, 20b, 218, 339-5p, 19b, 19a, 212, 590-3p, 320a, 320b, 33b, 33a, 96, 132, 106b, 106a, 93, 17, 543, 374b, 520d-3p, 216a, 373, 372, 130b, 506, 130a, 520a-3p
CDC25A (993) NM_001789	141, 485-5p, 520b, 195, 155, 424, 519d, 653, 520c-3p, 371-5p, 590-5p, 302b, 497, 302a, 302d, 302c, 494, 302e, 103, 15a, 100, 200a, 520c, 20a, 107, 24, 20b, 365, 21, 339-5p, 99b, 15b, 99a, 98, 106b, 106a, 93, 17, 382, 520d-3p, 16, let-7d, 184, 346, let-7e, 377, let-7b, let-7c, 216b, let-7a, 373, 372, let-7i, let-7f, 520a-3p, let-7g
RALA (5898) NM_005402	431, 539, 139-5p, 149, 186, 27b, 1297, 193b, 301a, 320d, 374a, 320c, 488, 301b, 155, 199a-5p, 153, 129-5p, 193a-3p, 133a, 133b, 197, 653, 519d, 32, 371-5p, 196b, 224, 140-5p, 328, 590-5p, 222, 196a, 223, 495, 221, 329, 124, 181d, 410, 181a, 20a, 128, 454, 24, 181c, 25, 20b, 181b, 21, 367, 219-5p, 362-3p, 486-5p, 363, 19b, 19a, 214, 590-3p, 448, 320a, 146b-5p, 320b, 26a, 106b, 92b, 92a, 106a, 93, 544, 17, 381, 199b-5p, 374b, 135a, 135b, 183, 205, 216a, 340, 130b, 506, 300, 26b, 130a, 499-5p, 203, 874
MUC5B (727897) NM_002458	383, 433, 125b, 125a-5p
RELA (5970) NM_021975	124, 101, 7, 185, 186, 520e, 520b, 383, 22, 362-3p, 320d, 488, 330-5p, 320c, 155, 320a, 421, 320b, 520d-3p, 138, 182, 520c-3p, 373, 372, 506, 302b, 302a, 326, 302d, 302c, 520a-3p, 329, 302e
ANGPT1 (284) NM_001146	144, 539, 139-5p, 149, 186, 190, 374a, 153, 129-5p, 429, 197, 371-5p, 224, 496, 494, 181d, 410, 200b, 200c, 411, 29a, 181a, 29b, 29c, 181c, 24, 1271, 181b, 146a, 486-5p, 376a, 376b, 376c, 125a-3p, 19b, 19a, 211, 137, 448, 590-3p, 146b-5p, 93, 543, 374b, 135a, 135b, 183, 182, 204, 340, 876-5p, 499-5p
CASP8 (841) NM_001080125	143, 187, 520b, 148a, 148b, 301a, 488, 150, 301b, 129-5p, 152, 519d, 520c-3p, 371-5p, 590-5p, 302b, 302a, 302d, 495, 302c, 302e, 411, 520e, 20a, 128, 29a, 454, 29b, 29c, 20b, 142-3p, 21, 339-5p, 19b, 19a, 590-3p, 106b, 106a, 93, 17, 543, 520d-3p, 10a, let-7e, 10b, let-7b, 373, 372, 340, 130b, 876-5p, 130a, 203, 520a-3p, let-7f
EXOC8 (149371) NM_175876	141, 431, 144, 539, 145, 186, 27a, 27b, 1, 1297, 320d, 374a, 320c, 23a, 150, 23b, 125a-5p, 199a-5p, 613, 491-5p, 424, 653, 196b, 497, 196a, 450a, 221, 494, 103, 181d, 15a, 410, 200a, 20a, 181a, 29a, 29b, 107, 29c, 181c, 20b, 181b, 486-5p, 339-5p, 376c, 342-3p, 211, 15b, 448, 590-3p, 136, 320a, 320b, 26a, 381, 382, 199b-5p, 374b, 206, 183, 378, 204, 182, 377, 216b, 340, 422a, 876-5p, 125b, 300, 26b, 873, 504
IFNGR1 (3459) NM_000416	448, 590-3p, 136, 129-5p, 433, 190b, 381, 1, 425, 362-3p, 486-5p, 216a, 216b, 371-5p, 373, 224, 300, 329
SAP130 (79595) NM_001145928	199a-5p, 410, 26a, 613, 185, 199b-5p, 338-3p, 1, 425, 24, 1297, 138, 206, 28-5p, 377, 31, 26b, 708
ANP32A (8125) NM_006305	181d, 431, 143, 30c, 30d, 30e, 34a, 149, 186, 30a, 30b, 181a, 454, 181c, 181b, 146a, 384, 486-5p, 449b, 212, 449a, 23a, 23b, 125a-5p, 590-3p, 154, 129-5p, 146b-5p, 132, 543, 425, 34c-5p, 138, 653, 371-5p, 340, 125b, 450a, 203, 495, 494, 873
HDAC1 (3065) NM_004964	539, 410, 9, 34a, 185, 485-5p, 24, 376c, 342-3p, 374a, 708, 449b, 211, 449a, 15b, 214, 590-3p, 18b, 135a, 34c-5p, 135b, 424, 28-5p, 204, 216a, 340, 874
EGFR (1956) NM_201284	218, 33b, 33a, 375, 140-5p, 544, 149, 542-3p, 29c
EGFR (1956) NM_201283	141, 204, 200a, 876-5p
LY75 (4065) NM_002349	141, 361-5p, 9, 384, 148a, 148b, 301a, 23a, 23b, 301b, 199a-5p, 421, 152, 429, 519d, 494, 181d, 101, 200b, 200c, 30d, 30e, 411, 30a, 181a, 454, 181c, 181b, 142-3p, 146a, 365, 218, 486-5p, 376a, 376b, 19b, 19a, 212, 590-3p, 136, 98, 146b-5p, 132, 106b, 93, 381, 543, 199b-5p, let-7d, 379, let-7e, let-7b, 204, let-7c, 205, 216b, let-7a, 373, 340, 130b, 876-5p, 300, 130a, 202, 499-5p, let-7i, let-7f, let-7g
FOS (2353) NM_005252	361-5p, 431, 141, 144, 433, 139-5p, 7, 149, 187, 384, 383, 148a, 194, 374a, 155, 154, 133a, 133b, 653, 196b, 222, 196a, 495, 221, 329, 181d, 101, 410, 30d, 29a, 181a, 29b, 181c, 29c, 181b, 22, 362-3p, 376b, 590-3p, 98, 381, 543, 382, 374b, 338-3p, 379, let-7d, let-7e, let-7b, let-7c, let-7a, 340, 208a, 300, 208b, 499-5p, 203, let-7i, let-7f, let-7g, 873
FNBP1L (54874) NM_001024948	141, 144, 9, 7, 1, 384, 194, 301a, 374a, 23a, 23b, 301b, 129-5p, 421, 613, 491-5p, 519d, 653, 371-5p, 224, 497, 495, 494, 103, 15a, 296-3p, 122, 200a, 20a, 107, 20b, 142-3p, 365, 362-3p, 376c, 15b, 590-3p, 137, 26a, 106b, 106a, 93, 17, 374b, 16, 206, 10a, 10b, 377, 182, 340, 505, 876-5p, 26b, 130a, 873
EGFR (1956) NM_201282	539, 488, 203
PIAS1 (8554) NM_016166	15a, 30c, 30d, 30e, 34a, 30a, 30b, 486-5p, 195, 342-3p, 320d, 320c, 449b, 15b, 449a, 214, 590-3p, 320a, 320b, 381, 491-5p, 16, 424, 34c-5p, 377, 375, 300, 497
TNK2 (10188) NM_001010938	15a, 7, 149, 24, 138, 424, 16, 184, 195, 224, 125a-3p, 328, 326, 330-5p, 497, 15b, 214
EXOC6 (54536) NM_019053	141, 361-5p, 30c, 410, 30d, 30e, 200a, 30a, 30b, 454, 542-3p, 1297, 217, 191, 301a, 125a-3p, 320d, 320c, 23a, 23b, 301b, 448, 137, 421, 320a, 320b, 26a, 381, 543, 758, 346, 375, 340, 130b, 140-5p, 26b, 300, 130a, 494, 504
HNF4A (3172) NM_000457	361-5p, 143, 34a, 185, 149, 485-5p, 1, 24, 384, 376c, 342-3p, 125a-3p, 330-5p, 449b, 449a, 150, 421, 613, 133a, 133b, 382, 197, 34c-5p, 206, 346, 216b, 328, 326
PIAS4 (51588) NM_015897	590-3p, 29a, 29b, 29c
RICTOR (253260) NM_152756	141, 144, 143, 139-5p, 9, 185, 186, 485-5p, 1, 148a, 148b, 192, 194, 335, 374a, 488, 150, 155, 154, 152, 613, 491-5p, 425, 424, 32, 196b, 196a, 495, 494, 181d, 200b, 200c, 200a, 128, 454, 181b, 1271, 215, 142-3p, 365, 217, 218, 342-3p, 19b, 19a, 211, 137, 590-3p, 448, 98, 96, 381, 543, 382, 374b, 299-3p, let-7d, 206, 378, let-7e, let-7b, 204, 377, let-7c, let-7a, 340, 130b, 422a, 300, 130a, 499-5p, let-7i, 203, let-7f, 503, 874, let-7g
SAP18 (10284) NM_005870	433, 539, 145, 520b, 148a, 190, 194, 301a, 374a, 150, 301b, 155, 153, 421, 152, 520c-3p, 302b, 302a, 302d, 496, 495, 302c, 494, 329, 302e, 101, 520e, 370, 454, 1271, 365, 362-3p, 19b, 19a, 212, 590-3p, 137, 136, 96, 190b, 132, 520d-3p, 374b, 135a, 135b, 184, 10a, 10b, 377, 205, 373, 372, 130b, 506, 130a, 203, 520a-3p
PAK1IP1 (55003) NM_017906	590-3p, 431, 141, 421, 433, 539, 145, 106b, 411, 200a, 106a, 93, 17, 20a, 425, 20b, 519d, 346, 140-5p, 505
MECP2 (4204) NM_001110792	448, 361-5p, 374a, 374b
MAX (4149) NM_145113	30e, 615-3p, 149, 485-5p, 1, 24, 22, 362-3p, 193b, 335, 339-5p, 376c, 708, 320d, 320c, 488, 214, 137, 320a, 320b, 193a-3p, 613, 381, 382, 206, 28-5p, 377, 31, 328, 300, 329, 494, 873
MAX (4149) NM_145114	127-3p, 421, 15a, 32, 539, 195, 133a, 133b, 186, 485-5p, 497, 15b, 23a, 23b
AKAP5 (9495) NM_004857	361-5p, 143, 185, 186, 520b, 1, 1297, 191, 335, 708, 330-5p, 23a, 23b, 301b, 155, 421, 129-5p, 613, 429, 425, 519d, 653, 520c-3p, 32, 590-5p, 302b, 222, 223, 302a, 326, 302d, 302c, 221, 302e, 181d, 200b, 410, 200c, 411, 520e, 370, 128, 20a, 29a, 181a, 454, 29b, 181c, 29c, 20b, 181b, 25, 146a, 21, 367, 218, 363, 211, 448, 590-3p, 136, 146b-5p, 26a, 106b, 92b, 106a, 93, 92a, 17, 544, 382, 543, 520d-3p, 206, 183, 204, 377, 182, 216b, 373, 340, 372, 300, 26b, 499-5p, 520a-3p
CYP19A1 (1588) NM_000103	539, 186, 520b, 1, 1297, 190, 194, 488, 23a, 23b, 18a, 18b, 613, 197, 425, 519d, 520c-3p, 32, 371-5p, 590-5p, 302b, 302a, 302d, 496, 302c, 103, 181d, 30c, 410, 30d, 30e, 520e, 30a, 30b, 181a, 107, 181c, 25, 181b, 20b, 21, 219-5p, 367, 363, 376c, 212, 448, 137, 590-3p, 136, 98, 26a, 190b, 132, 92b, 93, 92a, 544, 520d-3p, let-7d, 206, 183, let-7e, let-7b, 377, 182, let-7c, 216a, let-7a, 216b, 373, 372, 130b, 26b, 130a, 499-5p, let-7i, let-7f, let-7g, 873
NFATC3 (4775) NM_173165	137, 590-3p, 361-5p, 129-5p, 15a, 101, 410, 185, 370, 374b, 29a, 29b, 29c, 16, 424, 384, 371-5p, 195, 340, 328, 374a, 497, 15b, 494
CCL5 (6352) NM_002985	155, 146a, 599, 146b-5p, 33b, 33a, 335, 411, 758, 503
TCF4 (6925) NM_001083962	361-5p, 141, 139-5p, 145, 7, 186, 27a, 27b, 383, 148a, 190, 148b, 193b, 335, 301a, 374a, 708, 301b, 155, 129-5p, 421, 153, 152, 193a-3p, 519d, 653, 28-5p, 32, 590-5p, 223, 495, 124, 181d, 103, 101, 200b, 410, 30c, 200c, 200a, 128, 29a, 20a, 542-3p, 107, 454, 29b, 29c, 25, 20b, 367, 218, 376c, 19a, 211, 590-3p, 448, 137, 320a, 320b, 33b, 33a, 190b, 96, 106b, 93, 106a, 544, 17, 382, 374b, 299-3p, 135a, 135b, 138, 379, 183, 377, 204, 216b, 340, 130b, 506, 324-5p, 875-5p, 130a, 202, 203

Gene Symbol (Entrez Gene ID) Transcript ID	miRNAs
ECSIT (51295) NM_016581	143
NFATC3 (4775) NM_173163	361-5p, 101, 15a, 410, 185, 370, 29a, 29b, 29c, 384, 195, 339-5p, 374a, 15b, 150, 137, 590-3p, 129-5p, 18a, 18b, 374b, 16, 424, 371-5p, 340, 328, 497, 494
PTEN (5728) NM_000314	141, 144, 193b, 301a, 320d, 320c, 23a, 23b, 301b, 155, 154, 153, 152, 193a-3p, 519d, 28-5p, 103, 296-3p, 30c, 200b, 200c, 30d, 30e, 200a, 30a, 30b, 107, 454, 219-5p, 486-5p, 19b, 19a, 590-3p, 136, 320a, 320b, 26a, 92b, 92a, 374b, 10a, 10b, 505, 26b, 875-5p, 539, 139-5p, 185, 186, 485-5p, 1297, 148a, 190, 148b, 374a, 708, 18a, 18b, 429, 425, 653, 32, 328, 223, 496, 495, 494, 181d, 410, 455-5p, 20a, 29a, 181a, 29b, 542-3p, 181c, 29c, 20b, 181b, 25, 146a, 22, 365, 367, 363, 125a-3p, 214, 146b-5p, 190b, 106b, 93, 106a, 17, 543, 382, 338-3p, 205, 216a, 216b, 372, 340, 130b, 130a
IKBKB (3551) NM_001556	15a, 200b, 200c, 34a, 1, 146a, 22, 148a, 148b, 218, 195, 708, 19a, 15b, 214, 590-3p, 155, 448, 199a-5p, 136, 153, 152, 146b-5p, 613, 429, 199b-5p, 16, 424, 206, 653, 183, 28-5p, 377, 224, 497, 499-5p, 203, 874, 494
MAPKAPK2 (9261) NM_032960	137, 136, 320a, 320b, 433, 539, 9, 7, 24, 34c-5p, 183, 486-5p, 362-3p, 31, 335, 224, 506, 875-5p, 496, 495, 329
BTRC (8945) NM_033637	143, 433, 149, 186, 1, 193b, 195, 708, 199a-5p, 421, 613, 193a-3p, 491-5p, 424, 28-5p, 32, 31, 224, 497, 221, 495, 329, 103, 181d, 15a, 410, 181a, 107, 181c, 181b, 25, 362-3p, 367, 339-5p, 363, 125a-3p, 211, 212, 15b, 214, 136, 132, 92b, 92a, 543, 199b-5p, 16, 206, 182, 204, 505, 130b, 874, let-7f
MMP2 (4313) NM_004530	296-3p, 34a, 485-5p, 20a, 20b, 142-3p, 376c, 488, 449b, 449a, 125a-5p, 214, 137, 448, 136, 153, 421, 106b, 93, 106a, 17, 299-3p, 34c-5p, 424, 653, 519d, 130b, 125b, 328, 551a, 551b
TIFA (92610) NM_052864	144, 539, 149, 186, 485-5p, 27a, 27b, 191, 374a, 330-5p, 155, 199a-5p, 429, 140-5p, 196b, 328, 222, 196a, 326, 495, 494, 181d, 410, 200b, 30c, 200c, 30d, 30e, 30a, 30b, 128, 181a, 542-3p, 181c, 181b, 146a, 376a, 376b, 342-3p, 125a-3p, 212, 590-3p, 146b-5p, 134, 132, 543, 374b, 338-3p, 205, 499-5p, 873
TNFSF11 (8600) NM_003701	141, 144, 539, 145, 139-5p, 186, 190, 195, 335, 194, 301a, 374a, 488, 301b, 421, 129-5p, 429, 197, 425, 424, 653, 519d, 32, 31, 224, 328, 497, 450a, 496, 495, 329, 494, 124, 181d, 15a, 101, 200b, 410, 30c, 200c, 30d, 200a, 30a, 370, 30b, 181a, 29a, 20a, 29b, 454, 542-3p, 181c, 29c, 20b, 1271, 25, 181b, 22, 217, 362-3p, 367, 486-5p, 363, 342-3p, 19b, 19a, 15b, 448, 590-3p, 33b, 96, 33a, 190b, 132, 92b, 106b, 93, 106a, 92a, 544, 17, 543, 374b, 338-3p, 16, 10b, 378, 183, 377, 182, 205, 340, 130b, 505, 422a, 506, 324-5p, 130a, 203
CDKN2A (1029) NM_058195	590-3p, 365, 136, 134, 410, 9, 340, 544, 186, 125b, 128, 125a-5p
CDKN2A (1029) NM_058197	590-3p, 136, 134, 410, 9, 544, 186, 128, 365, 340, 125b, 23a, 125a-5p, 23b, 214
CHEK2 (11200) NM_001005735	134, 340, 381, 300, 495, 542-3p, 425
PAK2 (5062) NM_002577	144, 143, 433, 139-5p, 7, 185, 186, 520b, 1297, 383, 195, 301a, 708, 374a, 23a, 23b, 301b, 155, 129-5p, 429, 425, 424, 28-5p, 520c-3p, 32, 328, 222, 302b, 302a, 497, 196a, 496, 302d, 495, 221, 302c, 302e, 181d, 15a, 200b, 200c, 455-5p, 520e, 451, 181c, 181b, 25, 362-3p, 376a, 376b, 342-3p, 15b, 212, 137, 590-3p, 136, 26a, 132, 92a, 543, 520d-3p, 374b, 16, let-7c, 377, 216a, 216b, 373, 372, 26b, 520a-3p
KLRC3 (3823) NM_007333	590-3p, 410, 425
CD58 (965) NM_001779	155, 15a, 599, 200b, 539, 200c, 382, 429, 374b, 29b, 135a, 135b, 16, 216a, 195, 374a, 15b
DNMT3A (1788) NM_022552	144, 143, 599, 101, 296-3p, 410, 30c, 200b, 30d, 139-5p, 200c, 30e, 186, 27a, 30a, 370, 27b, 30b, 29a, 29b, 29c, 335, 194, 374a, 330-5p, 488, 211, 212, 150, 129-5p, 132, 193a-3p, 543, 429, 374b, 377, 204, 216a, 340, 224, 876-5p, 875-5p, 551a, 551b, 495
CDK1 (983) NM_001786	181d, 143, 410, 411, 7, 186, 181a, 181c, 181b, 146a, 217, 362-3p, 376a, 335, 194, 590-3p, 154, 129-5p, 146b-5p, 543, 382, 31, 371-5p, 208a, 208b, 499-5p, 203, 495, 329, 494

Gene Symbol (Entrez Gene ID) Transcript ID	miRNAs
CASP2 (835) NM_032983	361-5p, 145, 185, 186, 485-5p, 520b, 1, 383, 190, 335, 374a, 320d, 708, 320c, 449b, 449a, 429, 519d, 28-5p, 520c-3p, 31, 495, 494, 329, 181d, 200b, 200c, 122, 34a, 455-5p, 451, 20a, 542-3p, 1271, 20b, 146a, 362-3p, 339-5p, 376c, 342-3p, 19b, 19a, 448, 320a, 146b-5p, 320b, 96, 190b, 106b, 93, 106a, 17, 544, 382, 520d-3p, 34c-5p, 10a, 206, 183, 10b, 377, 551a, 203, 551b, 520a-3p, 873
CFLAR (8837) NM_003879	519d, 106b, 93, 106a, 17, 149, 20a, 150, 504, 20b
CASP2 (835) NM_032982	185, 186, 485-5p, 1, 383, 190, 374a, 708, 320d, 320c, 449b, 449a, 429, 519d, 28-5p, 31, 495, 494, 329, 181d, 200b, 200c, 122, 34a, 455-5p, 451, 20a, 542-3p, 1271, 20b, 146a, 362-3p, 339-5p, 342-3p, 320a, 146b-5p, 320b, 190b, 96, 106b, 93, 106a, 17, 299-3p, 34c-5p, 10a, 206, 10b, 183, let-7e, 346, let-7b, 377, 551a, 551b, 203, let-7f, 873
CFLAR (8837) NM_001127184	590-3p, 34a, 194, 381, 186, 300, 449b, 495, 449a, 34c-5p
MAPT (4137) NM_001123066	181d, 361-5p, 320a, 320b, 539, 132, 34a, 185, 186, 197, 181a, 181c, 181b, 34c-5p, 383, 342-3p, 320d, 210, 320c, 449b, 449a, 212
TNFSF4 (7292) NM_003326	124, 181d, 141, 143, 101, 200b, 539, 200c, 200a, 485-5p, 181a, 181c, 1271, 181b, 146a, 148a, 148b, 486-5p, 376c, 374a, 125a-5p, 590-3p, 146b-5p, 96, 18a, 18b, 381, 543, 429, 138, 205, 216b, 224, 125b, 506, 300, 874
IL20 (50604) NM_018724	103, 15a, 200b, 539, 186, 107, 1297, 362-3p, 195, 342-3p, 374a, 15b, 590-3p, 155, 448, 154, 153, 98, 26a, 381, 374b, 16, 424, let-7d, let-7e, let-7b, let-7c, let-7a, 340, 300, 26b, 497, let-7i, 503, let-7f, let-7g
STAT3 (6774) NM_139276	124, 181d, 410, 485-5p, 29a, 20a, 181a, 454, 29b, 29c, 181c, 181b, 20b, 21, 301a, 342-3p, 125a-3p, 320d, 320c, 211, 301b, 125a-5p, 320a, 129-5p, 320b, 106b, 106a, 93, 544, 17, 519d, 204, 372, 130b, 125b, 506, 590-5p, 130a, 499-5p, 495, 329, 874
CRK (1398) NM_016823	141, 361-5p, 145, 186, 27a, 27b, 520b, 191, 193b, 192, 194, 449b, 449a, 490-3p, 193a-3p, 133a, 133b, 519d, 653, 520c-3p, 31, 328, 302b, 302a, 302d, 302c, 329, 302e, 34a, 200a, 520e, 370, 181a, 20a, 181c, 20b, 142-3p, 215, 362-3p, 212, 136, 132, 106b, 106a, 93, 17, 381, 520d-3p, 34c-5p, 183, 373, 372, 208a, 208b, 300, 499-5p, 203, 520a-3p, 874
SMAD6 (4091) NM_005585	144, 143, 539, 7, 186, 520b, 1297, 374a, 488, 330-5p, 23a, 23b, 155, 429, 425, 653, 519d, 520c-3p, 32, 371-5p, 196b, 302b, 302a, 196a, 326, 302d, 495, 302c, 329, 302e, 103, 410, 200b, 200c, 520e, 29a, 20a, 29b, 107, 29c, 25, 20b, 362-3p, 367, 363, 210, 590-3p, 136, 98, 33b, 134, 26a, 33a, 92b, 106b, 106a, 93, 92a, 381, 17, 374b, 520d-3p, 379, let-7d, let-7e, let-7h, 377, let-7c, 216a, let-7a, 373, 340, 372, 300, 26b, 499-5p, let-7i, 520a-3p, let-7f, let-7g
TRAF6 (7189) NM_004620	124, 141, 200b, 410, 200c, 200a, 146a, 194, 374a, 320c, 448, 136, 154, 320a, 421, 146b-5p, 320b, 490-3p, 429, 374b, 378, 196b, 422a, 506, 196a, 202, 496, 873
TLX2 (3196) NM_016170	34a, 449b, 449a, 34c-5p
STAT1 (6772) NM_007315	155, 448, 590-3p, 421, 144, 146b-5p, 599, 152, 455-5p, 185, 382, 20b, 34c-5p, 146a, 519d, 148a, 140-5p, 26b, 223, 203, 495, 494
ZFYVE9 (9372) NM_007323	155, 204, 223, 211, 203, 425
ZNF423 (23090) NM_015069	145, 7, 186, 195, 335, 374a, 488, 330-5p, 23a, 23b, 153, 429, 425, 424, 32, 224, 328, 326, 497, 494, 181d, 296-3p, 15a, 200b, 410, 200c, 451, 181b, 25, 22, 217, 367, 486-5p, 363, 376c, 342-3p, 19b, 19a, 211, 15b, 214, 136, 134, 374b, 16, 346, 204, 377, 216a, 216b, 506, 203, 503, 873
SH2D1B (117157) NM_053282	186, 1, 194, 320d, 488, 320c, 23a, 23b, 421, 613, 429, 653, 519d, 224, 223, 495, 181d, 200b, 30c, 30d, 200c, 30e, 30a, 30b, 181a, 128, 181c, 181b, 20b, 146a, 22, 376c, 590-3p, 136, 320a, 146b-5p, 320b, 93, 381, 135a, 138, 135b, 206, 183, 377, 216a, 340, 422a, 505, 300, 203, 504
CALR (811) NM_004343	590-3p, 383, 143, 375, 216a, 539, 145, 31, 543, 125a-3p, 203
MALT1 (10892) NM_006785	433, 539, 485-5p, 520b, 1297, 190, 192, 374a, 199a-5p, 154, 613, 429, 653, 520c-3p, 371-5p, 590-5p, 302b, 302a, 496, 302d, 495, 302c, 329, 302e, 181d, 599, 410, 200b, 200c, 30e, 520e, 181a, 181c, 181b, 215, 146a, 21, 362-3p, 218, 376a, 376b, 19b, 19a, 137, 590-3p, 146b-5p, 190b, 26a, 543, 199b-5p, 520d-3p, 206, 373, 372, 876-5p, 875-5p, 26b, 130a, 520a-3p

(continued)

Table 2 (continued)

Gene Symbol (Entrez Gene ID) Transcript ID	miRNAs
IL29 (282618) NM_172140	448, 153, 218, 340, 544, 590-5p, 210, 30b, 19b, 19a, 24
CDK4 (1019) NM_000075	124, 136, 539, 9, 613, 1, 206, 183, 486-5p, 216b, 340, 196b, 506, 196a
MAP3K12 (7786) NM_006301	296-3p, 410, 30c, 30d, 122, 30e, 186, 370, 30a, 30b, 128, 20a, 454, 20b, 22, 217, 191, 190, 367, 301a, 125a-3p, 374a, 19b, 19a, 150, 301b, 590-3p, 199a-5p, 190b, 106b, 106a, 93, 17, 381, 199b-5p, 374b, 299-3p, 519d, 340, 140-5p, 130b, 125b, 300, 130a
JAK2 (3717) NM_004972	144, 433, 143, 9, 139-5p, 1297, 384, 193b, 374a, 320d, 320c, 23a, 23b, 155, 490-3p, 193a-3p, 133a, 133b, 197, 425, 32, 371-5p, 181d, 101, 410, 30c, 30d, 411, 370, 30b, 181a, 181c, 25, 181b, 367, 376a, 376b, 363, 211, 590-3p, 320a, 320b, 26a, 92b, 92a, 381, 543, 374b, 135a, 135b, 377, 204, 216a, 375, 216b, 300, 26b, 203
MAP4K1 (11184) NM_001042600	143
GNL3 (26354) NM_014366	143, 300, 374a, 374b
DDIT3 (1649) NM_004083	144, 98, 101, 96, 381, 299-3p, 542-3p, 24, 1271, let-7d, 142-3p, let-7b, let-7c, 216a, 376a, let-7a, 216b, 376b, 340, 224, 300, 150
TNFRSF4 (7293) NM_003327	346, 98
CRADD (8738) NM_003805	590-3p, 181d, 26a, 543, 186, 181a, 181c, 1297, 181b, 10a, 10b, 365, 26b, 495, 494, 23a, 23b
TICAM1 (148022) NM_182919	590-3p, 206, 30c, 30d, 145, 30e, 30a, 374a, 374b, 30b, 1
PRKCA (5578) NM_002737	590-3p, 154, 599, 186, 374a, 374b, 873
PRKDC (5591) NM_006904	155, 136, 141, 320a, 129-5p, 320b, 539, 9, 145, 200a, 455-5p, 381, 186, 218, 320d, 300, 488, 320c, 495, 203, 150, 874
PRMT1 (3276) NM_001536	455-5p, 328, 494
KLRC2 (3822) NM_002260	590-3p, 361-5p, 129-5p, 152, 599, 539, 374b, 197, 383, 377, 182, 148b, 190, 140-5p, 125b, 374a, 324-5p, 125a-5p
TNFSF10 (8743) NM_003810	361-5p, 200b, 200c, 139-5p, 122, 455-5p, 362-3p, 590-3p, 137, 154, 98, 153, 129-5p, 33b, 33a, 490-3p, 429, 197, let-7d, let-7e, let-7b, 377, let-7c, let-7a, 373, 372, 340, let-7i, 494, 329, let-7f, let-7g
IGF1R (3480) NM_000875	186, 520e, 520b, 448, 98, 146b-5p, 429, let-7d, let-7e, 182, let-7b, 520c-3p, let-7c, let-7a, 373, 505, 302b, 223, 302a, 302d, 302c, let-7i, 494, let-7f, 520a-3p, 302e, let-7g
HDAC9 (9734) NM_058176	590-3p, 410, 374a, 374b
CASP3 (836) NM_032991	144, 139-5p, 149, 1, 384, 190, 374a, 320d, 320c, 23a, 23b, 155, 153, 421, 613, 490-3p, 197, 28-5p, 140-5p, 222, 495, 221, 494, 329, 103, 101, 200b, 30c, 200c, 30d, 30e, 30a, 30b, 107, 362-3p, 376c, 342-3p, 590-3p, 137, 98, 320a, 320b, 190b, 543, 382, 374b, 138, let-7d, 206, let-7e, let-7b, 182, let-7c, let-7a, 203, let-7i, let-7f, let-7g
IL8 (3576) NM_000584	361-5p, 431, 185, 186, 520b, 374a, 23a, 23b, 125a-5p, 154, 129-5p, 429, 653, 519d, 520c-3p, 32, 328, 302b, 302a, 302d, 302c, 495, 494, 302e, 124, 181d, 296-3p, 410, 200b, 30c, 200c, 30d, 30e, 520e, 30a, 30b, 128, 20a, 25, 20b, 181b, 217, 367, 363, 376c, 19b, 19a, 448, 590-3p, 92b, 106b, 106a, 93, 92a, 17, 382, 374b, 520d-3p, 10a, 183, 10b, 182, 216b, 373, 340, 372, 876-5p, 125b, 506, 203, 520a-3p, 873, 504
MAP3K5 (4217) NM_005923	144, 101, 599, 296-3p, 200b, 30c, 539, 30d, 200c, 139-5p, 30e, 30a, 370, 30b, 20a, 454, 20b, 22, 217, 301a, 19b, 19a, 23a, 301b, 23b, 448, 155, 137, 590-3p, 199a-5p, 106b, 93, 106a, 17, 544, 199b-5p, 429, 425, 519d, 183, 371-5p, 340, 130b, 130a, 221, 495, 203, 494
IL6ST (3572) NM_002184	143, 520e, 27a, 27b, 520b, 1, 142-3p, 218, 376a, 376b, 590-3p, 613, 382, 520d-3p, 206, 520c-3p, 373, 372, 224, 302b, 223, 302a, 302d, 499-5p, 302c, 520a-3p, 302e, 873
IL1RL2 (8808) NM_003854	132, 212
PREX2 (80243) NM_024870	103, 136, 28-5p, 33b, 33a, 340, 7, 708, 497, 338-3p, 107
PLK1 (5347) NM_005030	181d, 486-5p, 101, 455-5p, 181a, 23a, 23b, 181b
LTB (4050) NM_002341	132, 212

Gene Symbol (Entrez Gene ID) Transcript ID	miRNAs
MAPKAPK5 (8550) NM_139078	137, 590-3p, 361-5p, 15a, 381, 186, 299-3p, 424, 16, 653, 383, 195, 376c, 300, 497, 495, 15b, 203, 503, 214
CISH (1154) NM_145071	181d, 361-5p, 433, 7, 181a, 181c, 24, 181b, 142-3p, 22, 21, 374a, 488, 98, 374b, 135b, let-7d, let-7e, 378, let-7b, let-7c, let-7a, 422a, 324-5p, 202, let-7i, let-7f, let-7g
TNFSF15 (9966) NM_005118	124, 431, 181d, 145, 186, 451, 181a, 181c, 181b, 383, 376a, 376b, 150, 190b, 381, 543, 299-3p, 653, 31, 140-5p, 506, 300, 495, 874, 504, 873
TNFSF9 (8744) NM_003811	433, 30c, 410, 30d, 122, 30e, 485-5p, 30a, 30b, 374a, 98, 33b, 33a, 381, 374b, let-7d, let-7e, let-7b, 377, 182, let-7c, let-7a, 300, let-7i, let-7f, let-7g
PSMB9 (5698) NM_148954	204, 433, 328, 125b, 222, 211, 29b, 125a-5p
FKBP1A (2280) NM_000801	433, 186, 195, 301a, 374a, 320d, 320c, 301b, 421, 424, 32, 224, 497, 495, 181d, 15a, 410, 30c, 30d, 30e, 34a, 30a, 30b, 181a, 454, 542-3p, 181c, 181b, 25, 142-3p, 367, 218, 363, 376c, 15b, 448, 590-3p, 137, 320a, 320b, 92b, 92a, 543, 374b, 338-3p, 135a, 16, 135b, 183, 130b, 130a
NCR3 (259197) NM_001145466	378, 296-3p, 330-5p, 326, 24
ABCB1 (5243) NM_000927	181d, 200b, 30c, 200c, 30d, 30e, 185, 186, 30a, 30b, 181a, 181c, 181b, 142-3p, 374a, 19b, 19a, 23a, 23b, 214, 590-3p, 155, 421, 129-5p, 381, 429, 374b, 182, 216a, 371-5p, 875-5p, 223, 202, 496, 495, 494, 873
CDC7 (8317) NM_001134419	15a, 410, 30c, 30d, 30e, 455-5p, 186, 30a, 30b, 29a, 29b, 29c, 215, 192, 195, 335, 125a-3p, 488, 211, 15b, 212, 590-3p, 199a-5p, 33b, 132, 133a, 381, 133b, 199b-5p, 429, 16, 34c-5p, 183, 204, 216a, 371-5p, 340, 875-5p, 300, 223, 499-5p
PPARD (5467) NM_006238	181d, 191, 185, 149, 223, 19b, 19a, 24, 138
VHL (7428) NM_000551	141, 143, 101, 410, 200a, 185, 29a, 20a, 1, 20b, 21, 376c, 335, 320d, 320c, 211, 212, 23a, 23b, 590-3p, 136, 320a, 320b, 132, 106b, 93, 106a, 613, 381, 17, 653, 519d, 206, 204, 216a, 340, 590-5p, 300, 223, 496, 499-5p
NKX2-5 (1482) NM_004387	384, 367, 32, 92b, 363, 92a, 25
VAV2 (7410) NM_001134398	431, 433, 599, 410, 34a, 7, 370, 27a, 27b, 454, 1297, 148a, 148b, 301a, 19b, 19a, 449b, 449a, 150, 301b, 152, 26a, 34c-5p, 182, 216a, 216b, 130b, 505, 26b, 130a, 495
PXN (5829) NM_001080855	137, 132, 145, 7, 24, 204, 216b, 335, 505, 211, 495, 212, 203
CCL7 (6354) NM_006273	143, 433, 410, 7, 384, 320d, 374a, 19b, 320c, 19a, 23a, 23b, 98, 320a, 320b, 374b, 135a, 135b, let-7d, let-7e, let-7b, let-7c, 216a, 216b, let-7a, 324-5p, 223, let-7i, let-7f, let-7g
ZAK (51776) NM_016653	431, 181d, 143, 599, 410, 9, 122, 149, 181a, 181c, 181b, 142-3p, 384, 367, 219-5p, 194, 330-5p, 19b, 488, 19a, 211, 214, 590-3p, 155, 421, 490-3p, 613, 543, 382, 135a, 135b, 204, 371-5p, 422a, 140-5p, 505, 328, 326, 495, 873
CD4 (920) NM_000616	181d, 15a, 143, 539, 132, 491-5p, 544, 181a, 181c, 424, 181b, 16, 383, 195, 194, 222, 497, 212, 15b, 221
SERPINE1 (5054) NM_000602	181d, 143, 30c, 539, 30d, 145, 30e, 30a, 30b, 181a, 454, 181c, 181b, 215, 22, 148a, 218, 148b, 486-5p, 193b, 192, 342-3p, 301a, 19b, 488, 19a, 150, 301b, 590-3p, 129-5p, 421, 152, 134, 26a, 193a-3p, 197, 425, 10a, 10b, 224, 196b, 130b, 26b, 130a, 196a, 494
MAPK7 (5598) NM_002749	124, 143, 410, 200b, 200c, 34a, 128, 24, 148a, 148b, 374a, 330-5p, 488, 449b, 449a, 199a-5p, 152, 199b-5p, 429, 374b, 34c-5p, 138, 183, 182, 506
CFL1 (1072) NM_005507	103, 182, 219-5p, 491-5p, 543, 107, 150
GAB1 (2549) NM_207123	141, 539, 7, 186, 27a, 27b, 520b, 384, 383, 194, 301a, 330-5p, 449b, 449a, 23a, 150, 301b, 23b, 421, 129-5p, 153, 18a, 18b, 429, 519d, 520c-3p, 222, 302b, 302a, 326, 302d, 302c, 221, 302e, 181d, 101, 410, 30c, 200b, 200c, 30d, 30e, 34a, 200a, 520e, 30a, 30b, 181a, 20a, 454, 181c, 20b, 181b, 142-3p, 376a, 376b, 590-3p, 106b, 93, 106a, 17, 543, 374b, 520d-3p, 34c-5p, 205, 373, 340, 372, 26b, 520a-3p
LCP2 (3937) NM_005565	141, 144, 200b, 200c, 200a, 186, 370, 128, 454, 542-3p, 142-3p, 365, 148a, 148b, 301a, 212, 301b, 137, 199a-5p, 129-5p, 152, 33b, 33a, 132, 543, 199b-5p, 429, 758, 425, 138, 182, 216b, 371-5p, 505, 130b, 130a, 495, 203

Gene Symbol (Entrez Gene ID) Transcript ID	miRNAs
HOXC9 (3225) NM_006897	141, 431, 599, 539, 410, 200a, 187, 370, 520b, 1297, 193b, 342-3p, 320d, 320c, 150, 23a, 214, 23b, 129-5p, 320a, 320b, 134, 26a, 193a-3p, 520d-3p, 184, 520c-3p, 373, 372, 302b, 26b, 302a, 302d, 495, 302c, 302e
LBP (3929) NM_004139	383, 216b
SOCS3 (9021) NM_003955	9, 185, 485-5p, 520b, 1, 190, 148b, 193b, 301a, 488, 301b, 155, 152, 193a-3p, 613, 653, 520c-3p, 222, 302b, 302a, 302d, 495, 302c, 221, 302e, 30c, 410, 30d, 30e, 455-5p, 520e, 30a, 30b, 20a, 454, 20b, 218, 367, 339-5p, 19b, 19a, 134, 106a, 93, 17, 520d-3p, 379, 206, 216b, 373, 372, 340, 130b, 130a, 551a, 203, 551b, 520a-3p, 874
EXOC4 (60412) NM_021807	30c, 30d, 30e, 186, 149, 30a, 30b, 1271, 215, 384, 148a, 217, 148b, 192, 194, 211, 214, 136, 421, 152, 33b, 134, 33a, 96, 382, 653, 182, 204, 503, 873
EGF (1950) NM_001963	590-3p, 199a-5p, 181d, 134, 433, 539, 145, 199b-5p, 181a, 24, 181c, 181b, 190, 216a, 488, 499-5p, 873
PTK2B (2185) NM_173176	590-3p, 613, 491-5p, 185, 186, 1, 206, 378, 340, 422a, 224, 19b, 19a, 23a, 150, 23b
BCL2 (596) NM_000633	181d, 15a, 433, 185, 181a, 1, 181c, 181b, 384, 142-3p, 383, 365, 219-5p, 218, 190, 195, 342-3p, 374a, 211, 15b, 23a, 23b, 301b, 448, 137, 590-3p, 136, 190b, 613, 135a, 16, 135b, 424, 206, 204, 205, 216a, 371-5p, 876-5p, 590-5p, 450a, 497, 499-5p, 203, 874
PPARD (5467) NM_177435	590-3p, 153, 129-5p, 599, 149, 24
SHC1 (6464) NM_001130040	124, 361-5p, 296-3p, 9, 186, 1271, 365, 218, 219-5p, 335, 339-5p, 330-5p, 211, 150, 448, 153, 134, 96, 18a, 18b, 491-5p, 197, 299-3p, 204, 216b, 371-5p, 340, 506, 324-5p, 326, 203, 873
PSMB5 (5693) NM_002797	155, 142-3p, 376c, 455-5p
DOCK1 (1793) NM_001380	144, 433, 143, 539, 185, 186, 1271, 146a, 191, 21, 219-5p, 486-5p, 194, 374a, 708, 150, 214, 590-3p, 155, 136, 154, 146b-5p, 96, 381, 543, 374b, 338-3p, 28-5p, 31, 224, 300, 496
MMP7 (4316) NM_002423	155, 590-3p, 137, 181d, 152, 599, 122, 544, 543, 181a, 542-3p, 181c, 181b, 346, 218, 194, 876-5p, 19b, 19a, 494
IL1F9 (56300) NM_019618	361-5p, 143, 410, 29a, 29b, 29c, 22, 362-3p, 339-5p, 374a, 23a, 23b, 155, 129-5p, 98, 381, 425, let-7d, let-7e, 182, 377, let-7b, let-7c, let-7a, 340, 224, 590-5p, 208a, 208b, 300, 223, 202, 499-5p, let-7i, let-7f, 329, let-7g
IL32 (9235) NM_001012718	362-3p, 874, 329
SIGIRR (59307) NM_021805	378, 326
BCL2L1 (598) NM_138578	296-3p, 30c, 30d, 30e, 30a, 30b, 486-5p, 342-3p, 330-5p, 212, 98, 421, 132, 133a, 491-5p, 133b, let-7d, 184, let-7e, 377, let-7b, let-7c, let-7a, 31, 371-5p, 140-5p, 326, let-7i, 495, let-7f, let-7g
TLR7 (51284) NM_016562	127-3p, 599, 433, 101, 539, 9, 29a, 542-3p, 454, 146a, 148a, 148b, 301a, 708, 19b, 488, 19a, 214, 301b, 590-3p, 146b-5p, 152, 18a, 18b, 758, 34c-5p, 28-5p, 183, 216a, 340, 130b, 130a, 494, 504
LCK (3932) NM_001042771	448, 421, 153, 33b, 33a, 132, 18a, 18b, 185, 27a, 27b, 299-3p, 183, 328, 202, 212, 23a, 873, 23b
LTB (4050) NM_009588	22, 134, 132, 376c, 212
TNFRSF12A (51330) NM_016639	346, 193a-3p, 125a-3p, 149, 19b, 19a
HIF1A (3091) NM_001530	361-5p, 144, 143, 433, 139-5p, 186, 520b, 1, 384, 148a, 148b, 335, 194, 301a, 374a, 488, 301b, 155, 199a-5p, 153, 152, 18a, 613, 18b, 133a, 133b, 758, 653, 519d, 520c-3p, 371-5p, 222, 302b, 302a, 223, 302d, 302c, 221, 494, 302e, 103, 410, 411, 520e, 370, 20a, 454, 107, 542-3p, 20b, 1271, 142-3p, 365, 217, 376a, 376b, 376c, 210, 19b, 19a, 212, 448, 590-3p, 98, 33b, 33a, 96, 132, 106b, 106a, 93, 17, 543, 199b-5p, 520d-3p, 374b, 338-3p, 135a, 135b, 138, 206, let-7d, 346, let-7e, let-7b, 182, let-7c, let-7a, 373, 340, 372, 130b, 130a, 203, let-7f, 520a-3p
XPO1 (7514) NM_003400	143, 139-5p, 186, 27a, 485-5p, 27b, 1297, 190, 194, 374a, 320d, 320c, 129-5p, 133a, 133b, 429, 32, 371-5p, 196b, 224, 590-5p, 196a, 302a, 329, 103, 30c, 30d, 30e, 451, 30a, 30b, 542-3p, 107, 25, 181b, 1271, 142-3p, 146a, 365, 21, 362-3p, 376a, 376b, 376c, 363, 19b, 19a, 590-3p, 320a, 33b, 320b, 146b-5p, 96, 26a, 33a, 190b, 381, 382, 374b, 338-3p, 379, 182, 205, 216a, 373, 340, 26b, 300, 873
ACIN1 (22985) NM_014977	153, 106b, 18a, 18b, 106a, 93, 17, 186, 374b, 20a, 24, 20b, 519d, 376a, 376b, 376c, 340, 224, 422a, 374a, 326, 495
IL2RG (3561) NM_000206	let-7d, let-7b, 98, 421, let-7a, 491-5p, 505, 185, 128, 873, 504
IL17A (3605) NM_002190	296-3p, 30c, 200b, 30d, 200c, 30e, 122, 186, 485-5p, 30a, 30b, 25, 146a, 383, 367, 218, 363, 488, 19a, 150, 590-3p, 136, 146b-5p, 92b, 92a, 543, 429, 378, 182, 32, 371-5p, 505, 876-5p, 495, 494
CREBBP (1387) NM_004380	431, 361-5p, 181d, 141, 200b, 410, 539, 30c, 200c, 145, 30d, 30e, 200a, 186, 30a, 30b, 181a, 181c, 181b, 191, 376c, 374a, 488, 330-5p, 23a, 23b, 590-3p, 153, 544, 381, 543, 429, 374b, 653, 379, 204, 205, 340, 300, 326, 203, 495, 494
CXCL1 (2919) NM_001511	141, 181d, 296-3p, 539, 410, 200a, 520e, 186, 27a, 27b, 181a, 520b, 128, 181c, 181b, 218, 376a, 376b, 363, 376c, 374a, 211, 590-3p, 421, 92b, 543, 520d-3p, 374b, 204, 520c-3p, 205, 371-5p, 216b, 373, 372, 505, 302b, 302a, 302d, 203, 302c, 494, 520a-3p, 873, 302e
RFXAP (5994) NM_000538	431, 200b, 200c, 122, 186, 27a, 27b, 20a, 29a, 29b, 454, 29c, 1297, 1271, 20b, 384, 362-3p, 218, 376c, 301a, 374a, 211, 301b, 137, 590-3p, 154, 199a-5p, 96, 26a, 106b, 106a, 93, 17, 543, 199b-5p, 429, 374b, 299-3p, 519d, 653, 378, 204, 140-5p, 505, 130b, 422a, 26b, 130a, 495, 494, 329
POU5F1 (5460) NM_002701	146b-5p, 433, 599, 106b, 106a, 93, 17, 20a, 299-3p, 20b, 384, 519d, 146a, 373, 335, 372, 339-5p, 302b, 302a, 302d, 150
CD74 (972) NM_001025158	653, 320a, 33b, 320b, 33a, 328, 485-5p, 320d, 320c, 24, 873, 16
IKBKG (8517) NM_001099856	134, 193a-3p, 34a, 185, 34c-5p, 193b, 140-5p, 125b, 324-5p, 449b, 449a, 503, 125a-5p
MAP3K14 (9020) NM_003954	539, 9, 122, 520e, 370, 20a, 520b, 454, 542-3p, 20b, 181b, 384, 362-3p, 301a, 301b, 214, 137, 155, 106b, 93, 106a, 133a, 17, 133b, 520d-3p, 299-3p, 519d, 346, 182, 520c-3p, 31, 373, 372, 130b, 302b, 302a, 130a, 302d, 302c, 520a-3p, 494, 329, 302e
CCL13 (6357) NM_005408	181d, 103, 33b, 33a, 544, 181a, 107, 181c, 181b, 379, 205, 32, 376c, 708, 324-5p, 19b, 19a, 23a, 23b
CD74 (972) NM_001025159	653, 320a, 33b, 320b, 33a, 328, 320d, 485-5p, 320c, 24, 16, 873
TNFRSF1B (7133) NM_001066	122, 454, 22, 148a, 148b, 301a, 488, 19b, 211, 19a, 301b, 98, 152, 491-5p, 520d-3p, 338-3p, let-7d, let-7e, 378, 204, let-7b, let-7c, let-7a, 422a, 130b, 130a, 495, let-7i, let-7f, let-7g
FCER1G (2207) NM_004106	30c, 30d, 30e, 194, 30a, 30b, 138
SUDS3 (64426) NM_022491	539, 9, 186, 384, 148a, 148b, 194, 335, 301a, 330-5p, 301b, 152, 429, 425, 653, 32, 224, 196b, 326, 196a, 496, 495, 181d, 30c, 30d, 30e, 200a, 30a, 370, 30b, 181a, 454, 542-3p, 181c, 24, 25, 181b, 218, 367, 363, 376c, 125a-3p, 212, 137, 136, 134, 26a, 132, 92b, 92a, 135a, 135b, 182, 216a, 372, 26b, 499-5p, 203, 873
HBEGF (1839) NM_001945	539, 145, 27a, 27b, 194, 708, 374a, 153, 491-5p, 758, 653, 32, 31, 140-5p, 495, 296-3p, 599, 410, 29a, 128, 29b, 542-3p, 29c, 1271, 25, 219-5p, 367, 376a, 376b, 376c, 363, 212, 98, 96, 132, 92b, 92a, 381, 382, 374b, 135a, 135b, 379, let-7d, let-7e, 183, 378, let-7b, 182, let-7c, let-7a, 340, 300, 202, 203, let-7i, let-7f, let-7g
TNFSF13B (10673) NM_006573	223
ATM (472) NM_000051	141, 431, 181d, 101, 599, 30c, 410, 200a, 181a, 454, 181c, 1297, 181b, 146a, 383, 217, 376a, 376b, 194, 339-5p, 301a, 374a, 211, 212, 214, 137, 421, 146b-5p, 26a, 190b, 132, 18a, 18b, 544, 543, 382, 374b, 204, 182, 26b, 203, 494, 873
BCL2A1 (597) NM_004049	181d, 182, 122, 376c, 411, 613, 381, 382, 300, 181c

(continued)

Table 2 (continued)

Gene Symbol (Entrez Gene ID) Transcript ID	miRNAs
IL6ST (3572) NM_175767	144, 143, 27a, 27b, 520b, 1297, 192, 421, 133a, 491-5p, 133b, 429, 758, 520c-3p, 224, 328, 302b, 302a, 223, 302d, 302c, 329, 494, 302e, 181d, 296-3p, 200b, 200c, 122, 455-5p, 520e, 370, 181a, 128, 181c, 181b, 142-3p, 215, 22, 217, 362-3p, 218, 125a-3p, 590-3p, 136, 146b-5p, 26a, 382, 520d-3p, 135a, 135b, 379, 378, 205, 373, 340, 372, 422a, 876-5p, 875-5p, 26b, 520a-3p, 873
KIAA0652 (9776) NM_001142673	15a, 539, 200c, 34a, 485-5p, 1, 454, 1297, 146a, 195, 335, 449b, 15b, 449a, 150, 214, 421, 98, 146b-5p, 26a, 613, 490-3p, 299-3p, 34c-5p, 16, 424, 184, 206, 378, 371-5p, 31, 422a, 505, 26b, 497, 551a, 551b, 503, 873
CARD10 (29775) NM_014550	155, 146a, 146b-5p, 185, 140-5p, 19b, 326, 330-5p, 19a, 338-3p, 150, 873
RAD50 (10111) NM_005732	124, 103, 181d, 433, 15a, 539, 122, 186, 181a, 128, 1, 107, 181c, 365, 190, 195, 194, 320d, 320c, 488, 15b, 212, 590-3p, 320a, 421, 134, 320b, 190b, 132, 424, 16, 206, 183, 340, 506, 497
S1PR3 (1903) NM_005226	149, 27a, 27b, 520b, 1297, 374a, 488, 449b, 449a, 23a, 150, 23b, 153, 129-5p, 429, 519d, 653, 520c-3p, 590-5p, 302b, 302a, 302d, 495, 302c, 494, 302e, 103, 200b, 30c, 200c, 30e, 34a, 520e, 30b, 20a, 107, 20b, 142-3p, 146a, 365, 218, 376a, 376c, 342-3p, 211, 146b-5p, 26a, 106b, 106a, 93, 17, 381, 520d-3p, 374b, 34c-5p, 204, 205, 373, 372, 340, 876-5p, 26b, 300, 499-5p, let-7i, 520a-3p, 874, let-7g
BRCA1 (672) NM_007299	141, 200b, 200c, 34a, 200a, 7, 186, 1, 24, 146a, 190, 218, 125a-3p, 320d, 320c, 449b, 15b, 212, 449a, 199a-5p, 153, 320a, 421, 146b-5p, 320b, 190b, 132, 613, 543, 429, 199b-5p, 34c-5p, 206, 205, 216b, 224, 494
NFATC1 (4772) NM_172387	124, 101, 143, 139-5p, 30e, 122, 455-5p, 542-3p, 218, 190, 194, 19b, 19a, 214, 125a-5p, 137, 190b, 381, 338-3p, 505, 125b, 506, 300, 223, 203, 503, 874
OAS1 (4938) NM_016816	137, 28-5p, 141, 148a, 152, 216b, 200a, 485-5p, 708, 374a, 374b, 873
NFATC1 (4772) NM_172388	124, 143, 101, 139-5p, 30e, 122, 455-5p, 542-3p, 190, 218, 194, 19b, 19a, 214, 125a-5p, 137, 190b, 381, 338-3p, 505, 125b, 506, 300, 223, 203, 503, 874
PTPN7 (5778) NM_002832	136, 98, 185, 425, 379, let-7d, let-7e, let-7b, let-7c, let-7a, 194, 499-5p, let-7i, let-7f, let-7g, 504
B2M (567) NM_004048	181d, 186, 20a, 181a, 454, 181c, 20b, 181b, 190, 339-5p, 301a, 15b, 150, 301b, 106b, 93, 106a, 17, 425, 424, 16, 519d, 205, 340, 130b, 130a, 497, 495
GNA13 (10672) NM_006572	361-5p, 141, 144, 433, 139-5p, 185, 186, 27a, 27b, 1297, 384, 191, 194, 320d, 320c, 155, 154, 153, 653, 371-5p, 31, 450a, 223, 495, 329, 122, 200a, 29a, 29b, 29c, 365, 217, 362-3p, 218, 125a-3p, 211, 136, 320a, 320b, 26a, 381, 135a, 135b, 183, 378, 182, 216b, 422a, 26b, 300, 875-5p, 203
BCL2L11 (10018) NM_138621	9, 149, 186, 384, 148a, 148b, 192, 301a, 708, 488, 150, 301b, 152, 32, 224, 222, 496, 221, 495, 124, 181d, 101, 30c, 30d, 30e, 30a, 370, 30b, 181a, 454, 24, 181c, 25, 181b, 215, 217, 486-5p, 367, 219-5p, 376a, 376b, 339-5p, 363, 19b, 19a, 590-3p, 92b, 92a, 382, 138, 10a, 10b, 377, 216b, 340, 130b, 208a, 506, 208b, 130a, 499-5p, 873
CYCS (54205) NM_018947	433, 139-5p, 34a, 186, 215, 367, 376a, 192, 376b, 363, 125a-3p, 449b, 449a, 23a, 23b, 590-3p, 153, 490-3p, 544, 34c-5p, 653, 378, 183, 377, 182, 32, 340, 140-5p, 328, 499-5p, 495
LEPR (3953) NM_002303	374a, 374b, 330-5p, 326, 150
PABPC1 (26986) NM_002568	181d, 144, 599, 101, 9, 139-5p, 186, 27a, 27b, 128, 181a, 1, 24, 181c, 181b, 146a, 218, 374a, 488, 155, 590-3p, 421, 129-5p, 146b-5p, 613, 133a, 133b, 382, 543, 374b, 206, 182, 204, 31, 340, 450a, 223, 496, 203, 494
TLR3 (7098) NM_003265	30c, 410, 539, 30d, 30e, 7, 30a, 374b, 30b, 758, 384, 219-5p, 218, 376a, 376b, 373, 376c, 224, 302b, 302a, 302d, 495, 302c, 302e
CXCL12 (6387) NM_000609	141, 144, 539, 9, 139-5p, 7, 185, 186, 520b, 1, 148a, 148b, 301a, 708, 23a, 301b, 23b, 153, 152, 133a, 133b, 429, 519d, 28-5p, 520c-3p, 302b, 222, 302a, 302d, 302c, 495, 221, 494, 302e, 101, 410, 200b, 200a, 520e, 20a, 128, 454, 542-3p, 20b, 19b, 19a, 137, 448, 590-3p, 136, 98, 106b, 106a, 93, 17, 520d-3p, 182, 216b, 373, 372, 130b, 208a, 208b, 130a, 499-5p, 520a-3p
WIPF1 (7456) NM_003387	141, 143, 539, 185, 186, 149, 374a, 23a, 23b, 153, 129-5p, 18a, 613, 18b, 429, 425, 653, 196b, 196a, 494, 124, 101, 200b, 30c, 410, 200c, 30d, 30e, 200a, 30a, 30b, 181a, 376a, 376b, 125a-3p, 19b, 19a, 212, 448, 590-3p, 136, 134, 132, 544, 374b, 135a, 135b, 206, 10a, 10b, 182, 216b, 340, 505, 506, 875-5p, 324-5p, 203
CKS1B (1163) NR_024163	124, 181d, 361-5p, 103, 539, 9, 485-5p, 20a, 29a, 181a, 107, 29b, 29c, 181c, 20b, 181b, 22, 383, 194, 150, 125a-5p, 136, 106b, 93, 106a, 17, 382, 197, 519d, 371-5p, 224, 506, 876-5p, 302b, 302a, 302d, 551a, 551b, 302c, 494
TOLLIP (54472) NM_019009	421, 144, 199-5p, 106b, 106a, 93, 7, 17, 544, 199b-5p, 20a, 128, 20b, 519d, 335, 499-5p, 212
CDT1 (81620) NM_030928	200b, 200c, 363, 224, 429
PIN1 (5300) NM_006221	200b, 200c, 140-5p, 370, 429, 488, 450a
ITGAX (3687) NM_000887	103, 431, 15a, 145, 186, 485-5p, 107, 195, 335, 339-5p, 330-5p, 15b, 150, 125a-5p, 214, 199a-5p, 491-5p, 338-3p, 425, 424, 16, 140-5p, 125b, 326, 497, 495
CHEK1 (1111) NM_001114121	146a, let-7d, let-7e, 383, 146b-5p, 449b, let-7i, 449a, let-7g
TAP1 (6890) NM_000593	653, 590-3p, 22, 28-5p, 361-5p, 26a, 340, 149, 708, 26b, 338-3p, 1297
CD3D (915) NM_000732	154, 24
SOCS1 (8651) NM_003745	433, 30c, 410, 30d, 30e, 186, 149, 30a, 30b, 215, 192, 374a, 210, 19b, 19a, 214, 155, 98, 544, 543, 374b, let-7d, let-7e, let-7b, let-7c, let-7a, 340, 372, 324-5p, 495, let-7i, let-7f, let-7g
ORC1L (4998) NM_004153	10a, 181d, 182, 455-5p, 339-5p, 376c, 125a-3p, 543, 181a, 181c, 504, 873, 181b
MCL1 (4170) NM_021960	361-5p, 144, 139-5p, 186, 27a, 520b, 1297, 383, 193b, 192, 374a, 320d, 488, 320c, 125a-5p, 153, 193a-3p, 133a, 133b, 197, 519d, 520c-3p, 32, 224, 302b, 302a, 496, 302d, 302c, 495, 302e, 101, 410, 520e, 20a, 128, 29a, 29b, 29c, 25, 20b, 215, 217, 367, 376c, 363, 448, 320a, 320b, 33a, 26a, 106b, 92b, 93, 106a, 92a, 381, 17, 382, 520d-3p, 374b, 373, 372, 130b, 125b, 300, 26b, 130a, 520a-3p, 873
APAF1 (317) NM_181869	431, 144, 143, 145, 186, 485-5p, 27a, 27b, 1297, 190, 335, 301a, 374a, 23a, 301b, 23b, 155, 429, 758, 196b, 590-5p, 222, 196a, 221, 101, 200b, 410, 200c, 454, 21, 367, 339-5p, 19b, 19a, 212, 590-3p, 136, 190b, 26a, 132, 381, 374b, 138, 379, 216a, 340, 130b, 26b, 300, 130a, 202, 874, 504
CREB1 (1385) NM_134442	590-3p, 653, 33b, 134, 33a, 301a, 130b, 27a, 130a, 27b, 454, 301b
ABL1 (25) NM_005157	361-5p, 141, 30c, 96, 30d, 30e, 200a, 106a, 17, 27a, 30a, 30b, 27b, 128, 1271, 10a, 10b, 335, 196b, 196a, 203, 494
TFDP1 (7027) NM_007111	431, 361-5p, 7, 185, 186, 148a, 148b, 194, 374a, 152, 491-5p, 758, 653, 28-5p, 371-5p, 224, 495, 494, 181d, 599, 101, 30c, 410, 30d, 30e, 30a, 30b, 128, 181a, 181c, 181b, 146a, 365, 339-5p, 212, 448, 590-3p, 146b-5p, 132, 93, 543, 374b, 338-3p, 379, 182, 340, 505, 499-5p, 873
EEF2K (29904) NM_013302	124, 296-3p, 145, 30e, 370, 30a, 30b, 20a, 181a, 20b, 22, 148a, 148b, 335, 320d, 320c, 488, 590-3p, 448, 136, 320a, 98, 152, 320b, 106b, 93, 106a, 17, 382, let-7d, let-7e, let-7b, let-7c, let-7a, 216b, 196b, 224, 506, 196a, 499-5p, 495, 203, let-7i, let-7f, 494, let-7g, 873
CNOT7 (29883) NM_013354	361-5p, 433, 9, 185, 186, 27a, 27b, 520b, 1, 148a, 148b, 335, 301a, 320d, 488, 320c, 301b, 129-5p, 421, 152, 613, 490-3p, 429, 519d, 520c-3p, 32, 590-5p, 302b, 222, 302a, 302d, 221, 495, 302c, 329, 302e, 599, 410, 200b, 30c, 30d, 200c, 30e, 520e, 30a, 30b, 128, 20a, 454, 1271, 20b, 25, 365, 367, 218, 363, 19b, 19a, 212, 590-3p, 136, 320a, 134, 320b, 96, 132, 106b, 92b, 93, 106a, 92a, 17, 544, 381, 520d-3p, 206, 377, 182, 375, 216b, 373, 372, 340, 505, 130b, 876-5p, 875-5p, 300, 130a, 499-5p, 520a-3p
APAF1 (317) NM_181861	431, 144, 143, 145, 186, 485-5p, 27a, 27b, 1297, 190, 335, 301a, 374a, 23a, 301b, 23b, 155, 429, 758, 196b, 590-5p, 222, 196a, 221, 101, 200b, 200c, 454, 21, 367, 339-5p, 19b, 19a, 212, 590-3p, 136, 26a, 190b, 132, 381, 374b, 138, 379, 216a, 130b, 300, 26b, 130a, 202, 874, 504
ORC3L (23595) NM_181837	191, 204, 144, 342-3p, 186, 495
AZU1 (566) NM_001700	185

Gene Symbol (Entrez Gene ID) Transcript ID	miRNAs
MADD (8567) NM_130475	431, 181d, 103, 15a, 491-5p, 185, 543, 299-3p, 181a, 107, 542-3p, 181c, 181b, 16, 424, 377, 486-5p, 195, 340, 19b, 497, 19a, 15b, 23a, 23b
MAP2K3 (5606) NM_145109	377, 421, 96, 339-5p, 18b, 491-5p, 590-5p, 19b, 19a, 449b, 449a, 1271
GRB2 (2885) NM_002086	124, 141, 433, 15a, 30c, 410, 30d, 30e, 200a, 185, 186, 27a, 30a, 30b, 27b, 128, 1271, 142-3p, 362-3p, 193b, 195, 376c, 320d, 320c, 15b, 590-3p, 137, 153, 320a, 320b, 96, 193a-3p, 16, 424, 378, 377, 182, 196b, 422a, 506, 196a, 497, 329, 873
PTPN22 (26191) NM_015967	431, 181d, 361-5p, 200b, 30c, 30d, 9, 200c, 145, 30e, 7, 186, 30a, 30b, 181a, 181c, 181b, 25, 190, 367, 219-5p, 193b, 363, 335, 320d, 320c, 23a, 23b, 448, 155, 590-3p, 136, 129-5p, 320a, 320b, 190b, 92b, 193a-3p, 92a, 429, 183, 182, 32, 340, 422a, 876-5p, 222, 221, 874
HNF1A (6927) NM_000545	320a, 320b, 34a, 299-3p, 542-3p, 34c-5p, 320d, 320c, 449b, 202, 449a, 503, 214
TNFRSF25 (8718) NM_003790	539, 544
IL2 (3558) NM_000586	181d, 361-5p, 410, 186, 181a, 181c, 181b, 190, 376a, 376b, 376c, 374a, 19b, 19a, 590-3p, 421, 98, 153, 190b, 132, 543, 374b, let-7d, let-7e, let-7b, let-7c, let-7a, 340, 505, 196b, 222, 196a, 499-5p, 221, let-7i, let-7f, let-7g
VAV1 (7409) NM_005428	124, 506
JAK3 (3718) NM_000215	144, 15a, 139-5p, 185, 485-5p, 195, 320d, 374a, 320c, 15b, 421, 320a, 320b, 374b, 424, 16, let-7e, let-7b, 505, 222, 497, 221, let-7i, 495, 504, let-7g
TNFRSF25 (8718) NM_001039664	127-3p, 200b, 200c
ARRB2 (409) NM_004313	155, 199a-5p, 181d, 296-3p, 491-5p, 185, 199b-5p, 181a, 181c, 181b, let-7e, 365, let-7b, let-7c, let-7a, 125a-3p, let-7i, 150, let-7f, let-7g
CCR5 (1234) NM_001100168	433, 7, 455-5p, 185, 186, 370, 485-5p, 1297, 215, 384, 21, 486-5p, 218, 148b, 192, 708, 211, 19a, 212, 150, 125a-5p, 448, 26a, 132, 18a, 18b, 544, 381, 382, 197, 377, 204, 205, 216a, 216b, 590-5p, 125b, 26b, 875-5p, 300, 203
CAPN2 (824) NM_001748	141, 144, 433, 9, 7, 186, 148a, 190, 148b, 194, 374a, 320d, 320c, 23a, 23b, 421, 129-5p, 152, 519d, 653, 196b, 590-5p, 495, 302c, 221, 124, 103, 101, 599, 20a, 107, 20b, 21, 19b, 19a, 212, 137, 590-3p, 320a, 320b, 190b, 132, 106b, 93, 106a, 17, 544, 876-5p, 875-5p, 499-5p
RHEB (6009) NM_005614	141, 144, 433, 539, 30c, 410, 30d, 30e, 200a, 185, 30a, 30b, 128, 542-3p, 1, 1297, 142-3p, 22, 365, 335, 194, 301a, 374a, 19b, 19a, 590-3p, 155, 137, 199a-5p, 154, 26a, 381, 133a, 133b, 199b-5p, 374b, 28-5p, 340, 224, 300, 26b, 203, 495, 874
PIK3CG (5294) NM_002649	137, 590-3p, 124, 421, 146b-5p, 143, 539, 139-5p, 122, 186, 370, 1, 542-3p, 142-3p, 206, 378, 204, 340, 422a, 224, 506, 875-5p, 203, 873
IL19 (29949) NM_153758	377, 411, 27a, 27b, 128, 221, 24
COL1A1 (1277) NM_000088	103, 143, 9, 185, 186, 29a, 107, 29b, 29c, 218, 376c, 335, 212, 590-3p, 154, 98, 129-5p, 132, 133a, 381, 133b, 338-3p, let-7d, let-7e, 182, let-7b, let-7c, 216a, 371-5p, let-7a, 196b, 328, 300, 196a, let-7i, 494, let-7f, let-7g
MDM4 (4194) NM_002393	340, 875-5p, 374a
CSF2 (1437) NM_000758	448, 590-3p, 144, 410, 30e, 613, 544, 30a, 374b, 1, 206, 346, 340, 876-5p, 374a, 223, 494
HMGB2 (3148) NM_001130689	361-5p, 539, 139-5p, 186, 1297, 384, 320d, 374a, 320c, 23a, 23b, 421, 153, 490-3p, 429, 519d, 371-5p, 496, 329, 181d, 200b, 410, 200c, 451, 20a, 181a, 181c, 20b, 181b, 217, 486-5p, 362-3p, 376c, 19b, 448, 590-3p, 320a, 320b, 33b, 26a, 33a, 106b, 93, 106a, 17, 381, 543, 374b, 135a, 135b, 377, 340, 208a, 300, 26b, 208b, 499-5p, 203, 873
ARHGEF11 (9826) NM_198236	144, 296-3p, 7, 20a, 128, 20b, 194, 374a, 488, 212, 214, 590-3p, 132, 106b, 93, 106a, 17, 491-5p, 381, 374b, 299-3p, 519d, 130b, 300, 496, 873
A2M (2) NM_000014	26a, 381, 187, 26b, 300, 1297
AIRE (326) NM_000383	129-5p, 143, 376c, 140-5p, 299-3p, 138
KLRC1 (3821) NM_002259	590-3p, 377, 182, 599, 190, 539, 139-5p, 381, 374a, 300, 374b, 197
STAT4 (6775) NM_003151	154, 141, 431, 320a, 320b, 132, 9, 122, 490-3p, 200a, 382, 299-3p, 384, 371-5p, 140-5p, 505, 320d, 320c, 210, 212, 150
TLR8 (51311) NM_138636	181d, 30c, 410, 30d, 30e, 30a, 27a, 30b, 27b, 128, 181a, 20a, 454, 181c, 181b, 22, 217, 218, 195, 376c, 590-3p, 448, 153, 129-5p, 106a, 17, 543, 758, 135a, 138, 16, 135b, 183, 494
FANCA (2175) NM_000135	181d, 454, 542-3p, 1297, 148a, 148b, 335, 301a, 23a, 23b, 301b, 199a-5p, 136, 152, 26a, 199b-5p, 758, 138, 378, 340, 422a, 130b, 140-5p, 324-5p, 26b, 130a, 503, 874
MAP3K7 (6885) NM_145333	141, 143, 539, 149, 520b, 195, 301a, 374a, 320d, 488, 320c, 153, 421, 129-5p, 424, 519d, 520c-3p, 196b, 224, 302b, 302a, 497, 196a, 302d, 302c, 329, 494, 302e, 181d, 103, 15a, 30c, 200b, 200c, 30d, 30e, 200a, 411, 520e, 30a, 370, 30b, 20a, 454, 107, 181b, 20b, 22, 217, 486-5p, 362-3p, 376b, 376c, 339-5p, 15b, 448, 590-3p, 137, 320a, 33b, 320b, 33a, 106b, 106a, 93, 381, 17, 382, 374b, 520d-3p, 138, 16, 10a, 10b, 377, 375, 373, 372, 300, 875-5p, 503, 520a-3p
TSC1 (7248) NM_000368	361-5p, 126, 433, 27a, 370, 451, 27b, 181a, 454, 542-3p, 25, 384, 142-3p, 367, 363, 335, 301a, 374a, 320d, 320c, 19b, 211, 19a, 301b, 98, 320a, 320b, 92b, 92a, 382, 543, 374b, 338-3p, let-7d, let-7e, 183, let-7b, 204, let-7c, 32, 31, let-7a, 130b, 130a, 202, let-7i, let-7f, let-7g
MAP4K4 (9448) NM_145686	141, 139-5p, 145, 186, 148a, 148b, 190, 449b, 449a, 23a, 150, 23b, 154, 153, 152, 490-3p, 429, 197, 758, 424, 224, 497, 494, 181d, 200b, 30c, 200c, 30d, 30e, 411, 200a, 34a, 370, 30a, 30b, 454, 1271, 25, 217, 590-3p, 98, 33b, 33a, 96, 190b, 544, 374b, 34c-5p, 10a, let-7d, 10b, let-7e, let-7b, 182, 377, let-7c, let-7a, 340, 506, 208a, 208b, 499-5p, let-7i, let-7f, let-7g
MAP3K7 (6885) NM_145331	141, 144, 143, 539, 149, 520b, 195, 301a, 374a, 153, 421, 129-5p, 424, 519d, 520c-3p, 224, 302b, 450a, 302a, 497, 302d, 302c, 494, 329, 302e, 181d, 103, 15a, 101, 200b, 30c, 200c, 30d, 30e, 200a, 520e, 30a, 30b, 20a, 454, 107, 181b, 20b, 22, 217, 362-3p, 376b, 376c, 339-5p, 15b, 212, 590-3p, 448, 33a, 132, 106b, 106a, 93, 17, 381, 520d-3p, 374b, 16, 10a, 10b, 377, 375, 373, 372, 875-5p, 300, 503, 520a-3p
CD83 (9308) NM_004233	141, 15a, 539, 410, 30d, 139-5p, 122, 30e, 200a, 186, 30a, 485-5p, 370, 29a, 29b, 29c, 1271, 383, 148a, 148b, 190, 218, 195, 194, 342-3p, 708, 214, 590-3p, 137, 199a-5p, 134, 190b, 96, 613, 381, 199b-5p, 299-3p, 183, 377, 300, 223, 504, 873
IFNAR1 (3454) NM_000629	361-5p, 141, 433, 15a, 599, 200a, 149, 30a, 27a, 370, 27b, 384, 195, 301a, 15b, 301b, 448, 153, 544, 382, 424, 16, 497, 499-5p, 203
DEFA1B (728358) NM_001042500	544
MMP3 (4314) NM_002422	15a, 520e, 520b, 20a, 29b, 20b, 365, 195, 15b, 214, 134, 106b, 18a, 106a, 18b, 93, 17, 520d-3p, 16, 424, 519d, 377, 520c-3p, 205, 31, 373, 372, 590-5p, 302b, 497, 302a, 302d, 302c, 520a-3p, 874, 302e
MEF2D (4209) NM_005920	103, 410, 30c, 30d, 30e, 455-5p, 30a, 30b, 107, 1271, 25, 365, 367, 363, 342-3p, 374a, 421, 92b, 18a, 92a, 18b, 374b, 299-3p, 182, 205, 216a, 32, 505, 223
EIF4B (1975) NM_001417	431, 139-5p, 145, 185, 383, 190, 193b, 195, 320d, 320c, 150, 129-5p, 18a, 193a-3p, 18b, 133a, 133b, 429, 424, 497, 495, 329, 103, 15a, 200b, 410, 200c, 411, 29b, 107, 24, 365, 217, 362-3p, 376a, 376b, 339-5p, 376c, 342-3p, 19b, 211, 19a, 15b, 590-3p, 448, 136, 320a, 320b, 190b, 16, 377, 204, 182, 216a, 422a, 503
PARP1 (142) NM_001618	539, 9, 7, 186, 520b, 148a, 148b, 335, 301a, 301b, 155, 152, 613, 429, 197, 519d, 520c-3p, 31, 302b, 222, 223, 302a, 302d, 496, 221, 302c, 302e, 103, 200b, 200c, 520e, 20a, 181a, 454, 107, 20b, 19b, 19a, 98, 33b, 33a, 106b, 93, 106a, 17, 520d-3p, 379, let-7d, let-7e, let-7b, let-7c, let-7a, 216b, 373, 372, 130b, 208a, 208b, 130a, 203, let-7i, let-7f, 520a-3p, let-7g
SMAD3 (4088) NM_005902	181d, 15a, 145, 181a, 181c, 181b, 195, 374a, 330-5p, 15b, 23a, 23b, 590-3p, 153, 490-3p, 544, 374b, 135a, 424, 16, 135b, 371-5p, 326, 497, 495
HSP90AA1 (3320) NM_001017963	361-5p, 410, 9, 411, 185, 186, 520e, 370, 520b, 1, 1271, 217, 148a, 148b, 134, 152, 26a, 96, 520d-3p, 206, 377, 520c-3p, 373, 340, 302b, 26b, 302a, 302d, 495, 302c, 520a-3p

(continued)

Table 2 (continued)

Gene Symbol (Entrez Gene ID) Transcript ID	miRNAs
CDC25B (994) NM_021873	124, 141, 15a, 200b, 200c, 200a, 370, 148a, 148b, 195, 211, 212, 15b, 214, 421, 152, 132, 429, 299-3p, 425, 424, 16, let-7d, 184, let-7e, let-7b, 204, 377, 205, let-7a, 506, 497, let-7i, 874, let-7g
RBBP7 (5931) NM_002893	181d, 431, 101, 539, 139-5p, 520e, 370, 181a, 520b, 20a, 181c, 20b, 181b, 384, 487b, 19b, 19a, 590-3p, 448, 155, 421, 153, 106b, 106a, 93, 544, 17, 543, 520d-3p, 10a, 653, 519d, 184, 10b, 520c-3p, 373, 372, 505, 222, 302b, 302a, 499-5p, 302d, 221, 302c, 203, 520a-3p, 494, 302e
CD19 (930) NM_001770	362-3p, 7, 335, 329
PRKCZ (5590) NM_002744	448, 148a, 367, 148b, 152, 455-5p, 708
TP53 (7157) NM_000546	431, 143, 296-3p, 539, 410, 185, 186, 27a, 485-5p, 27b, 24, 22, 218, 19b, 19a, 150, 125a-5p, 421, 98, 381, 491-5p, 338-3p, let-7d, let-7e, let-7b, let-7c, let-7a, 340, 125b, 300, let-7i, let-7f, 504, let-7g
TCEB2 (6923) NM_007108	204, 134, 599, 216b, 149, 125b, 485-5p, 211, 150, 135a, 873, 125a-5p, 135b
BAIAP2 (10458) NM_017451	346, 144, 539, 328, 485-5p, 197, 495, 203, 138
ITGAM (3684) NM_001145808	136, 539, 96, 185, 382, 186, 29b, 425, 377, 21, 335, 340, 342-3p, 224, 590-5p, 19b, 19a, 203, 23a, 23b
RAC1 (5879) NM_018890	361-5p, 186, 485-5p, 1, 194, 320d, 374a, 320c, 155, 129-5p, 613, 429, 197, 31, 224, 495, 494, 101, 100, 200b, 200c, 181a, 454, 542-3p, 146a, 142-3p, 365, 22, 217, 376a, 376b, 99b, 19b, 19a, 99a, 590-3p, 137, 136, 320a, 146b-5p, 320b, 33b, 33a, 381, 544, 382, 374b, 206, 346, 377, 182, 340, 876-5p, 300
MAPK1 (5594) NM_002745	361-5p, 141, 144, 539, 9, 7, 186, 1, 190, 192, 194, 320d, 374a, 320c, 488, 129-5p, 613, 197, 140-5p, 590-5p, 181d, 599, 101, 410, 34a, 200a, 181a, 181c, 181b, 215, 22, 365, 21, 217, 219-5p, 342-3p, 210, 19b, 19a, 212, 214, 137, 590-3p, 136, 320a, 320b, 190b, 132, 381, 543, 374b, 338-3p, 34c-5p, 206, 378, 340, 422a, 300, 499-5p, 203, 873
TRAF3 (7187) NM_003300	361-5p, 144, 200b, 200c, 9, 7, 411, 186, 542-3p, 1297, 25, 383, 217, 367, 190, 376a, 376b, 363, 590-3p, 448, 129-5p, 33b, 190b, 26a, 33a, 92b, 92a, 429, 653, 32, 26b, 495, 494
CTNNB1 (1499) NM_001098210	141, 101, 410, 539, 9, 200a, 370, 20a, 20b, 217, 335, 708, 19b, 19a, 212, 23a, 150, 23b, 214, 448, 590-3p, 129-5p, 33b, 33a, 132, 106b, 93, 106a, 381, 17, 519d, 28-5p, 377, 130b, 140-5p, 300, 222, 130a, 495, 221, 494
MDM2 (4193) NM_002392	141, 145, 200a, 185, 29a, 29b, 29c, 181c, 384, 383, 193b, 194, 23a, 23b, 590-3p, 193a-3p, 374b, 338-3p, 758, 379, 377, 373, 140-5p, 302b, 223, 302a, 302d, 496, 495, 302c, 221, 504
PDPK1 (5170) NM_002613	155, 361-5p, 181d, 129-5p, 15a, 200b, 9, 200c, 382, 27a, 429, 374b, 27b, 181a, 181c, 181b, 424, 146a, 346, 193b, 340, 590-5p, 125a-3p, 374a, 15b, 23a, 504, 23b
MAP3K8 (1326) NM_005204	144, 433, 539, 9, 139-5p, 186, 27a, 27b, 190, 374a, 488, 23a, 23b, 155, 153, 429, 519d, 32, 371-5p, 140-5p, 590-5p, 222, 223, 221, 494, 124, 103, 181d, 101, 200b, 410, 200c, 370, 181a, 20a, 128, 107, 24, 181c, 20b, 181b, 21, 362-3p, 363, 212, 15b, 448, 137, 590-3p, 26a, 190b, 132, 106b, 93, 106a, 17, 381, 382, 543, 374b, 338-3p, 299-3p, 135a, 135b, 183, 506, 26b, 300, 499-5p
TAPBP (6892) NM_003190	129-5p, 143, 15a, 410, 190b, 7, 455-5p, 34a, 185, 34c-5p, 204, 190, 31, 342-3p, 328, 590-5p, 222, 488, 449b, 211, let-7i, 221, 15b, 449a
ASAP1 (50807) NM_018482	431, 144, 143, 433, 539, 186, 485-5p, 27a, 27b, 520b, 383, 148a, 190, 148b, 194, 301a, 330-5p, 23a, 301b, 23b, 129-5p, 153, 421, 152, 18a, 18b, 429, 424, 653, 520c-3p, 224, 590-5p, 302b, 326, 302a, 302d, 302c, 302e, 101, 296-3p, 200b, 200c, 411, 200a, 520e, 128, 454, 542-3p, 29b, 29c, 146a, 22, 217, 21, 218, 362-3p, 376a, 376b, 590-3p, 448, 136, 98, 33b, 146b-5p, 33a, 190b, 544, 520d-3p, 138, let-7d, 183, let-7e, 182, let-7b, let-7c, let-7a, 373, 372, 130b, 208b, 130a, 499-5p, 202, 203, let-7i, 874, 503, let-7f, 520a-3p, let-7g
CCKBR (887) NM_176875	136, 152, 599, 24, 28-5p, 148a, 148b, 196b, 324-5p, 210, 223, 196a, 202, 874
KLRC3 (3823) NM_002261	155, 346, 217, 33b, 599, 33a, 371-5p, 411, 544, 494
MAP2K7 (5609) NM_145185	141, 129-5p, 421, 433, 9, 200a, 27a, 370, 27b, 128, 425, 505, 876-5p, 125b, 125a-5p

Gene Symbol (Entrez Gene ID) Transcript ID	miRNAs
CXCR2 (3579) NM_001557	433, 410, 145, 122, 34a, 1, 24, 1297, 20b, 22, 376c, 301a, 320d, 320c, 23a, 23b, 301b, 320a, 129-5p, 134, 33b, 320b, 190b, 33a, 26a, 613, 544, 34c-5p, 206, 10a, 10b, 373, 224, 26b, 302d, 495
EXOC3 (11336) NM_007277	485-5p, 495
NFKB1 (4790) NM_003998	15a, 539, 200b, 9, 200c, 30e, 186, 520e, 520b, 1297, 383, 219-5p, 195, 335, 19b, 19a, 211, 15b, 23a, 23b, 214, 590-3p, 199a-5p, 129-5p, 26a, 543, 199b-5p, 429, 338-3p, 424, 16, 103, 182, 204, 520c-3p, 216b, 373, 340, 302b, 26b, 302a, 497, 450a, 302d, 496, 302c, 494, 520a-3p
LEP (3952) NM_000230	141, 143, 30c, 30d, 9, 30e, 200a, 149, 30a, 27a, 27b, 30b, 20a, 20b, 146a, 218, 362-3p, 342-3p, 708, 330-5p, 211, 146b-5p, 106b, 490-3p, 93, 106a, 17, 197, 135a, 425, 519d, 28-5p, 204, 208a, 208b, 326, 495, 874
MAPK11 (5600) NM_002751	199a-5p, 98, 455-5p, let-7d, 184, let-7e, let-7b, let-7c, let-7a, 221, let-7i, let-7f, let-7g
PTPN2 (5771) NM_002828	433, 145, 139-5p, 186, 194, 23a, 23b, 125a-5p, 155, 153, 491-5p, 429, 758, 519d, 653, 371-5p, 590-5p, 302b, 223, 302a, 302d, 302c, 495, 329, 494, 302e, 101, 200b, 30c, 30d, 200c, 30e, 411, 520e, 30a, 30b, 20a, 20b, 365, 21, 362-3p, 125a-3p, 137, 448, 590-3p, 134, 106b, 93, 106a, 17, 381, 374b, 520d-3p, 10a, 10b, 377, 205, 373, 340, 372, 125b, 300, 203, 520a-3p, 874, 504
TRAF1 (7185) NM_005658	137, 154, 136, 185, 149, 29a, 128, 454, 29b, 29c, 24, 204, 182, 218, 340, 194, 376c, 125a-3p, 211, 150, 504, 214
LTA (4049) NM_001159740	590-3p, 384, 431, 129-5p, 205, 216a, 455-5p, 7, 186, 876-5p, 330-5p, 203, 138
HDAC2 (3066) NM_001527	181d, 410, 539, 145, 186, 24, 383, 195, 374a, 320d, 320c, 155, 590-3p, 137, 320a, 320b, 490-3p, 544, 133a, 382, 133b, 197, 424, 182, 377, 216a, 340, 875-5p, 223, 499-5p, 203, 494
TGFA (7039) NM_003236	7, 384, 148a, 148b, 301a, 708, 374a, 330-5p, 449b, 449a, 23a, 301b, 23b, 155, 129-5p, 152, 18a, 490-3p, 491-5p, 429, 28-5p, 224, 326, 496, 495, 494, 124, 181d, 101, 122, 34a, 370, 454, 218, 376a, 376b, 376c, 590-3p, 137, 544, 543, 374b, 34c-5p, 205, 340, 505, 130b, 506, 130a, 499-5p, 203
IL27 (246778) NM_145659	30c, 200c, 30d, 18a, 30e, 30a, 30b, 874
CD40 (958) NM_152854	103, 15a, 145, 370, 107, 195, 374a, 330-5p, 15b, 590-3p, 448, 199a-5p, 320a, 421, 320b, 381, 544, 199b-5p, 197, 135a, 424, 135b, 16, 10a, 10b, 371-5p, 340, 300, 326, 497
TRADD (8717) NM_003789	137, 320a, 320b, 18a, 18b, 149, 543, 485-5p, 31, 342-3p, 125a-3p, 320d, 320c, 214
RIPK1 (8737) NM_003804	141, 127-3p, 101, 599, 200a, 27a, 27b, 29b, 24, 29c, 142-3p, 384, 125a-3p, 488, 211, 590-3p, 421, 106b, 93, 544, 133a, 133b, 197, 519d, 204, 216b, 496, 203
AXIN2 (8313) NM_004655	144, 433, 143, 539, 139-5p, 27a, 27b, 1297, 384, 195, 487b, 301a, 374a, 449b, 449a, 301b, 155, 153, 18a, 18b, 429, 425, 424, 32, 371-5p, 222, 223, 497, 326, 495, 221, 124, 103, 101, 15a, 200b, 410, 200c, 411, 34a, 107, 454, 19b, 19a, 211, 212, 15b, 590-3p, 448, 26a, 132, 381, 544, 374b, 34c-5p, 16, 183, 204, 205, 216b, 340, 130b, 876-5p, 506, 300, 26b, 130a, 499-5p
AKT1S1 (84335) NM_001098633	124, 146b-5p, 190b, 539, 491-5p, 185, 142-3p, 146a, 378, 216a, 422a, 506, 488, 150
DNMT1 (1786) NM_001130823	448, 155, 153, 152, 539, 410, 185, 374b, 128, 379, 148a, 217, 377, 148b, 340, 140-5p, 342-3p, 374a, 222, 495, 221
GIT2 (9815) NM_057169	141, 145, 185, 195, 194, 301a, 708, 320d, 320c, 488, 23a, 23b, 301b, 421, 18a, 18b, 133a, 133b, 429, 653, 519d, 28-5p, 32, 495, 103, 599, 15a, 200b, 200c, 200a, 34a, 451, 20a, 128, 107, 542-3p, 454, 24, 25, 20b, 146a, 367, 363, 19b, 210, 19a, 320a, 320b, 106b, 92b, 92a, 93, 106a, 17, 544, 34c-5p, 379, 183, 182, 340, 130b, 130a, 499-5p, 203
HTRA2 (27429) NM_013247	15a, 410, 145, 485-5p, 20a, 1, 20b, 190, 195, 708, 374a, 15b, 590-3p, 199a-5p, 190b, 106b, 93, 106a, 17, 199b-5p, 374b, 138, 424, 16, 10a, 519d, 206, let-7e, 10b, 28-5p, 340, 497, 202
RPS6KB1 (6198) NM_003161	361-5p, 539, 139-5p, 145, 7, 186, 27a, 27b, 148a, 148b, 195, 335, 301a, 374a, 488, 330-5p, 23a, 301b, 23b, 155, 421, 153, 129-5p, 152, 490-3p, 429, 424, 653, 32, 497, 223, 329, 181d, 103, 296-3p, 15a, 410, 200b, 30c, 30d, 200c, 30e, 455-5p, 30a, 30b, 181a, 128, 107, 454, 24, 181c, 181b, 142-3p, 217, 218, 367, 486-5p, 376a, 376b, 376c, 342-3p, 15b, 590-3p, 33b, 33a, 381, 382, 543, 135a, 16, 135b, 379, 377, 216b, 340, 130b, 505, 876-5p, 300, 130a, 203

Gene Symbol (Entrez Gene ID) Transcript ID	miRNAs
LASP1 (3927) NM_006148	143, 145, 106b, 106a, 93, 17, 133a, 133b, 197, 20a, 128, 542-3p, 24, 20b, 519d, 146a, 182, 218, 31, 342-3p, 326, 330-5p, 203, 23a, 150, 873, 23b
CASP9 (842) NM_001229	155, 590-3p, 124, 154, 181d, 599, 96, 7, 454, 181b, 1271, 377, 182, 376a, 376b, 376c, 140-5p, 130b, 301a, 506, 125a-3p, 130a, 301b, 504
WEE1 (7465) NM_003390	141, 144, 539, 139-5p, 7, 185, 186, 27a, 27b, 520b, 1, 1297, 148a, 192, 195, 301a, 23a, 23b, 301b, 155, 153, 613, 758, 424, 519d, 520c-3p, 140-5p, 302b, 222, 302a, 497, 302d, 302c, 221, 495, 302e, 124, 103, 15a, 410, 520e, 128, 20a, 454, 107, 20b, 215, 22, 219-5p, 362-3p, 19b, 211, 19a, 15b, 26a, 106b, 106a, 93, 381, 17, 544, 520d-3p, 338-3p, 138, 16, 206, 377, 204, 373, 372, 130b, 506, 300, 26b, 875-5p, 130a, 520a-3p, 503
HCST (10870) NM_014266	362-3p, 125a-3p, 329
PLCG1 (5335) NM_002660	181d, 101, 200b, 139-5p, 200c, 34a, 455-5p, 485-5p, 370, 1, 181b, 1271, 218, 449b, 211, 449a, 150, 125a-5p, 129-5p, 96, 613, 429, 299-3p, 135a, 34c-5p, 135b, 10a, 206, 10b, 204, 182, 205, 590-5p, 125b, 874, 873
MAX (4149) NM_002382	361-5p, 30e, 7, 149, 1, 22, 383, 362-3p, 193b, 339-5p, 376c, 335, 320d, 708, 488, 320c, 214, 137, 320a, 320b, 613, 193a-3p, 381, 382, 138, 206, 28-5p, 377, 328, 300, 494, 329, 873
UIMC1 (51720) NM_016290	590-3p, 448, 153, 544, 27a, 27b, 128, 135a, 181c, 135b, 138, 653, 346, 217, 371-5p, 376c, 340, 505, 487b, 876-5p, 495, 203, 494, 504
IL2RB (3560) NM_000878	139-5p, 34a, 27a, 27b, 1, 24, 191, 194, 374a, 449b, 449a, 150, 125a-5p, 33b, 33a, 613, 543, 34c-5p, 206, let-7d, let-7e, let-7a, 340, 125b, 499-5p, let-7f
MAP4K2 (5871) NM_004579	145, 543, 488, 495, 494
NCOA1 (8648) NM_003743	361-5p, 144, 539, 7, 149, 186, 27a, 27b, 383, 148a, 190, 148b, 335, 301a, 374a, 449b, 449a, 23a, 301b, 23b, 421, 129-5p, 152, 18a, 18b, 424, 32, 371-5p, 223, 496, 495, 329, 181d, 30c, 410, 30d, 30e, 34a, 30a, 30b, 181a, 128, 454, 24, 181c, 181b, 25, 146a, 22, 486-5p, 362-3p, 367, 219-5p, 376c, 363, 342-3p, 19b, 19a, 212, 448, 590-3p, 137, 98, 146b-5p, 190b, 132, 92b, 92a, 544, 381, 543, 374b, 135a, 135b, 34c-5p, 138, let-7d, let-7e, let-7b, 377, 182, 205, let-7c, 216a, 216b, let-7a, 130b, 300, 875-5p, 130a, 203, let-7i, let-7f, let-7g
TREM2 (54209) NM_018965	431, 361-5p, 31, 132, 876-5p, 382, 542-3p, 212, 425
DIAPH1 (1729) NM_005219	124, 101, 15a, 143, 9, 145, 370, 27a, 27b, 24, 384, 195, 194, 342-3p, 320d, 320c, 488, 15b, 214, 590-3p, 155, 136, 320a, 320b, 381, 424, 16, 183, 377, 506, 300, 497, 495, 504
FANCD2 (2177) NM_033084	599, 410, 520e, 520b, 20a, 20b, 218, 23a, 23b, 106b, 106a, 93, 17, 382, 520d-3p, 519d, 520c-3p, 373, 372, 340, 505, 302b, 302a, 302d, 202, 302c, 520a-3p, 302e
PTK2 (5747) NM_005607	433, 539, 145, 139-5p, 7, 186, 520b, 1297, 384, 193b, 194, 150, 23a, 125a-5p, 23b, 199a-5p, 421, 193a-3p, 519d, 520c-3p, 140-5p, 196b, 590-5p, 302b, 222, 223, 302a, 196a, 302d, 495, 221, 302c, 302e, 181d, 410, 520e, 20a, 1271, 20b, 21, 486-5p, 590-3p, 137, 98, 26a, 96, 106b, 93, 106a, 381, 17, 543, 199b-5p, 520d-3p, 135a, 138, 135b, 379, 183, let-7e, let-7b, let-7c, let-7a, 373, 372, 340, 505, 125b, 300, 26b, 551a, let-7i, 551b, 203, 520a-3p
OAS1 (4938) NM_001032409	137, 148a, 152, 216b, 374a, 485-5p, 374b
RBBP8 (5932) NM_002894	20a, 454, 20b, 148a, 148b, 301a, 488, 19b, 19a, 301b, 590-3p, 136, 152, 18a, 18b, 106a, 17, 377, 205, 340, 130b, 222, 130a, 202, 495, 221

Table 3
List of miRNAs and corresponding MIMAT accession numbers used to design the CTLs qPCR panel layout. ***hsa-miR-1297, hsa-miR-371-5p, hsa-miR-485-5p, hsa-miR-499-5p, hsa-miR-542-3p, hsa-miR-613*** **were excluded from the plate layout since no assay was available for these miRNAs at the date of our experiment**

miRBase Accession Number	miRNA name	miRBase Accession Number	miRNA name	miRBase Accession Number	miRNA name
MIMAT0000062	hsa-let-7a	MIMAT0000242	hsa-miR-129-5p	MIMAT0000424	hsa-miR-128
MIMAT0000063	hsa-let-7b	MIMAT0000243	hsa-miR-148a	MIMAT0000425	hsa-miR-130a
MIMAT0000064	hsa-let-7c	MIMAT0000244	hsa-miR-30c	MIMAT0000426	hsa-miR-132
MIMAT0000065	hsa-let-7d	MIMAT0000245	hsa-miR-30d	MIMAT0000427	hsa-miR-133a
MIMAT0000066	hsa-let-7e	MIMAT0000250	hsa-miR-139-5p	MIMAT0000428	hsa-miR-135a
MIMAT0000067	hsa-let-7f	MIMAT0000252	hsa-miR-7	MIMAT0000429	hsa-miR-137
MIMAT0000068	hsa-miR-15a	MIMAT0000253	hsa-miR-10a	MIMAT0000430	hsa-miR-138
MIMAT0000069	hsa-miR-16	MIMAT0000254	hsa-miR-10b	MIMAT0000431	hsa-miR-140-5p
MIMAT0000070	hsa-miR-17	MIMAT0000255	hsa-miR-34a	MIMAT0000432	hsa-miR-141
MIMAT0000072	hsa-miR-18a	MIMAT0000256	hsa-miR-181a	MIMAT0000434	hsa-miR-142-3p
MIMAT0000073	hsa-miR-19a	MIMAT0000257	hsa-miR-181b	MIMAT0000435	hsa-miR-143
MIMAT0000074	hsa-miR-19b	MIMAT0000258	hsa-miR-181c	MIMAT0000436	hsa-miR-144
MIMAT0000075	hsa-miR-20a	MIMAT0000259	hsa-miR-182	MIMAT0000437	hsa-miR-145
MIMAT0000076	hsa-miR-21	MIMAT0000261	hsa-miR-183	MIMAT0000438	hsa-miR-152
MIMAT0000077	hsa-miR-22	MIMAT0000262	hsa-miR-187	MIMAT0000439	hsa-miR-153
MIMAT0000078	hsa-miR-23a	MIMAT0000263	hsa-miR-199b-5p	MIMAT0000440	hsa-miR-191
MIMAT0000080	hsa-miR-24	MIMAT0000264	hsa-miR-203	MIMAT0000441	hsa-miR-9
MIMAT0000081	hsa-miR-25	MIMAT0000265	hsa-miR-204	MIMAT0000443	hsa-miR-125a-5p
MIMAT0000082	hsa-miR-26a	MIMAT0000266	hsa-miR-205	MIMAT0000445	hsa-miR-126
MIMAT0000083	hsa-miR-26b	MIMAT0000267	hsa-miR-210	MIMAT0000446	hsa-miR-127-3p
MIMAT0000084	hsa-miR-27a	MIMAT0000268	hsa-miR-211	MIMAT0000447	hsa-miR-134
MIMAT0000085	hsa-miR-28-5p	MIMAT0000269	hsa-miR-212	MIMAT0000448	hsa-miR-136
MIMAT0000086	hsa-miR-29a	MIMAT0000271	hsa-miR-214	MIMAT0000449	hsa-miR-146a
MIMAT0000087	hsa-miR-30a	MIMAT0000272	hsa-miR-215	MIMAT0000450	hsa-miR-149
MIMAT0000089	hsa-miR-31	MIMAT0000273	hsa-miR-216a	MIMAT0000451	hsa-miR-150
MIMAT0000090	hsa-miR-32	MIMAT0000274	hsa-miR-217	MIMAT0000452	hsa-miR-154
MIMAT0000091	hsa-miR-33a	MIMAT0000275	hsa-miR-218	MIMAT0000454	hsa-miR-184
MIMAT0000092	hsa-miR-92a	MIMAT0000276	hsa-miR-219-5p	MIMAT0000455	hsa-miR-185
MIMAT0000093	hsa-miR-93	MIMAT0000278	hsa-miR-221	MIMAT0000456	hsa-miR-186
MIMAT0000095	hsa-miR-96	MIMAT0000279	hsa-miR-222	MIMAT0000458	hsa-miR-190
MIMAT0000096	hsa-miR-98	MIMAT0000280	hsa-miR-223	MIMAT0000459	hsa-miR-193a-3p
MIMAT0000097	hsa-miR-99a	MIMAT0000281	hsa-miR-224	MIMAT0000460	hsa-miR-194
MIMAT0000098	hsa-miR-100	MIMAT0000318	hsa-miR-200b	MIMAT0000461	hsa-miR-195
MIMAT0000099	hsa-miR-101	MIMAT0000414	hsa-let-7g	MIMAT0000462	hsa-miR-206
MIMAT0000100	hsa-miR-29b	MIMAT0000415	hsa-let-7i	MIMAT0000510	hsa-miR-320a
MIMAT0000101	hsa-miR-103	MIMAT0000416	hsa-miR-1	MIMAT0000617	hsa-miR-200c
MIMAT0000103	hsa-miR-106a	MIMAT0000417	hsa-miR-15b	MIMAT0000646	hsa-miR-155
MIMAT0000104	hsa-miR-107	MIMAT0000418	hsa-miR-23b	MIMAT0000680	hsa-miR-106b
MIMAT0000222	hsa-miR-192	MIMAT0000419	hsa-miR-27b	MIMAT0000681	hsa-miR-29c
MIMAT0000226	hsa-miR-196a	MIMAT0000420	hsa-miR-30b	MIMAT0000682	hsa-miR-200a
MIMAT0000227	hsa-miR-197	MIMAT0000421	hsa-miR-122	MIMAT0000684	hsa-miR-302a
MIMAT0000231	hsa-miR-199a-5p	MIMAT0000422	hsa-miR-124	MIMAT0000686	hsa-miR-34c-5p
MIMAT0000241	hsa-miR-208a	MIMAT0000423	hsa-miR-125b	MIMAT0000687	hsa-miR-299-3p

miRBase Accession Number	miRNA name	miRBase Accession Number	miRNA name	miRBase Accession Number	miRNA name
MIMAT0000688	hsa-miR-301a	MIMAT0001541	hsa-miR-449a	MIMAT0003327	hsa-miR-449b
MIMAT0000689	hsa-miR-99b	MIMAT0001545	hsa-miR-450a	MIMAT0003328	hsa-miR-653
MIMAT0000691	hsa-miR-130b	MIMAT0001625	hsa-miR-431	MIMAT0003329	hsa-miR-411
MIMAT0000692	hsa-miR-30e	MIMAT0001627	hsa-miR-433	MIMAT0003339	hsa-miR-421
MIMAT0000703	hsa-miR-361-5p	MIMAT0001629	hsa-miR-329	MIMAT0003389	hsa-miR-542-3p
MIMAT0000707	hsa-miR-363	MIMAT0001631	hsa-miR-451	MIMAT0003393	hsa-miR-425
MIMAT0000710	hsa-miR-365	MIMAT0002171	hsa-miR-410	MIMAT0003879	hsa-miR-758
MIMAT0000715	hsa-miR-302b	MIMAT0002172	hsa-miR-376b	MIMAT0003885	hsa-miR-454
MIMAT0000717	hsa-miR-302c	MIMAT0002175	hsa-miR-485-5p	MIMAT0004602	hsa-miR-125a-3p
MIMAT0000718	hsa-miR-302d	MIMAT0002177	hsa-miR-486-5p	MIMAT0004679	hsa-miR-296-3p
MIMAT0000719	hsa-miR-367	MIMAT0002806	hsa-miR-490-3p	MIMAT0004683	hsa-miR-362-3p
MIMAT0000720	hsa-miR-376c	MIMAT0002807	hsa-miR-491-5p	MIMAT0004687	hsa-miR-371-5p
MIMAT0000722	hsa-miR-370	MIMAT0002809	hsa-miR-146b-5p	MIMAT0004692	hsa-miR-340
MIMAT0000724	hsa-miR-372	MIMAT0002811	hsa-miR-202	MIMAT0004693	hsa-miR-330-5p
MIMAT0000726	hsa-miR-373	MIMAT0002816	hsa-miR-494	MIMAT0004763	hsa-miR-488
MIMAT0000727	hsa-miR-374a	MIMAT0002817	hsa-miR-495	MIMAT0004801	hsa-miR-590-3p
MIMAT0000728	hsa-miR-375	MIMAT0002818	hsa-miR-496	MIMAT0004903	hsa-miR-300
MIMAT0000729	hsa-miR-376a	MIMAT0002819	hsa-miR-193b	MIMAT0004911	hsa-miR-874
MIMAT0000730	hsa-miR-377	MIMAT0002820	hsa-miR-497	MIMAT0004922	hsa-miR-875-5p
MIMAT0000732	hsa-miR-378	MIMAT0002821	hsa-miR-181d	MIMAT0004924	hsa-miR-876-5p
MIMAT0000733	hsa-miR-379	MIMAT0002825	hsa-miR-520e	MIMAT0004926	hsa-miR-708
MIMAT0000736	hsa-miR-381	MIMAT0002834	hsa-miR-520a-3p	MIMAT0004929	hsa-miR-190b
MIMAT0000737	hsa-miR-382	MIMAT0002843	hsa-miR-520b	MIMAT0004953	hsa-miR-873
MIMAT0000738	hsa-miR-383	MIMAT0002846	hsa-miR-520c-3p	MIMAT0004954	hsa-miR-543
MIMAT0000752	hsa-miR-328	MIMAT0002853	hsa-miR-519d	MIMAT0004955	hsa-miR-374b
MIMAT0000753	hsa-miR-342-3p	MIMAT0002856	hsa-miR-520d-3p	MIMAT0004958	hsa-miR-301b
MIMAT0000756	hsa-miR-326	MIMAT0002870	hsa-miR-499-5p	MIMAT0004959	hsa-miR-216b
MIMAT0000758	hsa-miR-135b	MIMAT0002874	hsa-miR-503	MIMAT0004960	hsa-miR-208b
MIMAT0000759	hsa-miR-148b	MIMAT0002875	hsa-miR-504	MIMAT0005792	hsa-miR-320b
MIMAT0000761	hsa-miR-324-5p	MIMAT0002876	hsa-miR-505	MIMAT0005793	hsa-miR-320c
MIMAT0000763	hsa-miR-338-3p	MIMAT0002878	hsa-miR-506	MIMAT0005796	hsa-miR-1271
MIMAT0000764	hsa-miR-339-5p	MIMAT0003150	hsa-miR-455-5p	MIMAT0005886	hsa-miR-1297
MIMAT0000765	hsa-miR-335	MIMAT0003163	hsa-miR-539	MIMAT0005931	hsa-miR-302e
MIMAT0000770	hsa-miR-133b	MIMAT0003164	hsa-miR-544	MIMAT0006764	hsa-miR-320d
MIMAT0000773	hsa-miR-346	MIMAT0003180	hsa-miR-487b		
MIMAT0001075	hsa-miR-384	MIMAT0003214	hsa-miR-551a		
MIMAT0001080	hsa-miR-196b	MIMAT0003218	hsa-miR-92b		
MIMAT0001339	hsa-miR-422a	MIMAT0003233	hsa-miR-551b		
MIMAT0001341	hsa-miR-424	MIMAT0003258	hsa-miR-590-5p		
MIMAT0001412	hsa-miR-18b	MIMAT0003267	hsa-miR-599		
MIMAT0001413	hsa-miR-20b	MIMAT0003281	hsa-miR-613		
MIMAT0001532	hsa-miR-448	MIMAT0003283	hsa-miR-615-3p		
MIMAT0001536	hsa-miR-429	MIMAT0003301	hsa-miR-33b		

4 Notes

1. IPA software requires a fee; however, the same information can be obtained from other public databases free of charge, where pathways name can be different.
2. miRNA Target database is freely available on the web. The complete list of the different web sites is available at the following address: http://www.ncrna.org/KnowledgeBase/link-database/mirna_target_database. The microRNA.org web site allows to download the microRNA target predictions based on the miRanda algorithm and scored using mirSVR score as described below.
3. August 2010 is the (current) release available.
4. On the same site miRNA target prediction tables for *Mus Musculus*, *Rattus Norvegicus*, *Drosophila melanogaster*, and *Caenorhabditis elegans* can also be downloaded . In the same section it is also possible to select: “Good mirSVR score, Non-conserved miRNA”; “Non-good mirSVR score, Conserved miRNA”; “Non-good mirSVR score, Non-conserved miRNA.” We recommend using the list containing “Good mirSVR Score, conserved miRNA” since the good mirSVR Score gives the best degree of predicted target down-regulation at the mRNA or protein level [11]. Conserved miRNA refers to mature microRNA families included into the miR_Family_Info table from TargetScan, with a value different from zero in the “conservation” field.
5. This operation requires some programming skills.
6. The introduction of locked nucleic acids (LNAs) into oligonucleotide primers has increased their performance in amplification success under diverse conditions due to their higher affinity and specificity [12]. Indeed, amplification primers with LNA reduce background and allow quantification of very small microRNA levels.
7. You can find the specific LNA-PCR primer set for the miRNA of your interest by searching for the miRNA name and adding the assay to your plate, in a specific well position of choice. MicroRNAs are named using the “mir” prefix and a unique identifying number followed by different suffixes. Different precursor sequences are indicated by numbers; closely related mature sequences are indicated by letters. Moreover two miRNAs can originate from the same predicted precursor and in this case the suffixes -5p (from the 5′ arm) and -3p (from the 3′ arm) are used [13]. To generate the custom qPCR plate we selected all the assays available for each miRNA.
8. Each plate can include different types of control assays: interplate calibrators, for calibration between different PCR plate runs, and RNA-spike in assays, to detect specific RNA added to

the sample before isolation and cDNA synthesis. According to our experience it is suggested to include in your custom plate all these controls in order to check for RNA quality, cDNA synthesis, and presence of PCR inhibitors. Moreover, we suggest to include in the experimental design of the plate at least one well with no template control (NTCs) to define the background levels. Finally it is mandatory to include in the plate design one or more reference assays for data normalization. In our laboratory we used different miRNAs as endogen miRNA normalizers for miRNA expression analysis in CTLs: RNU6, RNU24, and let-7a. We identified miRNA let7-a as the most stable reference.

9. Whole blood should be collected in blood collection tubes containing the anticoagulant Lithium Heparin. Blood collection tubes should be stored at room temperature and must not be chilled or frozen before processing. The addition of 1 mM EDTA to PBS 1× pH 7.4 for the dilution of whole blood avoids the formation of leukocyte's aggregates.
10. PBMC can also be used to isolate CD8+ T cells, thus obtaining a more selected population. To extract RNA several kits are commercially available. Make sure that the method used guarantees the recovery of small RNA and use the same method for all the samples you will compare.
11. Before proceeding to qRT-PCR, RNA integrity should be checked by gel electrophoresis or by the Agilent 2100 Bioanalyzer.
12. For the study of miRNA expressed in CTLs, we successfully used 20 ng of total RNA extracted as described, as starting material for cDNA synthesis reaction.
13. The ExiLENT SYBR® Green master mix does not include passive reference dye such as ROX. Some PCR Instruments require a specific amount of the reference dye to be included into the PCR reaction to normalize signals from single wells and compare results from different plates. If the Real-time instrument requires this type of reference, follow the suppliers instructions to define ROX concentration. For our experiments with CTLs, we used the 7900HT Fast Real-Time PCR System and added 100× concentrated ROX solution (SIGMA).
14. Set threshold and baseline manually and apply the same settings for all plates. Spike-in and reference miRNAs could be present at higher expression levels. In our laboratory practice we sometimes apply different baseline settings for these highly expressed miRNAs. In these cases it is important to keep the same settings for all the other samples to be compared; threshold should be adjusted accordingly to capture the threshold cycle values (Ct) in the linear portion of the amplification curve.

15. It is necessary to perform inter-plate calibration before calculating the relative changes in miRNA expression; to this purpose check that the Cq value for the inter-plate calibrator in all the plates has a standard deviation ±0.5, otherwise eliminate the outliers. Calculate the calibration factor as the difference between plate average and average of all the plates and subtract it from all Cq values in the plate. Moreover check for the absence of amplification in the NTCs, ROX stability in all the wells, melting curves without multiple peaks, and detection signals over Spike-ins RNA.

References

1. Barad O, Meiri E, Avniel A et al (2004) MicroRNA expression detected by oligonucleotide microarrays: system establishment and expression profiling in human tissues. Genome Res 14:2486–2494
2. Callari M, Dugo M, Musella V et al (2012) Comparison of microarray platforms for measuring differential microRNA expression in paired normal/cancer colon tissues. PLoS One 7(9):e45105
3. Chen C, Tan R, Wong L et al (2011) Quantitation of microRNAs by real-time RT-qPCR. Methods Mol Biol 687:113–34
4. Mestdagh P, Feys T, Bernard N et al (2008) High-throughput stem-loop RT-qPCR miRNA expression profiling using minute amounts of input RNA. Nucleic Acids Res 36(21):e143
5. Yin JQ, Zhao RC, Morris KV (2008) Profiling microRNA expression with microarrays. Trends Biotechnol 26:70–76
6. Benes V, Castoldi M (2010) Expression profiling of microRNA using real-time quantitative PCR, how to use it and what is available. Methods 50:244–249
7. Mou G, Wang K, Xu D, Zhou G (2013) Evaluation of three RT-qPCR-based miRNA detection methods using seven rice miRNAs. Biosci Biotechnol Biochem 77:1349–53
8. Deo A, Carlsson J, Lindlöf A (2011) How to choose a normalization strategy for miRNA quantitative real-time (qPCR) arrays. J Bioinform Comput Biol 9:795–812
9. Betel D, Wilson M, Gabow A et al (2008) The microRNA.org resource: targets and expression. Nucleic Acids Res 36(Database issue): D149–153
10. Livak KJ, Schmittgen TD (2001) Analysis of relative gene expression data using real-time quantitative PCR and the 2–ΔΔCT method. Methods 25:402–408
11. Betel D, Koppal A, Agius P et al (2010) Comprehensive modeling of microRNA targets predicts functional non-conserved and non-canonical sites. Genome Biol 11(8): R90
12. Ballantyne KN, van Oorschot RAH, Mitchell RJ (2008) Locked nucleic acids in PCR primers increase sensitivity and performance. Genomics 91:301–305
13. Ambros V, Bartel B, Bartel DP et al (2003) A uniform system for microRNA annotation. RNA 9:277–279

Chapter 12

Proteomic Approaches by SELDI and MALDI-TOF/MS for CTL Analysis

Massimo Papale and Maria Teresa Rocchetti

Abstract

Extracellular stimuli activate, on target cells, a number of signal transduction processes regulating gene expression and the function and/or synthesis of the proteins. In order to highlight the slight changes of the quantity and quality of the proteome it is essential to optimize preparative strategies able to improve the signals of the less expressed proteins and to standardize the use of high-throughput techniques useful to detect them. We describe a complete workflow useful to enrich, from PBMC protein extracts and extrapolated to their subpopulations, the low-molecular-weight proteins and peptides and to detect them by SELDI-TOF protein profiling. The described protocol can also be applied to MALDI-TOF/MS instruments in order to obtain fast, reproducible, and high-quality protein profiles.

Key words SELDI-TOF/MS, MALDI-TOF/MS, CTL, PBMC, Proteomics, Biomarkers

1 Introduction

Proteins carry out the duties specified by the information encoded by the genome, thus being the chief actors within the cells [1]. The set of proteins expressed in a particular cell or cell type is known as its proteome and its characterization is the mission of the proteomics. The proteomic analysis of cell extracts may lead to the identification of a set of proteins correlated to the effect of extracellular stimuli or specific phases of maturation/differentiation [2, 3]. However, stimuli-correlated slight changes of the proteome may be difficult to visualize; thus highly sensitive techniques are strictly necessary to identify them. Proteomics analysis of CTLs revealed, in fact, that the overall proteome of the activated vs. quiescent cells is almost comparable when analyzed by 2D-PAGE [4]. Although the analysis of CTLs by 2D-PAGE may provide a clear picture of the protein content of a cell type, including the analysis of the different protein isoforms, and their variation under particular conditions (i.e., extracellular stimuli), this approach remains laborious, less reproducible, and often not sensitive enough to identify slight changes of the proteome.

Elena Ranieri (ed.), *Cytotoxic T-Cells: Methods and Protocols*, Methods in Molecular Biology, vol. 1186, DOI 10.1007/978-1-4939-1158-5_12, © Springer Science+Business Media New York 2014

Most importantly, 2D-PAGE does not allow a satisfactory visualization of the low-molecular-weight proteins or peptides (less than 10 kDa) [5], which are often involved in the regulation, and or induction of intracellular signalling. The study of the low-molecular-weight proteome and peptidome can in fact provide a variety of information about protein synthesis, processing, and degradation since peptides include either intact small molecules, such as hormones, cytokines, and growth factors, or products of protein processing or, finally, degradation products of proteolytic activity, all processes that may be activated by extracellular stimuli. The use of high-throughput proteomic screening approaches such as SELDI and Clinprot/MALDI can allow the rapid analysis of thousands of biological samples and they have been widely used to identify potentially disease-correlated biomarkers [6, 7]. Here, we describe a workflow useful to analyze by the CM10 (weak cationic exchanger) ProteinChip array the PBMC protein extracts by means of SELDI-TOF in order to obtain fast and reproducible and high-quality profiles of peptides and low-molecular-weight proteins. This workflow has been evaluated also on MALDI-TOF/MS/MS (Autoflex III, Bruker Daltonics) as a valid alternative to the clinprot/MALDI protein profiling to generate reproducible and accurate protein profiles.

2 Materials

All solutions were prepared by using ultrapure water (sensitivity of 18 MΩ cm at 25 °C) and analytical grade reagents. All reagents were prepared at room temperature (unless indicated otherwise). Diligently follow all waste disposal regulations when disposing waste materials.

2.1 PBMC Isolation

1. Heparinized blood (HB) dilution solution (1× PBS pH 7.4 plus 1 mM EDTA).
2. Ficoll-Hypaque density gradient solution.
3. Phosphate-buffered saline (PBS).

2.2 Protein Extraction

1. Lysis buffer: 1 M Tris–HCl, pH 7.4, 1 M NaCl, 1.5 % NP-40 in water solution (*see* **Note 1**).
2. Bradford reagent.

2.3 SELDI Profiling

1. ProteinChip reader PCS400 (Personal or Enterprise model) (BIORAD, USA).
2. ProteinChip OQ calibration Kit (BIORAD).
3. Protein Standard I (Bruker Daltonics, Germany).
4. ProteinChip Cassette-Compatible Bioprocessor (BIORAD).

5. CM10 ProteinChip array (BIORAD) (*see* **Note 2**).
6. CM10 washing/binding buffer: 100 mM Sodium acetate, pH 4 (*see* **Note 3**).
7. Saturated sinapinic acid (SPA) solution [5 mg SPA dissolved in 200 µl of a solubilization solution (0.5 % trifluoroacetic acid (TFA)/50 % acetonitrile (ACN) (v/v)].

2.4 MALDI Profiling

1. Autoflex III Smartbeam MALDI-TOF/MS/MS (Bruker Daltonics, Germany).
2. Protein Standard I (Bruker Daltonics).
3. ProteinChip Cassette-Compatible Bioprocessor.
4. Lucid ID access pack (BIORAD/Bruker Daltonics) (*see* **Note 4**).
5. CM10 ProteinChip array.
6. CM10 washing/binding buffer.
7. Saturated sinapinic acid solution.

3 Methods

All procedures were carried out at room temperature unless otherwise specified. Always wear powder-free laboratory gloves when handling all apparatus and solution used in their preparation to prevent any protein contamination.

3.1 Human Peripheral Blood Mononuclear Cell (PBMC) Isolation

1. Dilute fresh heparinized blood (v/v 1:2) in HB dilution solution and mix well.
2. Gently transfer each 25 ml of diluted blood in a 50 ml conical centrifuge tubes containing 15 ml Ficoll-Hypaque density gradient solution in order to obtain two separate layers.
3. Centrifuge at 460 × *g* for 25 min without breaks.
4. Collect the leukocytes at the interphase layer and transfer them to another 50 ml tubes up to 25 ml (*see* **Note 5**).
5. Wash the cell suspensions with 50 ml 1× PBS and centrifuge at 250 × *g* for 12 min.
6. Discard the supernatant, resuspend the cells in PBS, and repeat the wash centrifuging for 10 min at 175 × *g*.
7. Remove the supernatant and store the cell pellet at −80 °C until use (*see* **Note 6**).

3.2 Protein Extraction

1. Add 500 µL of lysis buffer containing 10 µl of endonuclease and 5 µl of protease inhibitor to the cell pellet.
2. Pass the suspension 25–30 times through a 27 G needle with syringe and then leave on ice for 30 min, vortexing for 1 min every 10 min.

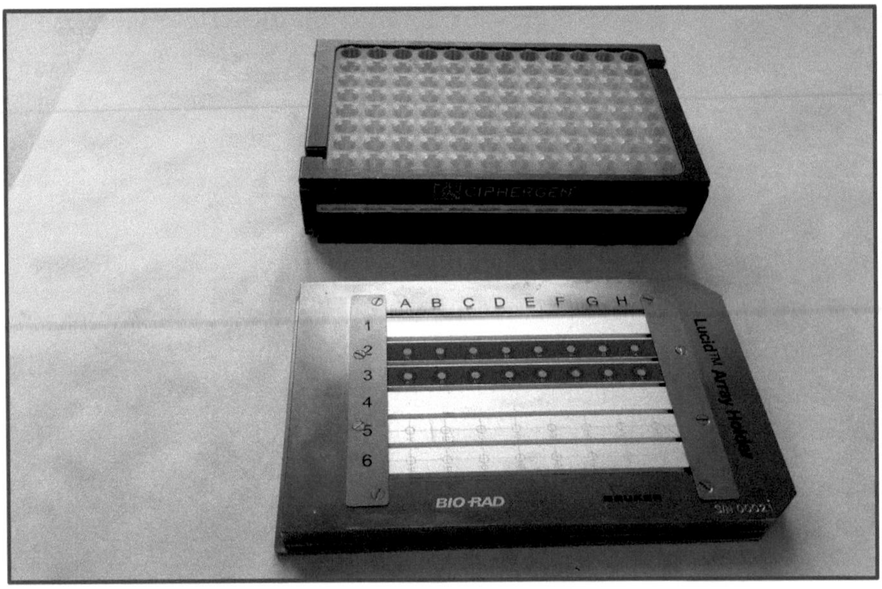

Fig. 1 *Upper*: ProteinChip Bioprocessor for the samples preparation; *lower*: LUCID array holder for the analysis of the ProteinChip by MALDI-TOF/MS

3. Centrifuge the cell lysate at 10,000 × *g* at 4 °C for 20 min. Transfer the supernatant to a clean vial.
4. Assay the protein concentration by Bradford method.

3.3 Protein Capturing by ProteinChip Array

1. Insert the ProteinChip in the ProteinChip Bioprocessor (Fig. 1) and wash two times with 150 μl CM10 washing/binding buffer.
2. Dilute 10 μg of the protein extracts in CM10 binding buffer to a final volume of 100 μl and then add the sample to the ProteinChip surface (*see* **Note** 7).
3. Incubate the sample on an orbital shaker for 30 min at maximum RPM.
4. Discard the supernatant containing the unbound proteins.
5. Add 150 μl CM10 binding buffer, incubate on an orbital shaker at maximum RPM for 5 min, and then remove the supernatant. Repeat the procedure two more times.
6. Perform a final wash with 150 μl ultrapure water, then remove the ProteinChip from the ProteinChip Bioprocessor, and let it dry on air for about 1 h.
7. Prepare saturated SPA solution, let it be on the bench for 30 min vortexing every 5 min, and then centrifuge at 13,000 × *g* for 5 min.
8. Dilute 1:1 the saturated SPA solution by adding the solubilization solution to obtain a 50 % working solution.

9. Add 1 μl of the SPA working solution on the top of the ProteinChip spots, let it dry, then add another μl, and let it dry.
10. Prepare the "protein standard I" (*see* **Note 8**).
11. For SELDI analysis deposit 1 μl of the resuspended standard solution on one spot of the ProteinChip array and let it dry.
12. For MALDI analysis deposit 1 μl of the resuspended standard solution between each spot of the ProteinChip array and let it dry.
13. Insert the ProteinChip into the instrument for the acquisition.

3.4 Protein Profiling Acquisition on SELDI-TOF/ MS

1. Open the ProteinChip Data Manager software (v 3.5).
2. Run the ProteinChip OQ calibration kit (*see* **Note 9**).
3. In the "Explorer panel" select the "protocol folder" and then, by right click, select "new."
4. Set the acquisition parameters (*see* **Note 10**) and save the new protocol.
5. Select the "protocol mode" tab.
6. In the "acquisition protocol" box select the saved protocol and then select the destination folder for your spectra.
7. Select 1:1 in the partition box (*see* **Note 11**).
8. Launch the acquisition by pressing "start running protocol."
9. Apply the same acquisition protocol to the spot/s containing the protein calibration standard I and the samples.
10. At the end of the acquisition, select the spectra of the calibration standard I and create a new calibration equation (*see* **Note 12**).
11. Open the folder in which you saved your spectra and then select the spectra to be calibrated. By right click select "Calibrate" and then "select calibration equation." A list of equations will appear. Select the calibration equation you want to use and then click "apply" to externally calibrate your spectra.
12. By right clicking in the "plot spectra" tab, select "plot selected spectra" option in order to visualize the acquired spectrum/s.
13. Use the detect peak function to identify the mass peaks in your spectrum/s (*see* **Note 13**).
14. When the "detection peak" box is opened set 5 time noise for "valley depth" and "peak height."
15. In the mass window set 3,000 as minimum mass and 30,000 as maximum mass and then press "save and detect" button to identity the mass peaks in your spectrum.
16. When acquiring more spectra from different groups normalize (*see* **Note 14**) and manage them by "expression difference mapping" (EDM) function in order to find differently expressed mass peaks (*see* **Note 15**).

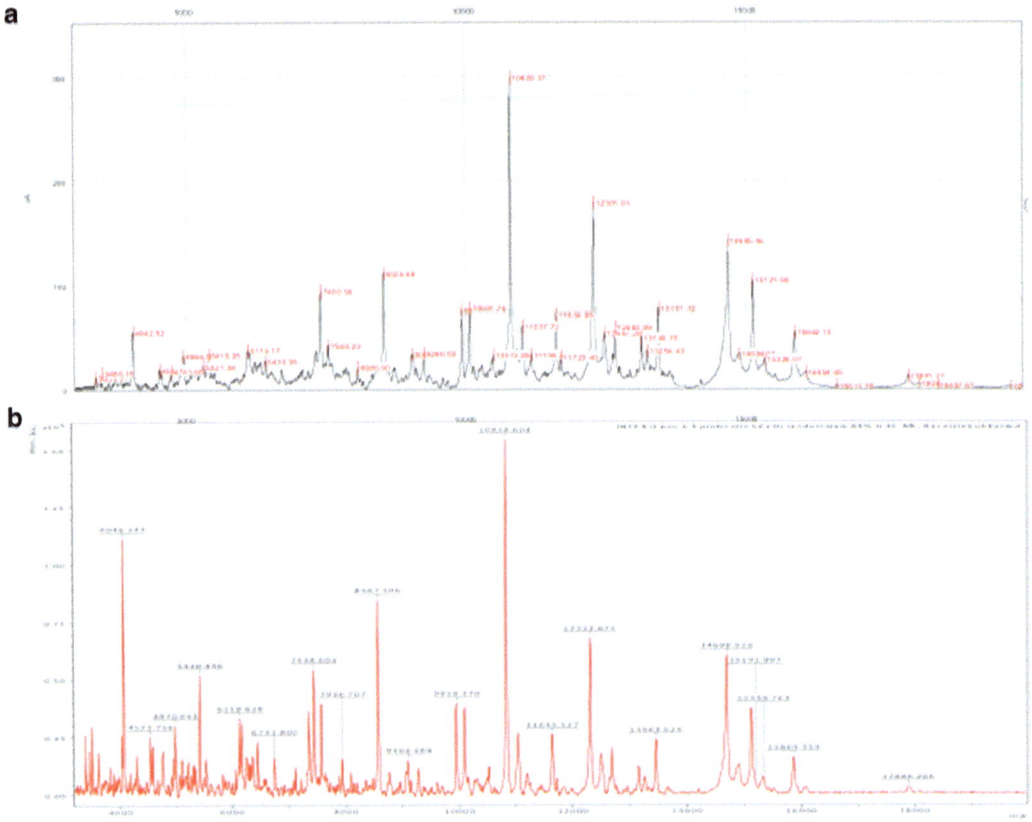

Fig. 2 Protein profile of a PBMC whole extract run on ProteinChip reader (**a**) and on Autoflex III Smartbeam MALDI-TOF-MS/MS (**b**). Note the improved resolution obtained by MALDI profiling in the low-molecular-weight region (3,000–6,000 *m/z*)

17. If you want to use external software for the analysis, use export spectra function and then define the format to which the dataset has to be exported (.xml or .csv).
18. A representative protein profile obtained by SELDI-TOF/MS is shown in Fig. 2a.

3.5 Protein Profiling Acquisition on MALDI-TOF/ MS

1. Open the FlexControl (v 3.3.64) software.
2. Insert the ProteinChip array into the LUCID array holder (Fig. 1), then insert the holder into the instrument, and let it perform routine controls before acquisition.
3. Calibrate the instrument by pointing the laser on the calibration spot between the sample spots of the ProteinChip array. Recall the calibration curve of the protein calibration standard I and then click "calibrate" button.
4. Set the acquisition protocol (*see* **Note 16**).
5. Set the detection parameters (*see* **Note 17**).
6. Set the mass range and the laser frequency (*see* **Note 18**).

7. Select the AUTOEXECUTE BOX and create a new acquisition protocol (*see* **Note 19**).
8. Set laser intensity at about 80 % (*see* **Note 20**) and run the saved acquisition protocol.
9. At the end of the acquisition select a destination folder and save your spectra.
10. Open the FlexAnalysis software (v 3.3.65) and recall your spectra.
11. Select the "process" button and then click on "smooth mass spectrum" and "subtract mass spectrum baseline."
12. Select the "method" button, choose the appropriate processing method in the list (*see* **Note 21**), and then select "find peaks" to identify the mass peaks in the MALDI spectrum.
13. If you have the ClinProTools™ software you can use it for post-acquisition analysis (*see* **Note 22**). Alternatively you can export the raw data (.xml or excel format) and use external software for the analysis.
14. A representative protein profile obtained by MALDI-TOF/MS is shown in Fig. 2b.

4 Notes

1. Leave one aliquot of lysis buffer at 4 °C for current use and store the remaining aliquots at −20 °C. Add endonucleases, phosphoprotease and protease inhibitor cocktail to lysis buffer according to the instruction of product information for cell lysate.
2. The commercially available ProteinChip arrays allow selective profiling of subsets of proteins according to their capability to bind the functionalized groups of each ProteinChip type: CM10 which binds proteins by weak cationic exchange is preferably used to capture basic proteins; Q10 which binds proteins through strong anionic exchange is used for acidic proteins; H50 which binds proteins through reverse hydrophobic interaction is generally used for capturing of hydrophobic proteins; IMAC 30 which is coupled to a number of metal ions (i.e., Cu^{2+}) binds proteins based on metal affinity and is finally used to select metal-binding proteins (e.g., enzymes).
3. The composition of the washing/binding buffer varies according to the ProteinChip to be used: Use 100 mM Tris–HCl pH 8.8 for Q10 ProteinChip; 100 mM sodium acetate, pH 4 for CM10; 10 % acetonitrile/0.1 % TFA for H50; the IMAC ProteinChip needs to be preloaded with Cu^{2+} and then neutralized by sodium acetate pH 4. Use 0.1 M Tris–HCl, pH 7.4 as binding/washing buffer for this PorteinChip array.

4. Lucid ID access pack includes Lucid array holder and stand and the instructions to configure the MALDI-TOF-MS (Autoflex series, Bruker Daltonics, Germany) for accommodating and analyzing SELDI ProteinChip arrays.
5. Be careful to avoid aspirating the plasma and Ficoll-Paque.
6. The protein extraction and analysis by SELDI and MALDI-TOF/MS can also be applied to $CD8^+$ T cells isolated from PBMC by negative selection using immunomagnetic system. Refer to the previous chapters for details on $CD8^+$ T cell isolation protocol.
7. Be aware to avoid the formation of air bubbles since it can interfere with the binding of the proteins to the ProteinChip surface.
8. Prepare the Protein Standard I according to the procedure described by the manufacturer's datasheet.
9. Run the ProteinChip OQ kit on your instrument according to the procedure described by the manufacturer's datasheet. Perform the ProteinChip OQ kit analysis bi-weekly to ascertain the stability of the instrument performance and improve the reproducibility of the results.
10. Set the following parameters in the acquisition protocol: Name: define a name for your acquisition protocol; template: select profiling high mass (25 kV) and then click *next*. In the acquisition setting panel define 3,000–30,000 as mass range; select 2,500 as matrix attenuation and 800 as sampling rate. In the shot sequences box define 1 as warming shot at 6,600 nj energy and 7 as Data Shots at 6,000 nj.
11. Set 1:1 in the partition box if you want to acquire the entire spectrum; reduce the partition (i.e., 1:2; 1:3; 1:4) if you want to try different acquisition protocols on the same spot.
12. Select the spectrum to be used for the creation of the calibration equation. By right clicking select "calibrate" and then "internal calibration." In the internal calibration dialog click "match calibrants to peaks" button. The software will auto-assign the calibrant's name to the corresponding mass peaks. Click "Calibrate" button and then select "Save calibration Equation" to assign a name to the calibration equation.
13. The peak detection uses the default values for baseline, filtering, noise, and spot correction that are reported in the analysis setting box (magnifier icon). These parameters are optimized for protein profiling analysis. Do not modify them.
14. Select the "η" icon, then define 3,000–30,000 as min and max M/Z, and then select APPLY to normalize all the spectra.
15. The EDM function allows to identify clusters of mass peaks (common mass peaks between two or more groups) in multiple mass spectra and to evaluate their significant association

(p-value < 0.05) within a specific group by applying the Mann-Whitney (for two groups) or the Kruskal-Wallis (for more than two groups) tests. Further the data sets may be analyzed by Biomarker Pattern Software (BPS) that uses CART algorithm to build a decision tree based on the combination of differently expressed mass peaks. Refer to the ProteinChip Data Manager and BPS handbooks for details.

16. In the SPECTROMETER dialog box set 20.00 kV for ion source 1; 18.70 kV for ion source 2; 6.5 kV for LENS; 50 ns for pulsed ion extraction; DEFLECTION for matrix suppression; and 1,500 Da for suppression.
17. Select the DETECTION dialog BOX and then set 3,000–30,000 Da for detection; MEDIUM RANGE as detection mode; "LINEAR 48X" as detection gain; and "0.5 GS/s" as sample rate.
18. Select the SETUP dialog box and then set MEDIUM RANGE as mass range selection and 200 Hz as laser frequency.
19. In the AUTOEXECUTE dialog box select EVALUATION and then set 3,000–30,000 Da as mass range. In the PROCESSING METHOD box select EDIT NEW METHOD and then set the following parameters: CENTROID as peak detection algorithm; 4 as signal-to-noise ratio; 50 as min intensity threshold; 500 as maximum number of peaks; 3 m/z as peak width; 50 % as peak height and TopHat as method for baseline subtraction; save this processing method. In the PEAK RESOLUTION box set 500 as minimum peak resolution and six times above the threshold as max resolution. In the "ACCUMULATION" box set up the cumulative spectra as the sum of 20,000 satisfactory shots in 200 shot steps. In the MOVEMENT box select RANDOM WALK and set up 200 shot at raster spot. Of note, the number of satisfactory shots can be increased or reduced until an overall good-quality spectra is obtained.
20. The reported results have been obtained by setting the laser intensity at 84 %. Depending on the overall performance or usage of the laser, you may need to optimize the laser intensity until achieving a satisfactory protein profile.
21. The manufacturer sets a list of processing methods. Select the preset method for the detection of the protein mass peaks acquired in positive linear mode in the 3,000–30,000 Da mass range. If using the default processing parameters of this method, the number of identified peaks is not satisfactory, select EDIT PARAMETERS from the method menu, then recall the processing method having the optimized parameters defined in **Note 17**, and select again FIND PEAKS.
22. ClinProTools™ (CPT) software provides univariate and multivariate statistical tools for normally and not normally distributed data sets. For the statistics of single peaks, CPT uses the

Quick Classifier algorithm (QC) which is a univariate sorting algorithm while genetic algorithms (GA) and support vector machine (SVM) are advanced multivariate analysis tools useful to create classification models based on a combination of differently expressed mass peaks. Refer to the manufacturer for detailed information on CPT features.

References

1. Lodish H, Berk A, Matsudaira P, Kaiser CA, Krieger M, Scott MP, Zipurksy SL, Darnell J (2004) Molecular cell biology, 5th edn. WH Freeman, New York, NY
2. Richards J, Le Naour F, Hanash S, Beretta L (2002) Integrated genomic and proteomic analysis of signaling pathways in dendritic cell differentiation and maturation. Ann N Y Acad Sci 975:91–100
3. Hettinger J, Richards DM, Hansson J et al (2013) Origin of monocytes and macrophages in a committed progenitor. Nat Immunol 14(8):821–830
4. Jeong HC, Lee SY, Lee EJ et al (2007) Proteomic analysis of peripheral T-lymphocytes in patients with asthma. Chest 132(2): 489–496
5. Papale M, Rocchetti MT, Gesualdo L (2013) Clinical proteomics: the potentiality of urine analysis for understanding diabetic nephropathy. EMJ Neph 1:32–39
6. Papale M, Di Paolo S, Magistroni R et al (2010) Urine proteome analysis may allow noinvasive differential diagnosis of diabetic nephropathy. Diabetes Care 33(11):2409–15
7. Sui W, Dai Y, Zhang Y et al (2010) Proteomic profiling of uremia in serum using magnetic bead-based sample fractionation and MALDI-TOF MS. Ren Fail 32(10):1153–9

Chapter 13

Two-Dimensional Gel Electrophoresis Approach for CTL Phosphoproteome Analysis

Maria Teresa Rocchetti, Massimo Papale, and Loreto Gesualdo

Abstract

Phosphorylation of proteins plays a pivotal role in signal transduction processes, and it is a key regulator of many biological cell functions. Various strategies have been proposed for the study of phosphoproteome; most of them require a multi-step analysis and sophisticated equipment. Here we describe the two-dimensional polyacrylamide gel electrophoresis (2D-PAGE) analysis of PBMC phosphoproteome using as preliminary enrichment step a simple phosphoprotein isolation by lanthanum chloride. This strategy can be most certainly applied to study the phosphoproteome of CTLs isolated from PBMCs. The phosphoproteome analysis of PBMCs, as well as of CTLs, may help to reveal the signaling pathways essential to their biological role in health and disease.

Key words Phosphoproteome, Two-dimensional gel electrophoresis, Lanthanum chloride, PBMC, CTL

1 Introduction

Phosphorylation represents the most salient protein's posttranslational modification (PTM) [1] which modulates the stereochemistry and therefore the functional activity of proteins in cellular processes. Phosphorylation of proteins plays a key role in signal transduction events; it controls proliferation, differentiation, and apoptosis by a complex interplay between kinases and phosphatases. Up to 50 % of the proteins are estimated to be reversibly phosphorylated at some point during their life-span [2]. This transient nature of phosphorylation together with the various protein sites of modification and the possibility that more than one phosphate group could be added to a protein offer the cell a wide range of responses to the several changing conditions. Phosphoproteins' analysis is a challenging task essentially because of the low stoichiometry of phosphorylation and the low abundance of phosphoproteins within cells at any given time. In recent years, a number of analytical methods for phosphoproteome analysis have been proposed, each with

Elena Ranieri (ed.), *Cytotoxic T-Cells: Methods and Protocols*, Methods in Molecular Biology, vol. 1186,
DOI 10.1007/978-1-4939-1158-5_13, © Springer Science+Business Media New York 2014

its own strengths and limitations. Both, top-down and bottom-up proteomic approaches have been applied [3]. Generally, the most used top-down approach used gel-based proteomic analysis, where proteins can be detected by using a phospho-specific fluorescent dye [4] or by specific anti-phospho antibodies after gel-membrane blotting [5]. Instead, among the bottom-up approach the chromatographic separation of the total protein tryptic digest followed by shotgun tandem mass spectrometry analysis (LC-MS/MS) has been the most applied [6, 7]. Anyway, the common limitation which characterized these proteomic approaches is the high background of non-phosphorylated proteins/peptides which decrease the sensitivity of the phosphoprotein analysis. Therefore, enrichment of phosphoproteins/phosphopeptides from complex protein/peptide mixture became a prerequisite before analysis. At the best of our knowledge, no data are available on 2DE gel PBMCs' phosphoproteome analysis which uses a phosphoprotein enrichment strategy as preliminary step. Literature data focused on quantitative phosphoproteomic studies on T cells (i.e., T cells expanded ex vivo from mice or human blood, Jurkat human leukemic T cell line), complex multi-step bottom-up strategy mainly consisting of immunoprecipitation of phosphoproteins (mainly phosphotyrosine) followed by (1) total protein tryptic digestion, (2) chromatographic enrichment of phosphopeptides (such as immobilized metal ion affinity chromatography, IMAC, or metal oxide affinity chromatography, MOAC), and (3) quantitative liquid chromatography tandem mass spectrometry analysis (LC-MS/MS) [8–10].

Here the phosphoproteome analysis of PBMCs is described by a top-down approach: PBMCs' phosphoproteins were enriched by a straightforward and easily applicable one-step method, which consists in the precipitation of phosphorylated proteins by lanthanum ions [11], and their analysis by two-dimensional polyacrylamide gel electrophoresis (2D-PAGE). Defining the 2D map of the phosphoproteins and their isoforms (visible on the gel as spot trains) offers a useful tool for protein cataloguing which could reveal the signaling pathways essential to maintain the epigenetic, transcriptional, and metabolic programs of PBMCs helpful to study several disorders in which the immune system turned out to be activated (i.e., autoimmune diseases [12], cancer [13], neurological disorders [14]). Definitely, the procedure described can be applied to study the phosphoproteome of CTLs after their isolation from PBMCs and expansion of T cell numbers ex vivo.

2 Materials

All solutions were prepared by using ultrapure water (sensitivity of 18 MΩ cm at 25 °C) and analytical grade reagents. All reagents were prepared at room temperature (unless indicated otherwise). Diligently follow all waste disposal regulations when disposing waste materials.

2.1 PBMC Isolation

1. Ficoll-Hypaque density gradient solution.
2. Phosphate-buffered saline (PBS).
3. EDTA.

2.2 Protein Extraction

1. Lysis buffer: 1 M Tris–HCl, pH 7.4, 1 M NaCl, 1.5 % NP-40 in water solution. Leave one aliquot at 4 °C for current use and store the remaining aliquots at −20 °C. Endonucleases and phosphoprotease and protease inhibitor cocktail were added at current use (*see* **Note 1**).
2. Bradford reagent (BioRad Protein assay).

2.3 Phosphoprotein Isolation

1. Lanthanum chloride solution: 1 M $LaCl_3$ in water.
2. Potassium dihydrogen phosphate solution: 2 M KH_2PO_4 in water.
3. Washing solution: 8 M urea, 1 % CHAPS in water.
4. Elution solution: 25 % 4 M Imidazole in water/75 % (8 M urea, 2 M thiourea, 2 %CHAPS, 1 % DTT in water).
5. Acetone/20 % trichloroacetic acid (TCA) (9/1).
6. Sample buffer: 8 M urea, 4 % CHAPS, 40 mM Tris–base, 65 mM DTT, and 0.002 % w/v bromophenol blue (BBP). Leave one aliquot at 4 °C for current use and store the remaining aliquots at −20 °C.

2.4 Isoelectrofocusing (IEF) and Sodium Dodecyl Sulfate-Polyacrylamide Gel Electrophoresis (SDS-PAGE) Components

1. IEF instrument: Protean® IEF Cell (Bio-Rad Laboratories, Hercules, CA).
2. ReadyStrip™ IPG Strip 7 cm, pH 3–10 (Bio-Rad Laboratories).
3. Rehydration solution: 8 M urea, 2 % w/v CHAPS, 0.5 % ampholine (pH 3–10), 18 mM DTT, 0.002 % w/v bromophenol blue (BBP). Leave one aliquot at 4 °C for current use and store the remaining aliquots at −20 °C (*see* **Note 2**).
4. Equilibration buffer: 75 mM Tris–HCl, pH 8.8, 6 M urea, 30 % v/v glycerol 87 %, 2 % w/v SDS, 0.002 % w/v BBP (*see* **Note 3**).
5. DTT, IAA (*see* **Note 4**), mineral oil.
6. SDS-PAGE instrument: Mini-PROTEAN® Tetra System (Bio-Rad Laboratories).
7. Resolving gel buffer: 1.5 M Tris–HCl, pH 8.8. Store at 4 °C.
8. 30 % acrylamide/piperazine diacrylamide (PDA, Bio-Rad laboratories) solution (12.5 %/2.6 % acrylamide/PDA): Add 3.2 g of PDA to 300 mL of 40 % acrylamide, make up to 400 mL with water, and mix for about 30 min in the dark. Filter through a 0.45 μm Corning filter and store at 4 °C in a bottle wrapped with aluminum foil (*see* **Note 5**).
9. Sodium dodecyl sulfate: 10 % solution in water.

10. Ammonium persulfate: 10 % solution in water (in a vial wrapped with aluminum foil).
11. *N*, *N*, *N*, *N'*-tetramethyl-ethylenediamine (TEMED) (Bio-Rad laboratories). Store at 4 °C.
12. 0.5 % w/v agarose solution in water.
13. SDS-PAGE running buffer (10×): 25 mM Tris base, 192 mM glycine, 1 % w/v SDS make up to 1 L of water and store at +4 °C (*see* **Note 6**).
14. Molecular weight standards: PeppermintStick™ Phosphoprotein Molecular Weight Standards (Invitrogen™).
15. Fixing solution: 40 % ethanol, 10 % acetic acid in water solution.
16. Sypro® Ruby gel dye (Invitrogen™).
17. Destaining solution: 10 % methanol, 7 % acetic acid in water solution.
18. Preserving solution: 1 % acetic acid in water solution.
19. Glass or plastic (PP) container.

3 Methods

All procedures were carried out at room temperature unless otherwise specified. Always wear powder-free laboratory gloves when handling IPG strip, gel, and all apparatus and solution used in their preparation to prevent protein contamination (keratins!). Further, to avoid contamination filter all aqueous solution, cover all recipients to use, and work under the fume hood.

3.1 Human Peripheral Blood Mononuclear Cell (PBMC) Isolation

1. Dilute 28–30 mL of fresh heparinized blood with PBS 1× pH 7.4/1 mM EDTA in ratio 1:2 and mix well.
2. Place 15 mL of Ficoll-Hypaque into three 50 mL conical centrifuge tubes and gently transfer 25 mL of the diluted blood onto the Ficoll-Paque so that they form two separate layers.
3. Centrifuge at room temperature at 460 × *g* for 30 min without breaks.
4. Using a sterile pipet, collect the leukocytes at the interphase layer and transfer them to another 50 mL tube up to 25 mL. Try to avoid aspirating the plasma and Ficoll-Paque.
5. Wash the cell suspensions with PBS up to 50 mL in each tube and centrifuge for 12 min at 250 × *g* and room temperature.
6. Discard the supernatants, resuspend the cells with physiological saline solution (0.9 % NaCl), and repeat the wash centrifuging for 10 min at 175 × *g* and room temperature.

   Remove the supernatant and store at −80 °C until use.

3.2 Protein Extraction from PBMCs

In our experience, a mean of 3×10^7 PBMCs yield about 1–2 mg of solubilized proteins. As well, about 3×10^7 $CD8^+$ T cells are necessary to obtain the same protein yield. $CD8^+$ T cells can be isolated by negative selection using immunomagnetic system, as described in detail in the previous chapter, and further expanded to gain the suitable number of cells.

1. Add 500 μL of lysis buffer, 10 μL of endonuclease, and 5 μL of protease inhibitor to the cell pellet (*see* **Note 1**). Disperse the pellet by pipetting up and down and transfer it in a clean vial. Then incubate on ice for 30 min, vortexing for 1 min every 5 min.
2. Centrifuge the cell lysate at 10,000 × *g* at 4 °C for 20 min. Transfer the supernatant to a clean vial.
3. Assay the protein concentration by Bradford method.

3.3 Phosphoprotein Isolation

1. Add 3 μL of 1 M LaCl3 solution to 1 mg/mL protein mixture and vortex for 1 min. Add the same volume of 2 M KH_2PO_4 to the protein mixture and vortex for a further 1 min.
2. Centrifuge the protein mixture for 1 min at 2,500 × *g*. Remove the supernatant.
3. Resuspend the pellet with 300 μL of washing solution. Centrifuge for 30 s at 2,500 × *g*. Remove the supernatant.
4. Resuspend the pellet with 300 μL of water. Centrifuge for 30 s at 2,500 × *g*. Remove the supernatant. Repeat this step three times.
5. Elute the phosphoproteins resuspending the pellet in 60 μL of elution solution. Incubate at room temperature for 10 min. Centrifuge for 1 min at 13,000 × *g*. Transfer the supernatant in a clean vial.
6. Add 120 μL of cold acetone/20 % TCA in water (9/1), vortex, and leave it at −20 °C overnight.
7. Centrifuge at +4 °C for 30 min at 15,000 rpm. Discard the supernatant and solubilize the phosphoproteins with about 30–40 μL of sample buffer.
8. Assay the protein concentration by Bradford method.

3.4 12 % Two-Dimensional Sodium Dodecyl Sulfate Polyacrylamide Gel Electrophoresis (2D-PAGE)

1. Rehydration of IPG strip: Add to 1 mL of rehydration buffer 2.8 mg of DTT and 13 μL of ampholine pH 3–10. Load 125 μL of rehydration buffer as a line along the edge of a channel in a clean dry disposable rehydration/equilibration tray (Fig. 1a). Take care not to introduce any bubbles. Remove the cover sheet from the IPG strip using forceps, and place the IPG strip, gel side down, onto the buffer. Overlay the IPG strip with 1 mL of mineral oil to prevent evaporation of buffer. Cover the rehydration/equilibration tray and leave it on Protean® IEF Cell overnight to rehydrate.

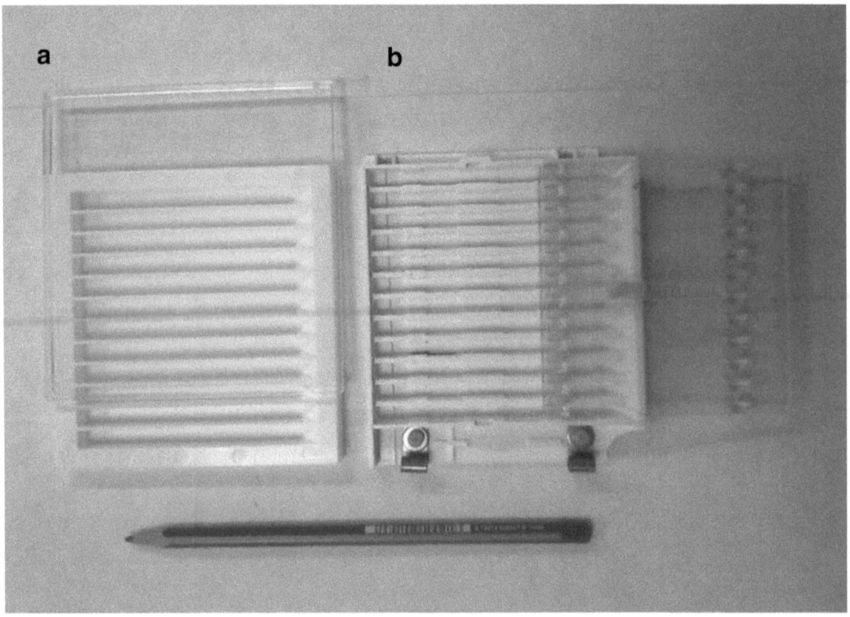

Fig. 1 (**a**) Rehydration/equilibration tray. (**b**) Focusing tray

2. IEF: Place a wet paper wick at each end of the channel to cover the wire electrode. Load 10–200 μg of phosphoproteins (max 30 μL) along the edge of a channel in the focusing tray (Fig. 1b). Transfer the rehydrated IPG strip from the rehydration/equilibration tray to the focusing tray maintaining the gel side down and observing the correct polarity. Cover the IPG strip with 1 mL of mineral oil, cover the focusing tray, and place it into the PROTEAN IEF cell. Run the electrophoresis using the following standardized protocol: 20 °C, 50 μA/IPG strip, 250 V for 1 h (linear slope), 500 V for 3 h (linear slope), 4,000 V for 4 h (linear slope), and 4,000 V for 4 h (slow slope).
3. Strip equilibration: Remove the IPG strip from the focusing tray and transfer them gel side up into a channel of the rehydration/equilibration tray. Add 1.25 mL of 130 mM DTT equilibration buffer for 15 min at room temperature under gentle shaking. Remove DTT solution and add 1.25 mL of 270 mM IAA equilibration buffer for 15 min at room temperature under gentle shaking in the dark. Remove the IPG strip from the tray and place it on the top of polyacrylamide gel.
4. 12 % polyacrylamide gel: Mix 2.5 mL of resolving buffer, 4 mL of acrylamide mixture, and 3.3 mL water in a 20 mL conical flask. Add 100 μL of 10 % SDS, 50 μL of 10 % ammonium persulfate, and 6.5 μ L of TEMED, and cast gel within an 8.2 cm × 8.2 cm × 1.5 mm vertical gel cassette (*see* **Note 5**). Allow 0.5 cm space for IPG strip loading and gently overlay with isopropanol. After allowing a minimum of 1 h for

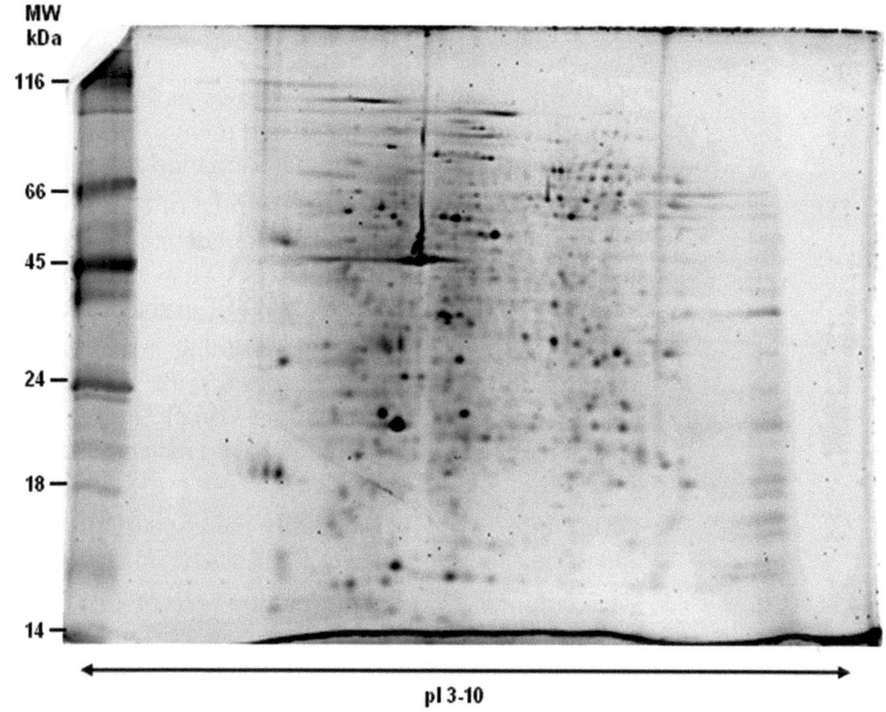

Fig. 2 Two-dimensional gel electrophoresis of PBMCs' phosphoproteins. *MW* molecular weight, *pI* isoelectric point

polymerization, remove the overlay and rinse the gel surface with water (*see* **Note 7**).

5. SDS-PAGE: Fill up the 0.5 cm space over the gel with warm 0.5 % agarose solution and immediately slip the equilibrated IPG strip into the agarose layer over the top surface of the gel. Apply 2 μL of phosphoprotein markers on a piece of paper and place it on the surface of the gel just beyond the end of the IPG strip. Place the gel cassette in the Mini-PROTEAN® Tetra System, plug in the electrode connectors to a power supply, and run at 50 V for 30 min and 200 V till the dye front reaches the end of the gel.
6. Fix the gel. After SDS-PAGE running, remove the gel from cassette with the help of a spatula and soak it in 250 mL of fixing solution for 3 h (*see* **Note 8**).
7. Stain the gel. Rinse the gel with small amount of water, add 100 mL of SYPRO® Ruby solution, and incubate the gel in the dark with gentle agitation overnight at 4 °C.
8. Destain the gel. Remove the staining solution and incubate with 250 mL of destaining solution in the dark with gentle agitation for 1 h. Repeat this procedure once more.
9. Preserve the gel. Remove the destaining solution and wash the gel with 100 mL of 1 % acetic acid solution for 30 min prior to imaging (Fig. 2) (*see* **Note 9**).

4 Notes

1. Thaw the aliquots of endonucleases and phosphoprotease–protease inhibitor cocktail and add them to lysis buffer following the instruction of product information for cell lysate.
2. Prepare a stock solution (i.e., 20 mL) of 8 M urea, 2 % w/v CHAPS, and 0.002 % w/v bromophenol blue (BBP), aliquot in 1 mL or less, and store at −20 °C. Thaw the aliquot and add fresh ampholine (pH 3–10) and DTT at the point of use.
3. Prepare the equilibration buffer adding first urea, Tris–HCl, and glycerol. Urea can be dissolved faster warming to about 37 °C. Add SDS and BBP after complete urea dissolution. Wear a mask when weighing SDS, and manage it gently; this is a very irritating fine powder.
4. Divide into two equal amounts the equilibration buffer and add in one aliquot fresh DTT and in the other one fresh IAA.
5. We recommend to filter all solution (except TEMED) used to make the polyacrylamide gel. Avoid air bubbles during the procedure. Unpolymerized acrylamide is a neurotoxin and care should be exercised to avoid skin contact.
6. To run the gel dilute ten times with water the SDS-PAGE running buffer.
7. Gels not used immediately can be stored for future use at 4 °C for up 2 weeks in an appropriate gel storage solution (0.375 M Tris–HCl, pH 8.8, 0.1 % SDS in water solution). In our laboratory we make gels fresh; we pipette a film of water over the top gel surface, seal the gel cassette with parafilm, store the gel at 4 °C, and use it within 24 h.
8. Cut the upper corner of the gel in correspondence to the IPG strip anode to orient the 2D gel map.
9. After image acquisition an image of two-dimensional gel map is obtained. To standardize the 2DE gel map of a biological sample, at least three technical replicates of more than one biological sample are required. The 2D images are analyzed by a dedicate software (Image Master 2D Platinum, Melanie, etc.) which allows the automatic spot detection and provides information from gel pattern such as spot number and position, background, and spot density. The images obtained from technical and biological replicate are matched to provide a reference gel with a specific number and position of spots (indicated as mean ± SD). The 2DE technique is often used in comparative analysis; the software can detect and graphically display quantitative changes in spot patterns (i.e., the gels of the healthy control group versus the gels of disease group)

providing a list of spots differentially expressed between them which can be subsequently identified by mass spectrometry analysis (i.e., MALDI-TOF-MS/MS, ESI-MS/MS).

Acknowledgment

The study was supported by the Grant of the Italian Ministry of Research and Education (FIRB2010-CAROMICS) to L.G. and E.R.

References

1. Fardilha M, Esteves SL, Korrodi-Gregorio L et al (2010) The physiological relevance of protein phosphatase 1 and its interacting proteins to health and disease. Curr Med Chem 17:3996–4017
2. Reinders J, Sickmann A (2005) State-of-the-art in phosphoproteomics. Proteomics 5: 4052–4061
3. Wu S, Lourette NM, Tolic N et al (2009) An integrated top-down and bottom-up strategy for broadly characterizing protein isoforms and modifications. J Proteome Res 8: 1347–1357
4. Schulemberg B, Goodman TN, Aggeler R et al (2004) Characterization of dynamic and steady-state protein phosphorylation using a fluorescent phosphoprotein gel stain and mass spectrometry. Electrophoresis 25: 2526–2532
5. Kaufmann H, Bailey JE, Fussenegge M (2001) Use of antibodies for detection of phosphorylated proteins separated by two-dimensional gel electrophoresis. Proteomics 1:194–199
6. Jerry DH, Surendra D, David LT (2013) Informatics of protein and posttranslational modification detection via shotgun proteomics. Methods Mol Biol 1002:167–179
7. McDonald WH, Yates JR 3rd (2002) Shotgun proteomics and biomarker discovery. Dis Markers 18:99–105
8. Cao L, Ding Y, Hung N et al (2012) Quantitative phosphoproteomics reveals SLP-76 dependent regulation of PAG and Src family kinases in T cells. PloS One 7:e46725
9. Iwai LK, Benoist C, Mathis D et al (2010) Quantitative phosphoproteomic analysis of T cell receptor signaling in diabetes prone resistant mice. J Proteome Res 9:3135–3145
10. Ruperez P, Gago-Martinez A, Burlingame AL et al (2012) Quantitative phosphoproteomic analysis reveals a role for serine and threonine kinases in the cytoskeletal reorganization in early T cell receptor activation in human primary T cells. Mol Cell Proteomics 11:171–186
11. Pink M, Verma N, Polato F et al (2011) Precipitation by lanthanum ions: a straightforward approach to isolating phosphoproteins. J Proteomics 75:375–383
12. Mesko B, Poliska S, Nagy L (2011) Gene expression profiles in peripheral blood for the diagnosis of autoimmune diseases. Trends Mol Med 17:223–233
13. Zhang Z, Li Y, Guan X, Yang X et al (2012) Human leukocyte antigen class I on peripheral blood mononuclear cells as a non-invasive biomarker for esophageal cancer. Dis Esophagus 25:273–278
14. Pasinetti GM, Fivecoat H, Ho L (2010) Personalized medicine in traumatic brain injury. Psychiatr Clin North Am 33:905–913

Chapter 14

Targeting the JAK/STAT Pathway in Cytotoxic T lymphocytes (CTL) by Next Generation Sequencing (NGS)

Maddalena Gigante, Sterpeta Diella, and Elena Ranieri

Abstract

Next Generation Sequencing (NGS), together with our evolving knowledge of genes and disease, is likely to change the current practice of medicine and public health by facilitating more accurate, sophisticated, and cost-effective genetic testing. Here, we propose a new molecular approach by using MiSeq Sequencing System (Illumina) to investigate the presence of mutations/variants in genes of JAK/STAT pathway involved in different cytotoxic T lymphocytes (CTL)-mediated immune disorders and to develop and validate new and less expensive molecular protocol based on Next Generation Sequencing.

Key words Mutation, NGS, Cytotoxic T lymphocytes

1 Introduction

Next Generation Sequencing (NGS), together with our evolving knowledge of genes and disease, is likely to change the current practice of medicine and public health by facilitating more accurate, sophisticated, and cost-effective genetic testing. Here, we propose a new molecular approach by using MiSeq Sequencing System (Illumina). Primary objectives of the present methodology will be to investigate the presence of genetic abnormalities in genes of JAK/STAT pathway involved in different cytotoxic T lymphocytes (CTL)-mediated immune disorders and to develop and validate new and less expensive molecular protocol based on Next Generation Sequencing. Cytotoxic T cells or natural killer cells have played important roles in the setting of infectious disease and cancer. Though many immune components that participate in these processes are known, the underlying mechanisms remain poorly defined. Cytokines and their receptors play an essential role in T cell proliferation and activation. Although cytokine receptors lack intrinsic kinase activity, they are associated with cytoplasmic protein tyrosine kinases (PTKs) that phosphorylate downstream signaling molecules such as the signal transducers and activators of

Elena Ranieri (ed.), *Cytotoxic T-Cells: Methods and Protocols*, Methods in Molecular Biology, vol. 1186,
DOI 10.1007/978-1-4939-1158-5_14, © Springer Science+Business Media New York 2014

transcription (STATs). Activated STATs, in turn, translocate to the nucleus and regulate gene expression [1]. The Janus kinase (JAK) family of non-receptor PTKs includes critical elements in cytokine signaling. To date, four JAKs (JAK1, JAK2, JAK3, TYK2) and seven STATs (STAT1, STAT2, STAT3, STAT4, STAT5a, STAT5b, STAT6) have been described and fully characterized [2]. Mutations in *JAK3* gene have been associated with autosomal recessive severe combined immunodeficiency (SCID), a condition in which T cell development and B cell function are severely reduced, indicating that this kinase is essential for the correct development of mature lymphoid lineages [3, 4]. Moreover, the association of constitutive activation of JAK/STAT pathway with proliferation of T cell leukemia/lymphoma cells [5] and the presence of activating mutations in the *JAK3* pseudokinase domain in the acute megakaryoblastic leukemia (AMKL) cell line [6] suggest a role for altered *JAK3* expression and/or function in the development of human cancer. An association between JAK/STAT pathway and Renal Cell Carcinoma (RCC), a highly immunogenic tumor, was demonstrated by our group [7, 8] and by Kolenko et al. [9]. Finally, activating mutations in STAT3 were recently identified in 40 % of patients with large granular lymphocytic leukemia, a disorder characterized by the presence of abnormal CD3+CD8+CD57+ lymphocytes corresponding to activated effector cytotoxic T lymphocytes (CTLs) [10]. Our capability to couple specific phenotypes to genetic variation is now unprecedented, as high-resolution genome wide approaches are able to uncover novel relationships and rare variants. Next Generation Sequencing (NGS) has the advantage to harvest all the genetic variations, both small variants (single base substitution, small INDELs) and structural variants, and to identify also rare variants in genes belonging to a functionally relevant pathway and the whole spectrum of variability associated with a specific clinical/phenotypic spectrum. Since serially testing each gene of pathway by Sanger sequencing would be time consuming and expensive, we propose a multi-gene protocol based on NGS for a panel of 11 selected genes (JAK1, JAK2, JAK3, TYK2, STAT1, STAT2, STAT3, STAT4, STAT5A, STAT5B, STAT6) already known to be involved in JAK/STAT pathway and immune mechanisms. The development and validation of a protocol based on NGS may act as a model for tracing the new way of genomic laboratory medicine and have a strong potential also for clinical and diagnostic applications. Considering the key role of JAKs/STATs pathway in immune mechanisms, here, we set up a protocol using Next Generation Sequencing (NGS) for targeted analysis of JAK/STAT pathway genes and validate it by comparing the results with standard Sanger method. A training set of samples was used to optimize the entire process, and a second set was used to validate and independently evaluate the performance of the workflow. By this validation we are able to evaluate if our NGS protocol is able to ensure appropriateness, with high sensitivity and specificity, if it is cheaper, faster, and with a higher reproducibility than the Sanger reference method. Although in the first instance our protocol has a major impact on the studied genes, the implications may extend beyond, acting as a model for the new course of genomic medicine.

2 Materials

1. DNA purification kit (Life Technologies, Qiagen, Hilden, Germany).
2. *primer3* software (http://frodo.wi.mit.edu/cgi-bin/primer3/primer3_www.cgi).
3. NCBI/Primer-BLAST software (http://www.ncbi.nlm.nih.gov/tools/primer-blast/).
4. Human JAKs/STATs gene flanking intronic forward and reverse primers.
5. TaqGold (Life Technologies).
6. PCR Thermocycler.
7. Big Dye Terminator v3.1 cycle sequencing kit (Life Technologies).
8. 3130 Genetic Analyzer (Life Technologies).
9. SeqScape program (Life Technologies).
10. Design Studio (Illumina) software.
11. TruSeq Custom Amplicon Library Preparation Kit (Illumina).
12. TruSeq Custom Amplicon Library Preparation Guide (CATALOG: FC-130-9005DOC).
13. ACD1 and ACP1: Amplicon Control DNA 1 and Amplicon Control Oligo Pool (Illumina).
14. OHS2: Oligo Hybridization for Sequencing Reagent 2 (Illumina).
15. ELM4: Extension Ligation Mix 4 (Illumina).
16. PMM2: PCR Master Mix 2 (Illumina).
17. TDP1: TruSeq DNA Polymerase (Illumina).
18. SW1: Stringent Wash 1 (Illumina).
19. UB1: Universal Buffer 1 (Illumina).
20. LNB1 Library Normalization Beads 1 (Illumina).
21. HT1 Hybridization Buffer (Illumina).
22. LNA1 Library Normalization Additives 1 (Illumina).
23. LNW1 Library Normalization Wash 1 (Illumina).
24. LNS2 Library Normalization Storage Buffer 2 (Illumina).

25. EBT Elution Buffer with Tris (Illumina).
26. TruSeq Custom Amplicon Library Preparation Index Kit (Illumina).
27. CAT Custom Amplicon oligo Tube (Illumina).
28. i5 Index Primers, A501–A508 (Illumina).
29. i7 Index Primers, A701–A712 (Illumina).
30. 10 N NaOH.
31. 96-well skirted PCR plates, 0.2 ml, polypropylene.
32. Eppendorf microcentrifuge tubes (screw top recommended).
33. Conical tubes, 15 ml.
34. Adhesive aluminum foil seal.
35. Microseal "A" adhesive seals.
36. PCR Eight-Tube Strips.
37. Agarose gel.
38. Agilent 2100 Bioanalyzer.
39. DNA molecular weight markers.
40. MiSeq Sequencing System (Illumina).
41. Filter plate with lid (Iluumina).
42. Adapter collar (Illumina).
43. MIDI plates.
44. AMPure XP Beads (Beckman Coulter).
45. 96 well magnet plate (Beckman Coulter).

3 Methods

3.1 Human DNA Isolation and Sample Selection

The collection and handling of human blood should be performed in accordance to institutional rules and guidelines. Assume all blood products contain infectious material.

1. Isolate Genomic DNA from human peripheral blood leukocytes using standard DNA Purification Kit according to manufacturing' instructions (Life Technologies, Qiagen).
2. Measure DNA concentration and purity with NanoDrop and Agilent 2100 Bioanalyzer (Agilent Technologies, Santa Clara, CA, USA), providing highly accurate concentration measures of extremely small samples and sensitive quality analysis of DNA samples.
3. A training set of DNA samples (15–20), previously fully Sanger sequenced for selected genes of JAK/STAT pathway, should be used to optimize the entire process and a second set (10–15) should be used to validate and independently evaluate the performance of the workflow.

4. The use of samples that were previously fully Sanger sequenced allows the development of a set of known variants to be used as surrogate markers. This set should include known SNPs and different types of mutations (missense, nonsense, and indels) to reflect the range of variants expected to be identified by NGS.
5. To analyze the performance of the developed variant prioritization pipeline (VPP), a set of 10–15 additional samples, for which no molecular analysis has been performed before, should be selected.

3.2 Design Custom Oligo Probes

1. Use DesignStudio software (Illumina), an easy-to-use online software tool, to design oligo probes of targeting genomic regions of interest.
2. Initiate a project by entering target regions of the genome into DesignStudio software. Perform probe design automatically using an algorithm that considers a range of factors, including GC content, specificity, probe interaction, and coverage.
3. Candidate amplicons should be visualized and assessed using estimated success scores. Probes could be filtered with user defined tags, and then added to, or removed from the design project.
4. Optimize the assay in-house, with additional primers designed to target regions that were not well captured.
5. The final assay includes 385 amplicons targeted the protein-coding sequence of 11 selected genes (JAK1, JAK2, JAK3, TYK2, STAT1, STAT2, STAT3, STAT4, STAT5A, STAT5B, STAT6) involved in JAK/STAT pathway with an overhang at exon boundaries to capture splice site variants (Table 1).
6. After visualization and Quality Control (QC) oligonucleotide probes are synthesized and pooled into a tube (Custom Amplicon Tube, CAT) containing all the probes necessary to generate the attempted amplicons per reaction.
7. Sample-specific indices will be then added to each library by PCR using common primers from TruSeq Amplicon index Kit (*see* Subheading 3.3).

3.3 Amplicon Library Preparation Workflow

1. Prepare your libraries using TruSeq Custom Amplicon Library Preparation Kit and TruSeq Custom Amplicon Library Preparation Index Kit (Illumina) and the protocol detailed in the user guide (Illumina, CATALOG: FC-130-9005DOC). In summary, the workflow includes the following seven steps (Fig. 1):
   (a) *Hybridization of oligo-pool* (Total duration: 1 h 35 min). During this step, a custom pool containing upstream and downstream oligos specific to your targeted regions of interest is hybridized to your genomic DNA samples (*see* **Note 1**).

Table 1

Characteristics of 11 genes included in the assay

Gene symbol	Gene product	Genomic locus	Reference sequence	Number of exons	Coding cDNA ?length (bp)	Number of amplicons	Disease association
JAK1	Tyrosine-protein Kinase JAK1	1p32.3–p31.3	NM_002227.2	25	3,465 bp	35	Variants associated with different type of tumors
JAK2	Tyrosine-protein Kinase JAK2	9p24	NM_004972.3	25	3,399 bp	36	Leukemia acute myeloid (AML) Myelofibrosis Polycythemia Vera Thrombocythemia 3
JAK3	Tyrosine-protein Kinase JAK3	19p13.1	NM_000215.3	24	3,375 bp	37	Severe combined immunodeficiency T– B+ Renal Cell Carcinoma Leukemia Lymphoma
TYK2	Non-receptor tyrosine-protein kinase TYK2	19p13.2	NM_003331.4	25	3,564 bp	34	Autosomal recessive hyper IgE syndrome due to TYK2 deficiency Juvenile rheumatoid factor-negative polyarthritis Oligoarticular juvenile arthritis
STAT1	Signal transducer and activator of transcription 1	2q32.2	NM_007315.3	25	2,253 bp	36	Mendelian susceptibility to mycobacterial diseases due to partial STAT1 deficiency Candidiasis, Familial Chronic Mucocutaneous, Autosomal Dominant
STAT2	Signal transducer and activator of transcription 2	12q13.3	NM_005419.3	24	2,556 bp	37	Variants associated with different type of tumors
STAT3	Signal transducer and activator of transcription 3	17q21.31	NM_003150.3	24	2,310 bp	44	Autosomal dominant hyper IgE syndrome
STAT4	Signal transducer and activator of transcription 4	2q32.2-q32.3	NM_001243835.1	24	2,247 bp	27	Behcet disease Juvenile rheumatoid factor-negative polyarthritis Oligoarticular juvenile arthritis
STAT5A	Signal transducer and activator of transcription 5A	17q11.2	NM_003152.3	20	2,385 bp	30	Variants associated with different type of tumors
STAT5B	Signal transducer and activator of transcription 5B	17q11.2	NM_012448.3	19	2,364 bp	34	Laron syndrome with immunodeficiency Growth hormone insensitivity with immunodeficiency
STAT6	Signal transducer and activator of transcription 6	12q13	NM_001178078.1	22	2,544 bp	35	Variants associated with different type of tumors
Total					3,0462 bp	385	

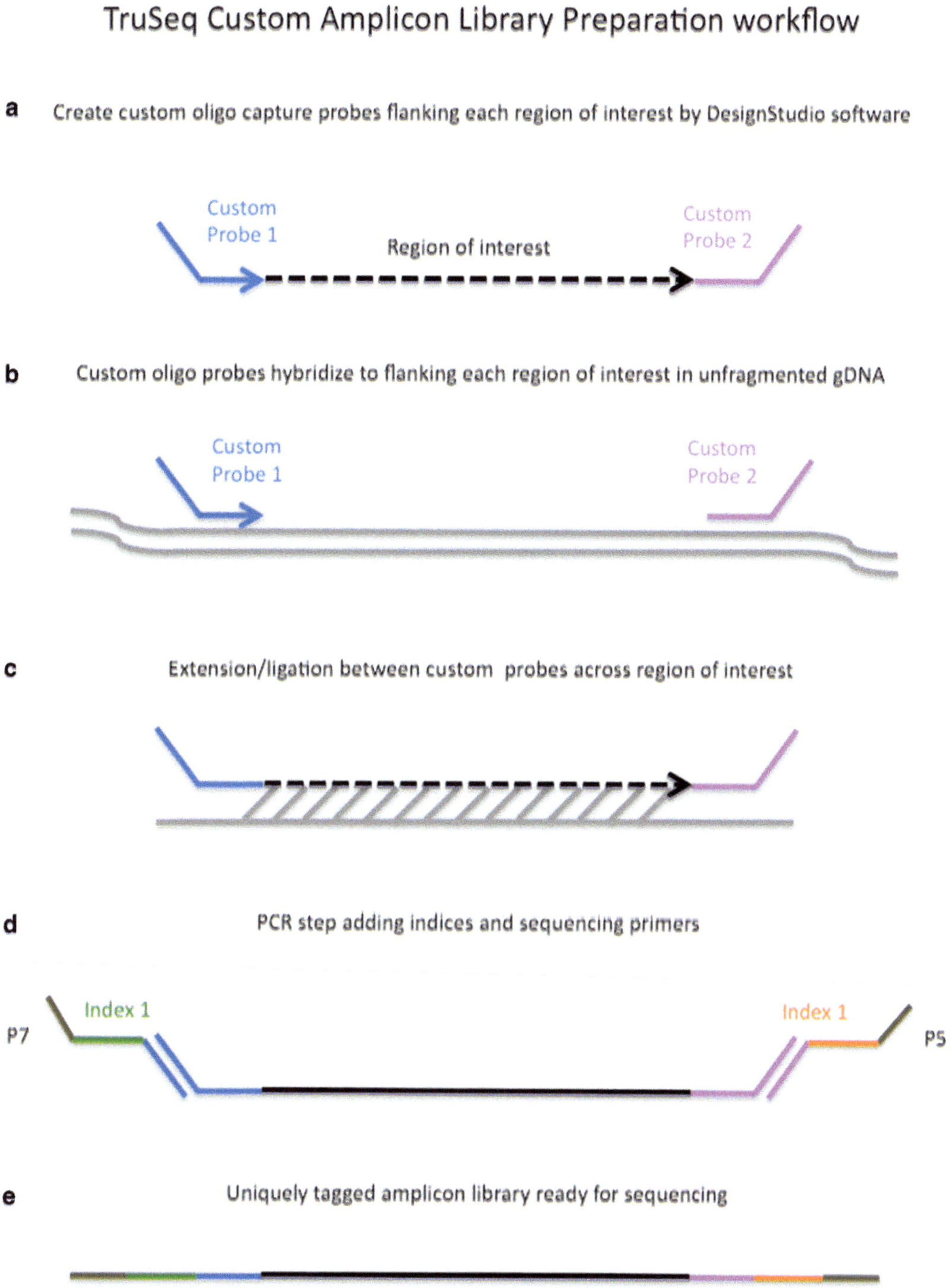

Fig. 1 TruSeq Custom Amplicon Library preparation workflow (modified by Illumina, CATALOG: FC-130-9005DOC)

Procedure

1. Make sure that concentrations and purity of your DNA samples are in agreement with those shown in the following table.

Type of DNA	Supported amplicon size	Input (Up to 15 μl)	A260/A280
High-quality genomic DNA	150, 175, 250, 425 bp	50 ng (minimum) 250 ng (recommended)	1.8–2.0

2. Use the provided controls of TruSeq Custom Amplicon Library Preparation Kit (ACD1/ACP1) in each batch of samples and add 5 μl of control DNA and 5 μl of TE or water to 1 well in the plate.
3. To each sample well to be used in the assay, add up to 15 μl of Genomic DNA (250 ng total).
4. Add 5 μl of control oligo pool ACP1 to the well containing control DNA ACD1.
5. Using a multichannel pipette, add 5 μl of CAT to the wells containing genomic DNA (*see* **Note 2**).
6. Using a multichannel pipette, add 35 μl of OHS2 (Oligo Hybridization for Sequencing 2) to each sample in the plate. When dispensing, gently pipette up and down 3–5 times to mix.
7. Seal the plate with adhesive aluminum foil and secure the seal with a rubber roller or sealing wedge.
8. Centrifuge to 1,000 × *g* at 20 °C for 1 min.
9. Place the plate in the preheated block at 95 °C and incubate for 1 min.
10. While the plate remains on the preheated block, set the temperature to 40 °C and continue incubating for 80 min.

(b) *Removal of unbound oligos* (Total duration: 20 min). This process removes unbound oligos from genomic DNA using a filter capable of size selection. Two wash steps using SW1 (Illumina) reagent ensure complete removal of unbound oligos. A third wash step using UB1 (Illumina) buffer removes residual SW1 and prepares samples for the extension ligation step.

Procedure

1. Assemble the filter plate assembly unit in the following order (from top to botton): lid, filter plate, adapter

collar and MIDI plate. Using a multichannel pipette, add 45 μl of SW1 (Stringent Wash 1) to each well. Cover the plate with the filter plate lid and centrifuge at 2,400 × g at 20 °C for 10 min.

2. After the 80 min incubation, confirm that the heat block has cooled to 40 °C. Remove the plate from the heat block and centrifuge to 1,000 × g at 20 °C for 1 min to collect condensation.
3. Using a multichannel pipette set to 65 μl, transfer the entire volume of each sample onto the center of the corresponding prewashed wells of the filter plate. Change tips after each column to avoid cross contamination.
4. Cover the plate with the filter plate lid and centrifuge at 2,400 × g at 20 °C for 2 min.
5. Wash the plate as using a multichannel pipette, adding 45 μl of SW1 to each sample well.
6. Cover the plate with the filter plate lid and centrifuge at 2,400 × g for 2 min (*see* **Note 3**).
7. Repeat the wash (**steps 5** and 6).
8. Discard all the flow-through (containing formamide waste and unbound oligos) collected up to this point in an appropriate hazardous waste container, then reassemble the filter plate.
9. Using a multichannel pipette add 45 μl of UB1 (Universal Buffer 1) to each sample well.
10. Cover the plate with the filter plate lid and centrifuge at 2,400 × g for 2 min.

(c) *Extension-Ligation of bound oligos* (Total duration: 50 min). This process connects the hybridized upstream and downstream oligos. A DNA polymerase extends from the upstream oligo through the targeted region, followed by ligation to the 5′ end of the downstream oligo using a DNA ligase. The extension-ligation results in the formation of products containing the targeted regions of interest flanked by sequences required for amplification.

Procedure

1. Using a multichannel pipette, add 45 μl of ELM4 (Extension-Ligation Mix 4) to each sample well of the plate.
2. The extension-ligation reaction takes place on the filter plate membrane.

3. Seal the plate with adhesive aluminum foil, and then cover with the lid to secure the foil during incubation. Incubate the plate in the preheated 37 °C incubator for 45 min.
4. While the plate is incubating, prepare the Indexed Amplification Plate (IAP) as described in the following section (**step 3** of PCR amplification section).

(d) *PCR amplification* (Total duration: 85–105 min). In this step, the extension-ligation products are amplified using primers that add sample multiplexing index sequences as well as common adapters required for cluster generation.

Procedure

1. Prepare fresh 50 mM NaOH.
2. Remove PMM2 and the index primers (i5 and i7) from −15 to −25 °C storage and thaw on a bench at room temperature.
3. Using a multichannel pipette, add 4 μl of i5 and i7primers to each column of the IAP plate (*see* **Note 4**).
4. For 96 samples, add 56 μl of TDP1 (TruSeq DNA Polymerase 1) to 2.8 ml of PMM2 (PCR Master Mix 2). Invert the PMM2/TDP1 PCR master mix 20 times to mix well. You will add this mix to the IAP plate in the following step.
5. When the 45 min extension-ligation reaction is complete, remove the filter plate from the incubator. Remove the aluminum foil seal and replace with the filter plate lid (*see* **Note 5**).
6. Centrifuge the filter plate at 2,400 × g for 2 min.
7. Using a multichannel pipette, add 25 μl of 50 mM NaOH to each sample well (*see* **Note 6**) and incubate the plate at room temperature for 5 min.
8. While the plate is incubating, use a multichannel pipette to transfer 22 μl of the PMM2/TDP1 PCR master mix to each well of the IAP plate containing index primers.
9. Transfer 20 μl of samples eluted from the filter plate to the corresponding column of the IAP plate. Gently pipette up and down 5–6 times to combine the DNA with the PCR master mix. Tips must be changed after each column to avoid index and sample cross contamination.
10. Cover the IAP plate with microseal film and centrifuge to 1,000 × g at 20 °C for 1 min.

11. Perform PCR on a thermal cycler using the following program and the recommended number (*X*) of PCR cycles:

    95 °C for 3 min

    - *X* cycles of:
      - 95 °C for 30 s
      - 66 °C for 30 s
      - 72 °C for 60 s
    - 72 °C for 5 min
    - Hold at 10 °C

12. The following table contains amplicon size, number of amplicons in your CAT (Custom Amplicon Tube), type of DNA input, and DNA input quantity to help you calculate the number of PCR cycles required.

Amplicon size DNA input (50–99 ng)	**150/175 bp**	**250 bp**	**425 bp**
Number of PCR cycles (*X*)			
<96 amplicons	32	33	33
97–384 amplicons	28	28	29
385–768 amplicons	26	27	28
769–1,536 amplicons	25	26	27

Amplicon size DNA input (100–250 ng)	**150/175 bp**	**250 bp**	**425 bp**
Number of PCR cycles (*X*)			
<96 amplicons	29	30	30
97–384 amplicons	25	25	26
385–768 amplicons	23	24	25
769–1,536 amplicons	22	23	24

(e) *PCR cleanup* (Total duration: 50 min). This process uses AMPure XP beads (Beckman Coulter) to purify the PCR products from the other reaction components.

Procedure

1. Prepare fresh 80 % ethanol from absolute ethanol.
2. After PCR amplification step, to confirm that the library successfully amplified, run an aliquot of the control and selected test samples on a 4 % agarose (5 μl) or on a Bioanalyzer (1 μl).
3. Prior to use, allow the beads to come to room temperature and vortex the beads until they are well dispersed.

4. Using a multichannel pipette, add the appropriate volume of AMPure XP beads (Beckman Coulter), corresponding to your amplicon size (60 μl for 150–175 bp; 45 μl for 250 bp and 35 μl for 425 bp).
5. Using a multichannel pipette set to 60 μl, transfer the entire PCR product from the IAP plate to a new plate.
6. Seal and shake the plate at 1,800 rpm for 2 min. Incubate at room temperature without shaking for 10 min.
7. Place the plate on a magnetic stand (Beckman Coulter) for 2 min or until the supernatant has cleared and with a multichannel pipette set to 100 μl, carefully remove and discard the supernatant. Change tips between samples.
8. Wash the beads with freshly prepared 80 % ethanol for two times.
9. Remove the plate from the magnetic stand and allow the beads to air-dry for 10 min.
10. Using a multichannel pipette, add 30 μl of EBT (Elution Buffer with Tris) to each well.
11. Seal and shake the plate at 1,800 rpm for 2 min.
12. Incubate at room temperature without shaking for 2 min.
13. Place the plate on the magnetic stand for 2 min or until the supernatant has cleared.
14. Using a P20 multichannel pipette and fine tips, carefully transfer 20 μl of the supernatant from the plate to a new MIDI plate and then centrifuge to 1,000 × *g* for 1 min.

(f) *Library normalization* (Total duration: 1 h 20 min). This step normalizes the quantity of each library to ensure more equal library representation in your pooled sample.

Procedure

1. Prepare fresh 0.1 N NaOH.
2. For 96 samples, add 4.4 ml of LNA1 (Library Normalization Additives 1) to a fresh 15 ml conical tube.
3. Use a P1000 pipette set to 1,000 μl to resuspend LNB1 (Library Normalization Beads 1) thoroughly by pipetting up and down 15–20 times, until the bead pellet at the bottom is resuspended, and transfer 800 μl of LNB1 to the 15 ml conical tube containing LNA1.
4. Using a multichannel pipette, add 45 μl of the combined LNA1/LNB1 to each well of the MIDI plate containing libraries.

5. Seal and shake the MIDI plate on a microplate shaker at 1,800 rpm for 30 min.
6. Place the MIDI plate on a magnetic stand for 2 min or until the supernatant has cleared and using a multichannel pipette set to 80 μl remove the supernatant.
7. Remove the plate from the magnetic stand and wash the beads with 45 μl of LNW1 (Library Normalization Wash 1) for two times.
8. Remove the plate from the magnetic stand and add 30 μl of 0.1 N NaOH
9. Seal and shake the plate on a microplate shaker at 1,800 rpm for 5 min.
10. During the 5 min of elution, prepare a new 96-well PCR plate and add 30 μl LNS2 (Library Normalization Storage buffer 2) to each well.
11. Using a multichannel pipette set to 30 μl, transfer the supernatant from the first plate to the second plate. Change tips between samples to avoid cross contamination.
12. Seal the plate and then centrifuge to 1,000×g for 1 min (*see* **Note 7**).

(g) *Library pooling and MiSeq sample loading* (Total duration: 10 min). In preparation for cluster generation and sequencing, equal volumes of normalized library are combined, diluted in hybridization buffer, and heat denatured prior to sequencing on the MiSeq.

Procedure

1. Determine the samples to be pooled for sequencing, based on the number of targeted regions and desired coverage, using the following table (Illumina; CATALOG: FC-130-9005DOC) [11].

Amplicons per CAT[a]	Desired mean coverage[b]	Suggested maximum Samples per MiSeq run	
		MiSeq v2[b]	MiSeq v3[b]
16	150×	96	96
	500×	96	96
48	150×	96	96
	500×	96	96
96	150×	96	96
	500×	96	96
384	150×	96	96
	500×	48	80

(continued)

Amplicons per CAT[a]	Desired mean coverage[b]	Suggested maximum Samples per MiSeq run	
		MiSeq v2[b]	MiSeq v3[b]
768	150×	72	96
	500×	24	40
1,536	150×	36	60
	500×	12	20

[a]Custom Amplicon Tube; [b]MiSeq Reagent Kit version

2. Using a P20 multichannel pipette, transfer 5 μl of each library to be sequenced from the plate, column by column, to a PCR eight-tube strip.
3. Combine and transfer the contents of the PCR eight-tube strip into a fresh Eppendorf tube.
4. Create your Diluted Amplicon Library by combining the volumes of HT1 (Hybridization buffer) and Pooled Amplicon Library based on your MiSeq Reagent Kit version.
5. Mix Diluted Amplicon Library by vortexing the tube and using a heat block, incubate the tube at 96 °C for 2 min.
6. After the incubation, invert the tube 1–2 times to mix and immediately place in the ice water bath for 5 min.
7. Load Diluted Amplicon Library into a thawed MiSeq reagent cartridge in the Load Samples reservoir.

3.4 Sequence Libraries on MiSeq and Analyze Data

1. In parallel to library preparation, a sample sheet, to identify each sample and its corresponding index, should be prepared. To prepare your sample sheet, use the Illumina Experiment Manager, a wizard-based application that allows the recording of your sample ID, workflow, indices, and other parameters applicable to your 96-well plate. The Illumina Experiment Manager can be run on any Windows platform. You can download the Illumina Experiment Manager from the Illumina website.
2. TruSeq Custom Amplicon Library must be sequenced on a MiSeq sequencing system. For more details on using the MiSeq instrument or setting up your run, see the MiSeq System User Guide (Illumina, part # 15027617).
3. Analyze data with MiSeq Reporter software. MiSeq Reporter processes the base calls generated by the MiSeq sequencing system. It is an on-instrument software and produces information such as alignment and structural variants. For TruSeq Custom Amplicon libraries, it produces aligned reads in the

BAM format and outputs variant calls in .vcf files. For more information, see the MiSeq System User Guide or MiSeq Reporter's online help (www.illumina.com/help/miseq_reporter/default.htm).

4. Analyze data with Illumina Amplicon Viewer. The Illumina Amplicon Viewer has been designed and developed for off-instrument visualization and analysis of TruSeq Custom Amplicon data. Amplicon Viewer allows you to view data (including coverage, Q-score, variant calls, etc.) from multiple MiSeq amplicon runs simultaneously and interactively. DesignStudio might need to cover a large contiguous region with multiple amplicons, and the Illumina Amplicon Viewer opens the reconstituted contiguous region with combined coverage and variants appropriately. You can also export custom reports based on selected samples/targets/variants.
5. Annotation of variants should be performed using 1000 Genomes and NCBI and ESP6400 databases by GATK2 tool or using Variant Studio software (Illumina).
6. Previously unreported DNA variants should be evaluated: (1) by looking at their frequency in controls; (2) by looking at segregation; (3) by comparative sequence analysis among different species; (4) by applying different prediction softwares (PolyPhen, Fruitfly, Genscan, ESE finder).

4 Notes

1. To ensure consistency across samples, use a multichannel pipette where possible. Calibrate pipettes periodically.
2. Always use fresh pipette tips between samples and between dispensing index primers.
3. If the SW1 does not drain completely after 2 min, the plate can be centrifuged again for up to 10 min. Significantly incomplete drainage of SW1 compromises target enrichment specificity.
4. Tips must be changed after each row to avoid index cross contamination.
5. Removing the aluminum foil seal before centrifugation is recommended to ensure the reaction supernatant drains into the waste plate effectively.
6. Ensuring that pipette tips come in contact with the membrane, pipette the NaOH up and down 5–6 times. Tips must be changed after each column.
7. The final library pool consists of single-stranded DNA, which does not resolve well on an agarose gel or Bioanalyzer chip. qPCR can be used for quality control if desired.

Acknowledgments

This work was supported in part by grant "Premio di ricerca Gianluca Montel, 2011/2012" from University of Foggia, awarded to Maddalena Gigante and Progetto Strategico Regione Puglia grant (E.R., 2008), Ministero dell'Istruzione, dell'Università e della Ricerca (MiUR) FIRB, CAROMICS grant (E.R., 2011). The authors thank Illumina Fiel Application Scientist for technical support.

References

1. Leonard WJ, O'Shea JJ (1998) JAKS and STATs: biological implications. Annu Rev Immunol 16:293–322
2. Ghoreschi K, Laurence A, O'Shea JJ (2009) Janus kinases in immune cell signaling. Immunol Rev 228:273–287
3. Schumacher RF, Mella P, Badolato R et al (2000) Complete genomic organization of the human JAK3 gene and mutation analysis in severe combined immunodeficiency by single-strand conformation polymorphism. Hum Genet 106:73–79
4. Pesu M, Candotti F, Husa M et al (2005) JAK3, severe combined immunodeficiency, and a new class of immunosuppressive drugs. Immunol Rev 203:127–142
5. Witthuhn BA, Silvennoinen O, Miura O et al (1994) Involvement of the Jak-3 Janus kinase in signaling by interleukins 2 and 4 in lymphoid and myeloid cells. Nature 370:153–157
6. Kiyoi H, Yamaji S, Kojima S et al (2007) JAK3 mutations occur in acute megakaryoblastic leukemia both in Down syndrome children and non-Down syndrome adults. Leukemia 21:574–576
7. Cavalcanti E, Gigante M, Mancini V et al (2010) JAK3/STAT5/6 pathway alterations are associated with immune deviation in CD8 T cells in renal cell carcinoma patients. J Biomed Biotechnol 2010:935764
8. de Martino M, Gigante M, Cormio L et al (2013) JAK3 in clear cell renal cell carcinoma: mutational screening and clinical implications. Urol Oncol 31(6):930–937
9. Kolenko V, Wang Q, Riedy MC et al (1997) Tumor-induced suppression of T lymphocyte proliferation coincides with inhibition of Jak3 expression and IL-2 receptor signaling: role of soluble products from human renal cell carcinomas. J Immunol 159:3057–3067
10. Koskela HL, Eldfors S, Ellonen P et al (2012) Somatic STAT3 mutations in large granular lymphocytic leukemia. N Engl J Med 366(20):1905–1913
11. TruSeq Custom Amplicon Library Preparation Guide (CATALOG: FC-130-9005DOC)

Chapter 15

Experimental Model for Studying the Involvement of Regulatory Cytotoxic T Cells in Bone Resorption

Giacomina Brunetti, Angela Oranger, Silvia Colucci, and Maria Grano

Abstract

T cells may affect the activity of osteoclasts, the bone resorbing cells. In particular, recently authors focalize their attention on $CD8^+$ T cells, demonstrating that murine pre-osteoclasts can recruit naïve $CD8^+$ T cells and induce them to differentiate in regulatory cytotoxic T cells (Tc_{REG}), which in turn may suppress osteoclast formation and activity. Thus, here we describe the methodological approach needed to obtain Tc_{REG} and to evaluate Tc_{REG} effects on murine osteoclast activity and formation in an in vitro experimental model.

Key words T cells, Osteoclastogenesis, $FoxP3^+CD8^+$ T cells, TRAP staining, Resorption assay

1 Introduction

In the last decade, it has been recognized that skeletal homeostasis is dynamically influenced by the immune system. This emerging field, called osteoimmunology [1], arose from observation demonstrating that lymphocyte-derived cytokines are potent mediators of osteoclast differentiation and activity [1]. Osteoclastogenesis requires macrophage colony stimulating factor (MCSF) and receptor activator factor of nuclear factor kB ligand (RANKL) [2], which act on cells of the monocyte–macrophage lineage, inducing their fusion to form polynucleated active resorbing cells. Osteoclast activity and numbers are increased by cytokines produced by activated effector $CD4^+$ T cells leading to increased bone erosion in inflammatory bone diseases such as arthritis, periodontitis, metastatic bone cancers, and osteoporosis [1, 3–9]. In contrast, activated cytotoxic $CD8^+$ T cells profoundly suppressed osteoclastogenesis [10].

Among effector $CD4^+$ T cells, which are dominant during the inflammatory phase, there are the regulatory T cells (T_{REG}) that have the ability to suppress both the aberrant activation of self-reactive lymphocytes [11, 12] as well as the osteoclast formation [13].

Elena Ranieri (ed.), *Cytotoxic T-Cells: Methods and Protocols*, Methods in Molecular Biology, vol. 1186,
DOI 10.1007/978-1-4939-1158-5_15, © Springer Science+Business Media New York 2014

The transcription factor FoxP3 is a marker of T_{REG}, as well as CD25, the α-chain of the IL-2 receptor [1, 11, 12]. Recently, a subset of regulatory T cells has been characterized also among $CD8^+$ T cells, the $FoxP3^+/CD25^+/CD8^+$ T cells (Tc_{REG}), which have not been extensively studied due in part to their low abundance in lymphoid tissue (0.2–2 % of CD8 T cells) [14]. However, few recent findings have indicated that Tc_{REG} may regulate the immune system [15–17] and suppress osteoclast activity [14]. In detail, RANKL treatment of bone marrow macrophages induces chemokine expression and MHC class I presentation pathway during osteoclastogenesis, leading to osteoclasts and their precursors act as antigen presenting cells preferentially for $CD8^+$ T cells [18]. The priming of naïve $CD8^+$ T cells by osteoclasts, in the presence of an antigen, induces their differentiation in Tc_{REG} [14, 19], which in turn produce cytokines suppressing osteoclast formation and activity [14]. Thus, in this chapter we describe the methodological approach needed to obtain Tc_{REG} and to evaluate Tc_{REG} effects on murine osteoclast activity and formation in an in vitro experimental model.

2 Materials

All the materials used must be sterile; in all the steps it is important to have a refrigerated benchtop centrifuge, a sterile hood, a CO_2 incubator, and a light microscope.

2.1 Macrophage Isolation Components

1. Bone marrow from C57BL/6 male mice that are 3–6 months of age (*see* **Note 1**).
2. Chloroform.
3. 70 % ethanol.
4. Sterile forceps, treated and not treated tissue culture dishes (10 cm), 50 mL tubes, syringes equipped with a 26-gauge needle, serological pipettes.
5. Alpha Minimal Essential Medium (αMEM) containing 2 % Amphotericin, 1 % Streptomycin, and 1 % Penicillin supplemented or not with 10 % heat inactivated Fetal Bovine Serum (FBS).
6. Recombinant Mouse Macrophage-Colony Stimulating Factor (M-CSF).
7. 0.05 % Trypsin-EDTA.

2.2 Splenocyte Isolation Components

1. OT-I/Rag as apex mice (Taconic) (*see* **Note 2**).
2. Sterile forceps, serological pipettes, tissue culture dishes (10 cm), 2 mL syringes, 50 mL tubes.

3. Cell strainer (40 μm Nylon filter).
4. 10× Ammonium-Chloride-Potassium (ACK) lysing buffer: Dissolve 82.9 g NH_4Cl, 10 g $KHCO_3$, and 372 mg Na_2-EDTA in 1 L deionized water. Adjust the pH of the solution to 7.2. Sterilize the solution using a 0.2 μm filter. Before use, dilute the solution with an appropriate volume of sterile deionized water as to obtain a 1× ACK lysis buffer (i.e., add 90 mL sterile deionized water to 10 mL 10× ACK lysis buffer) (*see* **Note 3**).
5. Sterile phosphate buffered saline (PBS): Dissolve 80 g NaCl; 2.0 g KCl; 14.4 g Na_2HPO_4; 2.4 g KH_2PO_4 in 1 L of deionized water. It is important to adjust the pH to 7.2, sterilize the solution by autoclaving, let cool and add 2 % Amphotericin, 1 % Streptomycin, and 1 % Penicillin.

2.3 T Cell Enrichment Components

1. Splenocytes from OT-I/Rag as apex mice (Taconic) (*see* **Note 2**).
2. Buffer: Prepare a solution containing PBS (pH 7.2), 0.5 % bovine serum albumin (BSA), and 2 mM EDTA (*see* **Notes 4** and **5**).
3. Mouse Pan T Cell Isolation Kit composed of a cocktail of biotin-conjugated, monoclonal antibodies [anti-CD11b, -CD11c, -CD19, -CD45R (B220), -CD49b (DX5), -CD105, -MHC class II, and -Ter-119] and of Anti-Biotin MicroBeads (Miltenyi Biotec S.r.l., Bologna, Italia).
4. MiniMACS™ Magnetic separator (Miltenyi Biotec).
5. MACS MS Columns (Miltenyi Biotec).

2.4 CD8 T Cell Purification Components

1. T cell enriched suspension.
2. $CD8a^+$ negative Isolation Kit composed of a cocktail of biotin-conjugated, monoclonal antibodies [anti-CD4, -CD11b, -CD11c, -CD19, -CD45R (B220), -CD49b (DX5), -CD105, -MHC Class II, and -Ter-119] and microBeads conjugated to monoclonal anti-biotin antibodies (Miltenyi Biotec).
3. MiniMACS™ Magnetic separator (Miltenyi Biotec).
4. MACS MS Columns (Miltenyi Biotec).

2.5 Tc_{REG} Generation Components

1. Purified murine macrophages and $CD8^+$ T cells.
2. αMEM supplemented with 10 % FBS (*see* **Note 6**).
3. Recombinant Mouse MCSF.
4. Recombinant Mouse Receptor Activator of NF-kB Ligand (RANKL).
5. Albumin from chicken egg white [(OVA) A-5503; Sigma-Aldrich].
6. 24-well tissue culture-treated plates.

2.6 Fluorescence Activated Cells Sorting (FACS) Components

1. Flow cytometer.
2. FACS tubes.
3. FACS Buffer: Prepare a solution containing PBS (pH 7.2) and 0.5 % bovine serum albumin (BSA) (*see* **Note 5**).
4. FITC-conjugated anti-mouse CD8a antibody.
5. PE-conjugated anti-mouse CD25 antibody.
6. APC Anti-FoxP3 antibody and the package included Fixation/Permeabilization Solutions and Permeabilization Buffer (Miltenyi Biotec).
7. 1× Fixation/Permeabilization buffer: Fixation/Permeabilization Solution 1 must be diluted 1:4 with the Fixation/Permeabilization Solution 2.

   1× Permeabilization Buffer: 10× Permeabilization Buffer must be diluted 1:10 with deionized or distilled water before use (i.e., 1 mL of 10× Permeabilization Buffer plus 9 mL of deionized/distilled water).

2.7 Osteoclastogenesis Assay Components

1. 24-well adhesion plates for osteoclast differentiation.
2. 24-well osteo-assay plates for osteoclast resorption activity evaluation (Corning Incorporated, New York, USA).
3. αMEM supplemented with 10 % FBS, recombinant murine MCSF, and recombinant murine RANKL.

2.8 Tartrate-Resistant Acid Phosphatase–Positive (TRAP) Staining Components

Most of the required reagents are available in a commercial kit (Sigma-Aldrich, Milan, Italy).

1. TRAP Fixative Solution: Prepare it by combining 25 mL Citrate solution, 65 mL Acetone, and 8 mL 37 % Formaldehyde (*see* **Note 7**).
2. TRAP staining solution (*see* **Note 8**).
   (a) Prepare the *Diazoted Fast Garnet GBC Solution* into a brown tube by adding 0.5 mL Fast Garnet GBC Base Solution and 0.5 mL Sodium Nitrite Solution. Mix by gentle inversion for 30 s. Let stand for 2 min.
   (b) In a 100 mL beaker add the following components while mixing: 45 mL Deionized water pre-warmed to 37 °C; 1 mL *Diazotized Fast Garnet GBC Solution*; 0.5 mL Naphthol AS-Bl Phosphate Solution; 2 mL Acetate Solution; 1 mL Tartrate Solution.

2.9 Evaluation of Resorption Pits Formation Components

1. 10 % bleach solution.
2. Silver nitrate ($AgNO_3$) solution: dissolve 1 g $AgNO_3$ into 20 mL distilled water (*see* **Note 9**).
3. 100 V lamp.
4. Light microscope connected with a digital camera.

3 Methods

3.1 Preparation of Macrophage from Bone Marrow

1. Select C57BL/6 male mice (*see* **Note 2**).
2. Stun the mice with chloroform before their sacrifice.
3. Sacrifice mouse and place it on its back. Wet fur of sacrificed mouse using 70 % ethanol. Dissect through the skin, making a long cut down the length of the leg. Once the majority of the muscle has been cut away from the bone, cut the tibia just above the ankle joint and the femur as close to the hip socket as possible.
4. Place bones in a sterile tissue culture dish containing αMEM and cut the epiphysis.
5. Under sterile conditions, load with αMEM a 20-mL syringe equipped with a 26-gauge needle.
6. Using this syringe, flush out the bone marrow by forcing media through the bone cavity. Collect marrow in a sterile conical tube. Flush the bones from both ends. Bones will appear white when all of the marrow has been removed.
7. Pellet cells at 400 × *g* for 5 min at room temperature. Resuspend pellet in about 10 mL of αMEM + 10 % FBS (*see* **Note 10**).
8. Plate cells in a 10 cm not treated dish in the presence of 100 ng/mL MCSF to permit macrophage selection/adhesion. Rotate and distribute the cell suspension evenly on the surface of the culture dish.
9. Culture overnight at 37 °C in a water-saturated atmosphere containing 5 % CO_2.
10. Harvest and discard the non-adherent cells from the tissue culture plate. Wash the plate with culture media until all non-adherent cells have been removed in order to have as adherent fraction only macrophage.
11. Add to the adherent fraction αMEM + 10 % FBS + 100 ng/mL MCSF. In these conditions, macrophages proliferate, reaching confluence within 4–5 days.
12. Trypsinize and transfer macrophage into appropriate culture dishes for osteoclastogenesis experiments. In detail:
    (a) Discard culture medium from dish.
    (b) Add into the dish sterile PBS to remove serum residues.
    (c) Discard PBS from dish.
    (d) Add into the dish 0.05 % trypsin-EDTA and place it in a CO_2 incubator for 2–5 min at 37 °C (*see* **Note 11**).
    (e) Pipette vigorously many times to favor mechanical cell detachment.
    (f) Check that cells are detached.

(g) Neutralize trypsin with αMEM + 10 %FBS.

(h) Collect the solution containing detached cells into a 50 mL tube.

(i) Centrifuge cells at 400 × *g* for 5 min.

(j) Count cells and plate them for the osteoclastogenesis experiments.

3.2 Isolation of Splenocytes

1. Prepare 1× ACK lysis buffer (*see* **Note 12**).
2. Cut away the fur along the left side of the sacrificed mouse, about half-way between the front and back legs.
3. Cut open the body cavity.
4. Remove the spleen using the forceps (the spleen is the color of a kidney bean; it is longer and flatter than the kidney).
5. Place the spleen and 1 mL PBS directly in the Petri dish.
6. Under sterile conditions, remove the plunger from a 2 mL syringe and use the black rubber end to mash the spleen and release the splenocytes into the Petri dish. Use grinding circular movements to homogenize the tissue.
7. Place a 40 μm cell strainer on a 50 mL conical tube and transfer the homogenized cell suspension. Wash out the Petri dish a few times to maximize recovery of splenocytes. Make up to the full volume of the tube with PBS.
8. Centrifuge at 400 × *g* for 10 min at room temperature and aspirate supernatant. The resulting cell pellet should be red in color.
9. Discard supernatant and resuspend pellet in 1 mL 1× ACK lysis buffer. Incubate at RT for 5–10 min.
10. Centrifuge at 400 × *g* for 5 min and aspirate the supernatant. Take care not to lose cells as the pellet will be loose.
11. Resuspend cells in the appropriate buffer to a final known volume.
12. Count live cells using a hemocytometer and a light microscope. Proceed with T cell enrichment protocol.

3.3 T Cell Enrichment

3.3.1 Magnetic Labeling

1. Resuspend cell pellet in 40 μL of buffer per 1×10^7 total cells.
2. Add 10 μL of Pan T Cell Isolation Kit II (Biotin-Antibody Cocktail) per 1×10^7 total cells (*see* **Note 13**).
3. Mix well and incubate for 10 min in the refrigerator (2–8 °C) (*see* **Note 14**).
4. Add 30 μL of buffer per 1×10^7 total cells.
5. Add 20 μL of Anti-Biotin MicroBeads per 1×10^7 total cells (*see* **Note 15**).
6. Mix well and incubate for 15 min in the refrigerator (2–8 °C) (*see* **Note 14**).

7. Wash cells by adding 2 mL of buffer per 1×10^7 cells and centrifuge at $400 \times g$ for 10 min. Aspirate supernatant completely.
8. Resuspend up to 1×10^8 cells in 500 μL of buffer (*see* **Note 16**).
9. Proceed to magnetic separation (Subheading 3.3.2).

3.3.2 Magnetic Separation

1. Place column in the magnetic field of a MiniMACS™ Magnetic separator.
2. Prepare MS column by rinsing with 500 μL buffer.
3. Apply cell suspension onto the column. Collect flow-through containing unlabeled cells, representing the enriched T cells (*see* **Note 17**).
4. Wash column three times with 500 μL buffer (*see* **Note 18**). Collect unlabeled cells that pass through, representing the enriched T cells, and combine with the effluent from **step 3**. Proceed with CD8a⁺ negative selection.

3.4 CD8a⁺ Negative Selection

1. Pellet enriched T cells and resuspend them in 40 μL of buffer per 1×10^7 total cells.
2. Add 10 μL of CD8a⁺ negative isolation kit (Biotin-Antibody Cocktail) per 1×10^7 total cells (*see* **Note 13**).
3. Proceed as detailed before in **steps 3–9** in Subheading 3.3.1.
4. The resulting T cells are routinely >97 % pure when stained with anti-CD8a antibody and checked by FACS.
5. Use these cells to generate Tc_{REG}.

3.5 Generation of Tc_{REG}

1. Day 3 macrophages cultured in 20 ng/mL M-CSF and 30 ng/mL RANKL were seeded at 5×10^5 cells/mL/well in the presence of 5 μM OVA in 24-well tissue culture-treated plates.
2. After overnight incubation, medium was removed and adherent cells were washed with pre-warmed (37 °C) medium.
3. 2.5×10^5 freshly harvested splenic OT-I transgenic T cells purified by negative selection were added in 2 mL of complete T-cell media (RPMI, 10 % heat-inactivated FBS, penicillin-streptomycin-glutamine, nonessential amino acids, sodium pyruvate, HEPES, and 55 μM β-mercaptoethanol).
4. Following 48 h co-culture, T-cell aliquots were removed and stained intracellularly to assay for FoxP3 expression through FACS.

3.6 Intracellular Staining for Flow Cytometry Analysis

1. Prepare 1× Fixation/Permeabilization buffer and 1× Permeabilization Buffer.
2. Resuspend up to 1×10^6 nucleated cells per 90 μL of FACS buffer (*see* **Note 19**).
3. Add 10 μL of FITC-conjugated anti-mouse CD8a and 10 μL of the PE-conjugated anti-mouse CD25 antibody.

4. Mix well and incubate for 10 min in the dark in the refrigerator (2–8 °C) (*see* **Note 14**).
5. Wash cells by adding 2 mL of buffer per 1×10^6 cells and centrifuge at $400 \times g$ for 5 min at 4 °C. Aspirate supernatant completely.
6. Proceed immediately to the Intracellular staining with the Anti-FoxP3 antibody.
7. Resuspend 1×10^6 nucleated cells in 1 mL of cold, freshly prepared Fixation/Permeabilization Buffer (*see* **Note 20**).
8. Mix well and incubate for 30 min in the dark in the refrigerator (2–8 °C) (*see* **Note 14**).
9. Wash cells by adding 2 mL of cold FACS buffer per 1×10^6 cells and centrifuge at $400 \times g$ for 5 min at 4 °C. Aspirate supernatant completely.
10. Wash cells by adding 2 mL of cold 1× Permeabilization Buffer per 1×10^6 cells and centrifuge at $400 \times g$ for 5 min at 4 °C. Aspirate supernatant completely.
11. Resuspend up to 1×10^6 nucleated cells in 80 μL of cold 1× Permeabilization Buffer.
12. Mix well and incubate for 5 min in the refrigerator (2–8 °C) (*see* **Note 14**).
13. Add 10 μL of the APC Anti-FoxP3 antibody.
14. Mix well and incubate for 30 min in the dark in the refrigerator (2–8 °C) (*see* **Note 14**).
15. Wash cells by adding 2 mL of cold 1× Permeabilization Buffer per 1×10^6 cells and centrifuge at $400 \times g$ for 5 min at 4 °C. Aspirate supernatant completely.
16. Resuspend cell pellet 500 μl PBS.
17. Acquire the data using a flow cytometer and analyze the results by a suitable software (*see* **Note 21**).

3.7 Osteoclastogenesis Assays

1. Plate macrophages at 80,000/cm² in a 24-well adhesion and/or Osteo-Assay plate in the presence of 25 ng/ml MCSF to permit cell adhesion (day 0) (*see* **Notes 22** and **23**).
2. After 24 h, remove the medium and add Tc or pre-differentiated Tc_{REG}. Co-culture them in the presence of 25 ng/ml M-CSF and 30 ng/ml RANKL.
3. Re-feed every 48 h with M-CSF and RANKL and fresh media.
4. On day 7, stop cell culture and evaluate osteoclast formation and activity through TRAP staining or pit area quantification, respectively (*see* **Note 24**).

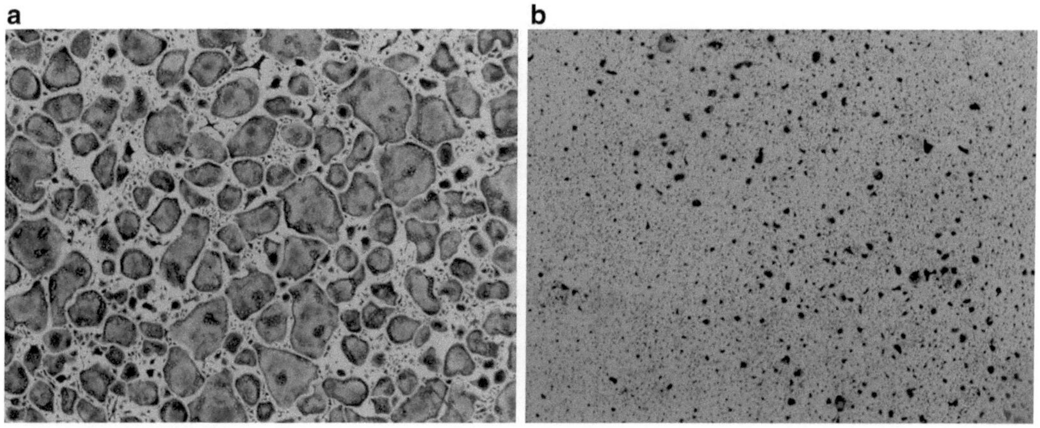

Fig. 1 TRAP staining observed in co-culture between macrophage and Tc or Tc_{REG}. Large multinucleated TRAP+ osteoclasts were observed in co-culture between macrophages and Tc (**a**), whereas no osteoclast were observed in co-culture between macrophages and Tc_{REG} (**b**)

3.8 Tartrate-Resistant Acid Phosphatase-Positive (TRAP) Staining

1. Prepare TRAP Fixative and staining solutions.
2. Discard the culture media from all wells or slides.
3. Fix cells by adding 0.5 mL Fixative Solution for 30 s into each well or slide.
4. Rinse thoroughly in deionized water: without allowing cells to dry.
5. Add 0.5 mL TRAP solution into each well and incubate for 1 h in 37 °C water bath protected from light.
6. Rinse wells thoroughly in deionized water.
7. Air dry and evaluate microscopically.

At the end of the culture period, mature OCs were identified as multinucleated $TRAP^+$ cells, containing three or more nuclei. $TRAP^+$ activity appears as purplish to dark red staining in the cytoplasm of mature osteoclasts or precursors. In Fig. 1, the typical result is reported: $TRAP^+$ osteoclast formation occurs in the presence of Tc cells, but not in the presence of Tc_{REG}.

3.9 Resorption Assay

1. Aspirate the media from the wells on day 7.
2. Add 100 μL of 10 % bleach solution and incubate for 5 min at room temperature to remove cells.
3. Wash wells with distilled water (pH = 7) for three times.
4. At this step you can decide to allow to dry the plate at room temperature for 3–5 h. However, to better display the resorbed area it is suggested to perform the following staining.
5. Add 0.5 mL $AgNO_3$ solution prepared as described in materials, and incubate for 30 min at room temperature, protecting the multiwell from light.

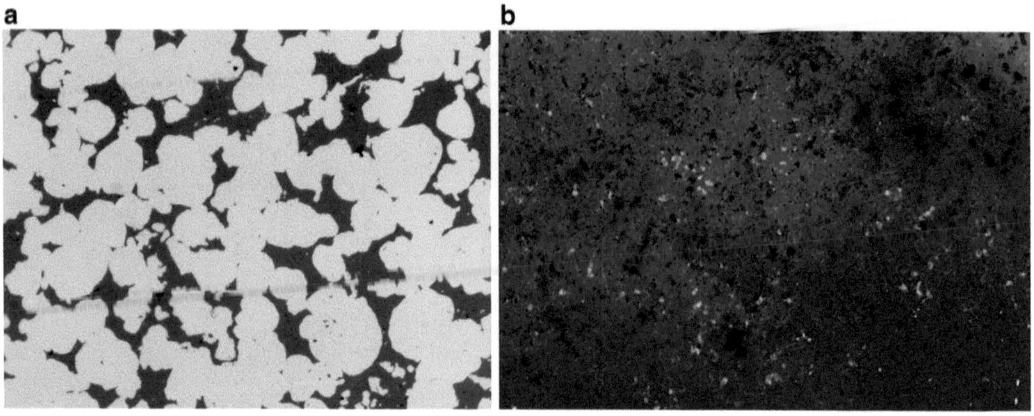

Fig. 2 Resorption pits observed in co-culture between macrophage and Tc or Tc_{REG}. Large pits were observed in co-culture between macrophages and Tc (**a**), whereas no pitting was observed in co-culture between macrophages and Tc_{REG} (**b**)

6. Discard the silver nitrate solution and rinse two times with distilled water.
7. Expose for 1 h to bright light (100 V).
8. Allow to dry at room temperature for 3–5 h and evaluate microscopically.

   The white zone corresponds to the resorptive area. In Fig. 2, the typical result is reported: osteoclast resorption occurs in the presence of Tc cells, but not in the presence of Tc_{REG}.
9. Quantify the resorption area using specific software or the freely available NIH ImageJ.

4 Notes

1. Use male mice to avoid the sex-dependent effect on osteoclastogenesis estrogen-mediated.
2. The use of OT-I/Rag as apex mice is recommended to investigate $CD8^+$ T-cell development, activation, memory, and tolerance.
3. 1× ACK solution is not stable: prepare 1× diluting the 10× just before use.
4. The presence of BSA into the wash buffer solution could cause foam formation. Thus prepare this solution using a gentle stirring.
5. Store the buffer at 2–8 °C.
6. Pre-warm at 37 °C the medium before use.
7. TRAP fixative solution can be stored at +4 °C and must be brought to room temperature (18–26 °C) before use. It is stable up to 2 months if stored tightly capped in refrigerator. Place in glass bottle and cap tightly.

8. TRAP solution must be prepared before use. It must be protected from light and warmed to 37 °C in a water bath. Check that temperature is at 37 °C before adding to the cells.
9. Silver nitrate solution must be prepared before use and must be protected from light also after its introduction into the multiwell.
10. Before plating cells, prepare the growth medium and place it in the incubator for 10–15 min. This equilibrates the pH of the medium.
11. Do not exceed 5 min of trypsinization. Over-trypsinization can result in cell lysis and loss of viability.
12. Ammonium chloride lysing reagent must be kept at room temperature.
13. Work fast, keep cells cold, and use precooled solutions. This will prevent capping of antibodies on the cell surface and non-specific cell labeling.
14. The recommended incubation temperature is 2–8 °C. Higher temperatures and/or longer incubation times may lead to non-specific cell labeling. In contrast, working on ice may require increased incubation times.
15. Volumes for magnetic labeling given below are for up to 1×10^7 total cells. When working with fewer than 1×10^7 cells, use the same volumes as indicated. When working with higher cell numbers, scale up all reagent volumes and total volumes accordingly (e.g., for 2×10^7 total cells, use twice the volume of all indicated reagent volumes and total volumes).
16. For higher cell numbers, scale up buffer volume accordingly.
17. Always wait until the column reservoir is empty before proceeding to the next step.
18. Perform washing steps by adding buffer aliquots only when the column reservoir is empty.
19. The suggested volume is for up to 1×10^6 nucleated cells. When working with fewer than 1×10^6 cells, use the same volumes as indicated except for the fixation step due to the impact on cell morphology. When working with higher cell numbers, scale up all reagent volumes and total volumes, accordingly (e.g., for 2×10^6 nucleated cells, use twice the volume of all indicated reagent volumes and total volumes).
20. When working with fewer cells, scale down the volume accordingly (e.g., for 5×10^5 cells use half the volume).
21. Due to fixation and permeabilization, cells can be smaller than viable cells. Thus, FSC/SSC settings of the flow cytometer might need to be adjusted.
22. To obtain osteoclasts from murine macrophages (from both bone marrow and splenocytes), it is important to plate 80,000

cells/cm². Higher or lower cell concentration could block osteoclastogenesis.

23. To measure resorption activity, the osteoclasts were grown on osteo-assay wells, rather than bone slices to avoid any confounding effects of TGFβ present in the bone.

24. Observe the osteoclast culture every day after replacing the culture medium. It could be possible to obtain large osteoclasts before or after 7 days, thus evaluate the best time in which to stop the culture.

References

1. Mori G, D'Amelio P, Faccio R, Brunetti G (2013) The interplay between the bone and the immune system. Clin Dev Immunol 2013(720504):1–9
2. Boyle WJ, Simonet WS, Lacey DL (2003) Osteoclast differentiation and activation. Nature 423:337–342
3. Kong YY, Feige U, Sarosi I, Bolon B, Tafuri A, Morony S, Capparelli C, Li J, Elliott R, McCabe S, Wong T, Campagnuolo G, Moran E, Bogoch ER, Van G, Nguyen LT, Ohashi PS, Lacey DL, Fish E, Boyle WJ, Penninger JM (1999) Activated T cells regulate bone loss and joint destruction in adjuvant arthritis through osteoprotegerin ligand. Nature 402:304–309
4. Colucci S, Brunetti G, Cantatore FP, Oranger A, Mori G, Quarta L, Cirulli N, Mancini L, Corrado A, Grassi FR, Grano M (2007) Lymphocytes and synovial fluid fibroblasts support osteoclastogenesis through RANKL, TNFalpha, and IL-7 in an in vitro model derived from human psoriatic arthritis. J Pathol 212:47–55
5. Teng YT, Nguyen H, Gao X, Kong YY, Gorczynski RM, Singh B, Ellen RP, Penninger JM (2000) Functional human T-cell immunity and osteoprotegerin ligand control alveolar bone destruction in periodontal infection. J Clin Invest 106:R59–R67
6. Brunetti G, Colucci S, Pignataro P, Coricciati M, Mori G, Cirulli N, Zallone A, Grassi FR, Grano M (2005) T cells support osteoclastogenesis in an in vitro model derived from human periodontitis patients. J Periodontol 76:1675–1680
7. Colucci S, Brunetti G, Rizzi R, Zonno A, Mori G, Colaianni G, Del Prete D, Faccio R, Liso A, Capalbo S, Liso V, Zallone A, Grano M (2004) T cells support osteoclastogenesis in an in vitro model derived from human multiple myeloma bone disease: the role of the OPG/TRAIL interaction. Blood 104:3722–3730
8. Roato I, Grano M, Brunetti G, Colucci S, Mussa A, Bertetto O, Ferracini R (2005) Mechanisms of spontaneous osteoclastogenesis in cancer with bone involvement. FASEB J 19:228–230
9. Faienza MF, Brunetti G, Colucci S, Piacente L, Ciccarelli M, Giordani L, Del Vecchio GC, D'Amore M, Albanese L, Cavallo L, Grano M (2009) Osteoclastogenesis in children with 21-hydroxylase deficiency on long term glucocorticoid therapy: the role of RANKL/OPG imbalance. J Clin Endocrinol Metab 94: 2269–2276
10. Choi Y, Woo KM, Ko SH, Lee YJ, Park SJ, Kim HM, Kwon BS (2001) Osteoclastogenesis is enhanced by activated B cells but suppressed by activated CD8(+) T cells. Eur J Immunol 31:2179–2188
11. Fontenot JD, Gavin MA, Rudensky AY (2003) Foxp3 programs the development and function of CD4+CD25+ regulatory T cells. Nat Immunol 4:330–336
12. Hori S, Nomura T, Sakaguchi S (2003) Control of regulatory T cell development by the transcription factor Foxp3. Science 299: 1057–1061
13. Zaiss MM, Axmann R, Zwerina J, Polzer K, Gückel E, Skapenko A, Schulze-Koops H, Horwood N, Cope A, Schett G (2007) Treg cells suppress osteoclast formation: a new link between the immune system and bone. Arthritis Rheum 56:4104–4112
14. Buchwald ZS, Kiesel JR, DiPaolo R, Pagadala MS, Aurora R (2012) Osteoclast activated FoxP3+ CD8+ T-cells suppress bone resorption in vitro. PLoS One 7:e38199
15. Sharabi A, Mozes E (2008) The suppression of murine lupus by a tolerogenic peptide involves foxp3-expressing CD8 cells that are required for the optimal induction and function of foxp3-expressing CD4 cells. J Immunol 181: 3243–3251

16. Kiniwa Y, Miyahara Y, Wang HY, Peng W, Peng G, Wheeler TM, Thompson TC, Old LJ, Wang RF (2007) CD8+ Foxp3+ regulatory T cells mediate immunosuppression in prostate cancer. Clin Cancer Res 13:6947–6958
17. Singh RP, La Cava A, Wong M, Ebling F, Hahn BH (2007) CD8+ T cell mediated suppression of autoimmunity in a murine lupus model of peptide induced immune tolerance depends on Foxp3 expression. J Immunol 178:7649–7657
18. Kiesel J, Miller C, Abu-Amer Y, Aurora R (2007) Systems level analysis of osteoclastogenesis reveals intrinsic and extrinsic regulatory interactions. Dev Dyn 236:2181–2197
19. Kiesel JR, Buchwald ZS, Aurora R (2009) Cross-presentation by osteoclasts induces FoxP3 in CD8+ T cells. J Immunol 182:5477–5487

Chapter 16

CTL and Transplantation: Tissue In Vivo Characterization

Federica Rascio, Chiara Divella, and Giuseppe Grandaliano

Abstract

During the course of an immune response in kidney transplantation, distinct functional subsets of effector and regulatory T cells are generated in the lymphoid compartment following the differentiation of T cells under the influence of specific cytokines. In addition to effector cells inflammation in a CXCR3-independent manner, a CXCR3-chemokine dependent pathway exacerbates these inflammatory processes in this scenario. Indeed, the upregulation of CXCR3 ligands mediates the mobilization of effector CTLs to the peripheral site of infection. The immediate upregulation of CXCR3 on CD4+ CTLs and CD8+ CTL following DC activation makes this an interesting proposal, as activated T cells are recruited into lymphoid and noncanonical lymphoid compartments. The importance of tissue in vivo characterization is emerged as a central topic in kidney transplantation.

In the following method we describe a protocol based on immunohistochemistry (IHC) and immunofluorescence/confocal microscopy along with strategies of overall signals quantification and positive cells quantification (Aperio, Adobe Photoshop). Through an in vivo approach, we focus on those changes that result relevant during immune response in transplantation. Although less quantitative than other methods, the information gained from IHC combined with microscopy provides a "picture" that can help to address our subsequent experiments. The advantage of this protocol consists in the possibility to evidence CTLs tissue accumulation and to investigate the different areas (tubular, glomerular, and interstitial) of the graft directly affected by CTLs-specific activity.

1 Introduction

Antigen-primed T-cell activation and the subsequent infiltration of activated T-cells, macrophages, and natural killer (NK) cells into the graft play a critical role in kidney transplantation.

Expression patterns of intragraft during a cytopathic allograft response seem substantially different from those seen in other causes of graft dysfunction and may provide timely and specific information of immune events relevant to graft rejection. The infiltration by cytotoxic T lymphocytes (CTLs) causes CTLs-associated transcripts (CATs) to appear in the tissues as a hallmark of severe injury. Granzyme B/GZMB, granzyme A/GZMA, and perforin/PRF1 are among the CATs often used as indicators of CTLs presence in tissues [1]. The presence of activated CTLs and expression

Elena Ranieri (ed.), *Cytotoxic T-Cells: Methods and Protocols*, Methods in Molecular Biology, vol. 1186,
DOI 10.1007/978-1-4939-1158-5_16, © Springer Science+Business Media New York 2014

of perforin (P) and/or GB have been described in acute rejection of kidneys [2, 3], while T cell infiltrates in well-functioning grafts do not express cytokines, GB, or P [4]. The effector transcription factor T-bet is another intragraft marker of acute rejection [5].

The induction of CD8+ CTLs is strongly linked to the upregulation of the chemokine receptor CXCR3. CD8+ T cells can differentiate to become CTLs which secrete IFN-γ along with other effector molecules and, once differentiated, these molecules upregulate chemokine receptors which guide them out of the lymphoid compartment and into sites of inflammation to enhance an adaptive immune response [6]. CXCR3 and its ligands (CXCL9, CXCL10, and CXCL11) are undoubtedly an inflammatory chemokine system, capable of coordinating DC-induced T cell responses in the inflamed periphery [7]. Accumulation of effector T cells at sites of autoimmune inflammation, strongly correlated with CXCR3 expression, characterize not only the autoimmune response in rheumatoid arthritis [8] but also infiltration of T cells into the kidney in systemic lupus erythematosus (SLE) [9, 10]. Although not studied in great detail yet, it is becoming increasingly clear that in immunological diseases CXCR3 chemokine system plays important roles in the migratory behavior and cellular interactions of T cells in the lymphoid compartment and within peripheral tissues, including noncanonical lymphoid tissue. Since kidney transplantation compliances share a similar immunological network along with the amount of graft CTLs infiltrating cells, in the following method we describe some strategies of tissue in vivo characterization in transplantation. Extensive similarities characterize CD4+ CTLs or CD8+ CTLs: perforin, granzymes, CXCR3 are shared between CD8+ CTLs and CD4+ CTLs. Thus, their accumulation in inflamed tissues may a priori be a hallmark of the presence of CD8+ CTLs, CD4+ CTLs, or NK cells and, although expression seems higher in CD8+ CTLs, requires additional information for its interpretation.

For this reason, in the following method we describe first some strategies of single immunostaining (IHC analysis) for individually CTLs-specific markers (e.g., Granzyme, perforin, CXCR3) detection in order to assure CTLs presence in tissue. Then, we describe a method of double immunostaining (combining CTLs markers with CD8+ or CD4+ markers) using confocal microscopy and strategies of cell quantification in order to provide additional knowledge of the frequency of each type of CTLs infiltrating cells in transplantation. The strength of the method consists in the possibility to use kidney biopsies from transplant patients as starting material and focus on those intragraft molecules, selected on the basis of existing evidences for this compliance or for similar immune-related diseases (e.g., kidneys in LES), which may characterize antigen-mediated T cell infiltration. This approach may be fruitful in the context of transplantation to study the local distribution of CTLs infiltrates and to better address the subsequent CTLs analysis.

2 Materials

All the procedures described below need previous preparation of formalin-fixed, paraffin-embedded sections. The paraffin tissue blocks can be stored at 4 °C for later use, while the sections on polylysine-coated slides can be stored at room temperature for years. Follow all waste disposal regulations when disposing of waste materials. All the techniques should be performed by personnel able to work with potential infectious material.

2.1 IHC Analysis

1. Patients' paraffin tissue blocks: paraffin-embedded sections (2 μm).
2. Xylenes and graded alcohol series.
3. Citrate buffer or EDTA buffer, Microwave or pressure.
4. H_2O_2 solution to block endogenous peroxidase activity.
5. Phosphate Buffered Saline (PBS).
6. Protein block serum-free (Dako).
7. Specific primary antibodies (customized).
8. Secondary biotinylated antibodies conjugated to HRP (customized).
9. DAB Chromogen solution.
10. Mayer's hematoxylin.
11. Glycerol for mounting.

2.2 Slide Digitation and Analysis

1. ScanScope Digital Slide Scanner (Aperio, Vista, CA, USA), Spectrum Server V10.2.2.2315 (Aperio).
2. ImageScope V10.2.1.2315 (Aperio).
3. Algorithms: **Positive Pixel Count v9**_v10.0.0.1805, **Nuclear v9**_v10.0.0.1798.

2.3 Indirect Immunofluorescence (IF) and Confocal Laser Scanning Microscope: Double Stainings

1. Patients' biopsies: paraffin-embedded tissue (2 μm), xylenes, and graded alcohol series.
2. Permeabilization: Triton X-100 solution.
3. Phosphate Buffered Saline (PBS).
4. Specific epitope demasking: microwave or pressure cooking with citrate buffer or EDTA buffer.
5. Appropriate protein blocking solution.

6. Mix of specific primary antibodies.
7. Wash in PBS.
8. Appropriate mix of secondary antibodies: FITC-conjugated (555 nm) and TRITC-conjugated (488 nm) antibodies (Alexa Fluor Molecular Probes, customized).
9. Washings with PBS.
10. TO-PRO3 for counterstained nuclei (Molecular probes, customized).
11. Mounting in Gel Mount (Biomeda Corp, Foster City, USA) and sealing with nail varnish.
12. Confocal microscope, Leica TCS SP2 (Leica, Wetzlar, Germany).

2.4 Images Analysis and Quantification

Adobe Photoshop version 6.0 (Adobe Systems Corporation, San Jose, CA, USA).

3 Methods

3.1 IHC Analysis on Paraffin-Embedded Sections

This method is able to detect the presence of your selected marker (e.g., CD8, Granzyme A/B, CXCR3, or T-bet) in kidney biopsies. Follow faithfully this procedure to reveal each antigen in single staining (Figs. 1 and 2).

1. This step requires an appropriate selection of kidney biopsies from patients enrolled for this study, with the auxilium of one or more pathologists, and technical ability to produce 2-μm thin kidney sections from paraffin tissue blocks using a microtome. A brief floating in a 37 °C water bath containing distilled water helps to stretch the tissue. Use a polylysine-coated slide suitable to retrieve each section. Allow the slides to dry overnight at room temperature until all the remaining water is evaporated (*see* **Note 1**).
2. Deparaffinize tissue sections through immersion in pure xylene for 15 min and rehydrate sections using graded alcohol series for few minutes: absolute alcohol (6 min), 95–90 % alcohol (1 min), 70 % alcohol (1 min), 50 % alcohol (1 min) (*see* **Note 2**). Rinse in running cold tap water. Keep the slides in tap water until you are ready to perform antigenic epitope demasking. At no time from this point onward should the slides be allowed to dry. Drying out will cause nonspecific antibody binding and therefore high background staining.
3. Perform antigenic epitope demasking using a heat-induced method by microwave or pressure-induced method by a pressure cooker. For the first method use citrate buffer 0.01 M pH = 6, while for the second method generally use EDTA buffer 0.01 M pH = 8 (*see* **Note 3**).

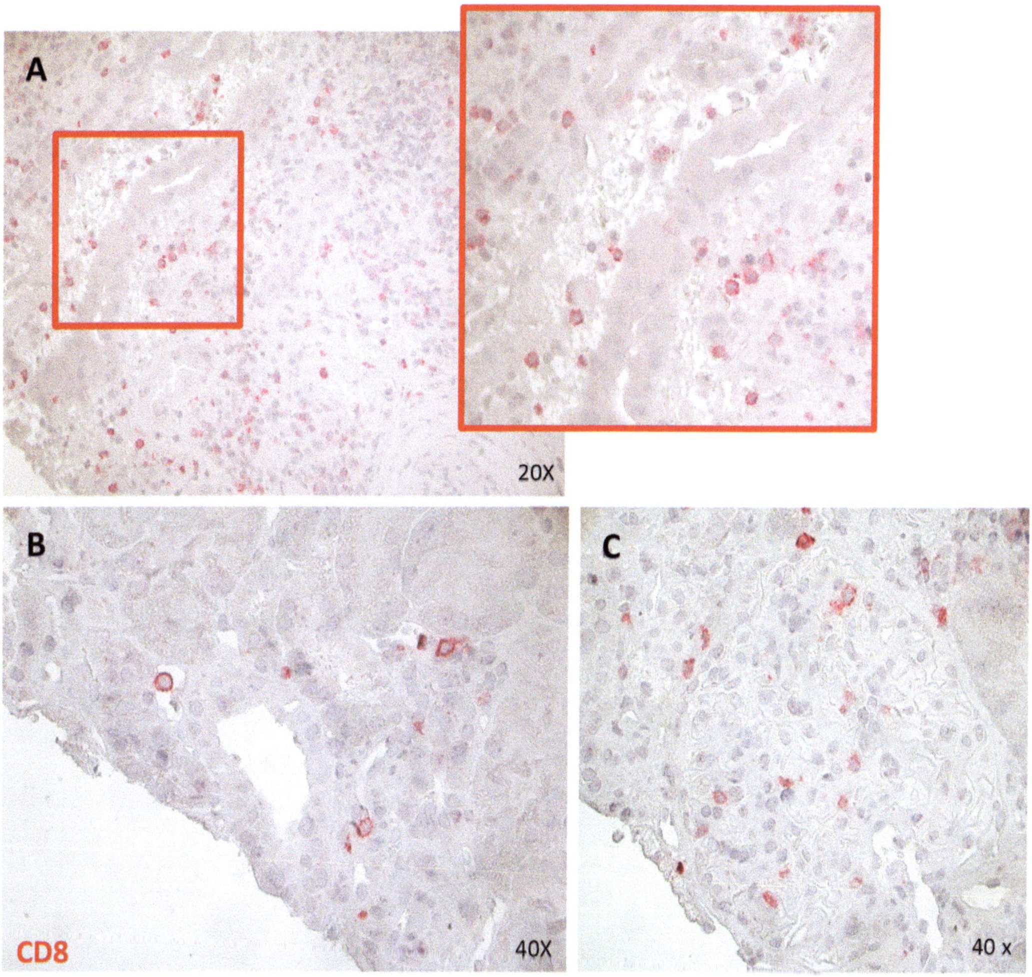

Fig. 1 Graft-infiltrating CD8+ cells in transplant patients with T cell-mediated rejection. Specific CD8-staining on paraffin-embedded kidney sections is detected by Permanent Red Chromogen Solution (*red*) and nuclei were counterstained by hematoxylin (*blue*) (**a**, ×20). The enlargement of the *red box* area in (**a**) shows more clearly CD8 positive cells. Sections acquired at a higher magnification (**b** and **c**, ×40)

For heat-induced epitope retrieval methods with microwave, the slides should be placed in a plastic rack in 100 ml of sodium citrate buffer 10 mM and subjected to three microwave (750 W) cycles of 5 min, and top up the volume of antigen retrieval buffer with distilled water in order to avoid evaporation during boiling. For pressure-induced epitope retrieval method with a pressure cooker, the slides should be placed in a metal rack such that their position allows for an even distribution of pressure. Add 2,000 ml of antigen retrieval buffer to the pressure cooker (200 ml EDTA 10× dissolved in 1,800 ml distilled water), as soon as the cooker has reached full pressure, time 1.30 min (*see* **Note 4**). Leave your slide container immersed in cold water until it becomes cool (*see* **Note 5**).

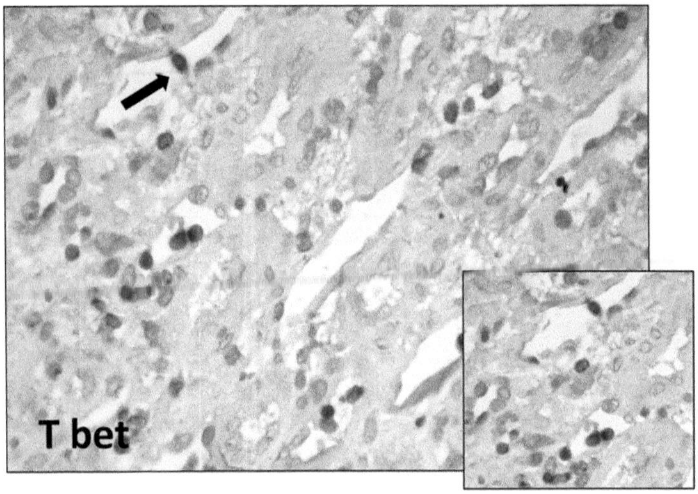

Fig. 2 Graft-infiltrating T-bet+ cells in transplant patients with acute rejection. Specific T-bet staining on paraffin-embedded kidney sections is detected by DAB (*brown*, ×40 magnification) and nuclei were counterstained by hematoxylin (*blue*). T-bet+ cells show a location predominantly into tubular lumen (*black arrow*)

4. If using peroxidase enzyme, block endogenous peroxidase activity by incubating sections with 0.3 % hydrogen peroxidase (H_2O_2) for 10 min (*see* **Note 6**). While if using AP, add two drops of Levamisole (Sigma) to the chromogen solution to suppress endogenous phosphatase activity.
5. Rinse 3×5 min PBS 1× with agitation.
6. After limiting your section with PAP-pen, add 100–150 μl blocking buffer (e.g., Protein blocking serum free 10 % fetal bovine serum in PBS, goat serum 5 % in PBS, or 2 % bovine serum albumin in PBS) onto the sections of the slides and incubate in a humidified chamber at room temperature for 1 h (*see* **Note 7**).
7. Drain off the blocking buffer from the slides. Add 100 μl appropriate diluted primary antibody (for example for Granzyme A, CD8, or CXCR3) to the sections and incubate in a humidified chamber at room temperature for 1 h (*see* **Note 8**). Rinse the slides in Wash buffer (Dako) for three times, 5 min each.
8. Apply 100 μl diluted biotinylated secondary antibody (HRP conjugates, EnVision+ System, Dako) to the sections and incubate on a humidified chamber at room temperature for 30 min. Wash slides as before (*see* **Note 9**).
9. Add 100 μl DAB substrate solution to the sections to reveal the color of antibody staining. Allow the color development for <5 min until the desired color intensity is reached. The reaction can be visualized by a brown precipitate. To stop

the chromogenic reaction, rinse the slides in distilled water (*see* **Note 10**).

10. Counterstain slides with Mayer's hematoxylin (blue) for 3 min. The nuclei can be visualized in blue. Rinse the slides in running tap water for 10 min (*see* **Note 11**).
11. Dry the tissue slides and coverslip tissue slides using mounting solution (Mounting medium Dako). The mounted slides can be stored at room temperature permanently. Observe the antibody staining under light microscopy (*see* **Note 12**).

3.2 Slide Digitation and Analysis

At the end of your immunohistochemical experiment, each slide should be analyzed for rapid and accurate quantification of detected signal. These algorithms represent useful tools for a reproducible and automated measurement of pathologic microscopic changes in kidneys affected by a disease process.

1. Digital images from the experimental glass slides are obtained using ScanScope Digital Slide Scanner (Aperio, Vista, CA, USA) at a 20× magnification (mag) and archived on the devoted Spectrum Server V10.2.2.2315 (Aperio).
2. Quality control of the scanned images and all further analyses are performed using ImageScope V10.2.1.2315 (Aperio).
3. Slides were analyzed by using one of the following algorithms: **Positive Pixel Count v9**_v10.0.0.1805, **Nuclear v9**_v10.0.0.1798, or Rare Event Detection v1_v10.0.0.1798. The **Positive Pixel Count algorithm** counts pixels of predetermined color, intensity, and saturation. The **Nuclear algorithm** is optimized to identify cell nuclei of declared size, color, roundness, or compactness (*see* **Note 13**). Look at Table 1 at the end of the chapter.

3.3 Indirect Immunofluorescence and Confocal Laser Scanning Microscope: Double Staining

This is the method for a type of immunohistochemistry, the indirect immunofluorescence labeling.

The primary antibodies do not have the fluorescent dye attached (as direct immunofluorescence), but the secondary antibodies, which carry the fluorophore, recognize the primary antibodies. Multiple secondary antibodies can bind a single primary antibody and this is the reason for more signal amplification than direct reaction. You can choose to perform a single indirect immunofluorescence for your selected markers instead of the simpler immunohistochemistry, previously described. However, it is more complex and time-consuming compared to immunohistochemical analysis. Thus, consider it useful especially in double staining, where you should to explore the co-distribution of the selected marker (e.g., CXCR3) and the antigens CD4 or CD8 in the same biopsies and, in turn, you may clearly visualize the co-localization of two different fluorophores (e.g., FITC and TRITC) by combination of two colors (yellow) (*see* **Note 14**).

Table 1

Parameters used in the image analysis algorithms (adapted from Aperio documentation)

Parameter	Description	Value range
Roundness	The ratio of the area of a nucleus to the area of a circle that fully encloses that nucleus	0–I (perfect circle)
Compactness	The ratio of area of a nucleus to the area of a circle with a circumference equal to the perimeter of that nucleus	0–I (perfect circle)
Elongation	The ratio of the min/max principal moments of the nuclei (a quantitative measure of the shape of a set of points)	0–I (perfect circle)
Nuclear size	Min/Max determines the nuclei size limits in μm^2	0 to user defined
Object pixels	Min/Max determines the object size limits in pixels	0 to user defined
Hue value	The color of the objects of interest, It is a number of a desired color indicated in radial value on an arbitrary color wheel, divided by 360	0–I
Hue width	Range of hues, centered on the Hue Value that will satisfy the hue detection process	0–360
Color saturation	The amount of color defined by the Hue Value. RGB values are represented as gray + color	0–I (fully saturated, no gray component)
Intensity	The measure of brightness of a pixel	0–255 (bright white)

Klapczynski M, Gagne GD, Morgan SJ, Larson KJ, Leroy BE, Blomme EA, Cox BF, Shek EW. Computer-assisted imaging algorithms facilitate histomorphometric quantification of kidney damage in rodent renal failure models. J Pathol Inform. 2012;3:20

1. Use preferably paraffin-embedded sections as starting material for higher quality of tissue then frozen sections. Follow the instructions described for IHC (**steps 1** and **2** in Subheading 3.1). Do not use this pretreatment if you work with frozen sections that are non-paraffin-embedded.
2. (Optional) Brief permeabilitation by a treatment with Triton X-100 solution (0.2 % in PBS) for 10 min Follow the indications in Subheading 3.1, **steps 4–6** (*see* **Note 15**).
3. Rinse 3 × 5 min PBS 1× with agitation.
4. Perform antigenic epitope demasking using a heat-induced method by microwave or pressure-induced method by a pressure cooker.
5. Add blocking buffer from slides.
6. Drain off the blocking buffer from slides. Add 100 μl mix of diluted first and second primary antibodies (for example for CXCR3/CD8+ double staining, prepare a mix of the two different antibodies respecting the dilution tested individually before) to the sections and incubate in a humidified chamber

at room temperature for 1 h. Wash slides with PBS for three times, 5 min each (*see* **Note 16**).

7. Wash in PBS, each 3 × 5 min.
8. Incubate sections in mix of two secondary antibodies, respectively to bind the first and the second primary antibodies. Wash slides with PBS for three times, 5 min each.
9. Wash in PBS, each 3 × 5 min.
10. Counterstain with TO-PRO3 (1:3,000 in PBS) for 10 min at room temperature (dark).
11. Coverslip with Gel/Mounting medium Dako, seal with nail varnish, and store slides in dark at +4 °C.
12. Images acquisition by confocal microscope Leica TCS SP2: first primary antibody staining sites (green), second primary antibody staining sites (red), double staining sites (yellow), counterstained nuclei (blue).

3.4 Image Processing and Quantification

After calibration of the monitor colors, images of trichrome-stained sections are captured with a 40× magnification objective and analyzed as RGB 24-bit images. Of each section examined, 30 adjacent fields are captured and a seamless widefield image (W-image) was reconstituted from these 30 frames on the Photoshop program.20. To ensure an accurate and identical total area is acquired from each section, a piece of black adhesive strap with a central square window measuring 5.0 mm ¥ 5.0 mm was stuck on the back of the examined section. The area of the square window represents the sum of the acquired fields and the total area of the reconstituted W-image. Of each biopsy, three W-images from three different anatomic planes are prepared using this method. Results are the sum of calculations of all three W-images.

A new set of actions is created from the "Action" palette to record the series of commands applied to the first W-image, which can be played back as one command to all subsequent W-images. The W-image size is first adjusted to 15 cm ¥ 15 cm and a resolution of 300 p.p.i. to obtain pixel dimensions of 1772 ¥ 1772 pixels per image. The contrast of the image is then adjusted automatically. Using the "Selective Color" command present under the "Image" drop-down menu, the red, magenta, cyan, and blue colors are adjusted after checking the "Relative" option in the "Selective Color" dialog box. From the color table, the red and magenta colors are chosen sequentially and their cyan component is reduced to −100 % and the magenta component expanded to +100 %. The cyan and blue colors are selected, their cyan component expanded to +100 % and their magenta component reduced to −100 %. Using the "Color Range" command present under the "Selection" drop-down menu, the blue color in the image is selected after providing a value of 100. The histogram of the selected color, which represents the signal tissue, counts the total area of positivity in pixels.

The cortical area of the entire biopsy is analyzed generally as a series of consecutive fields, avoiding the capsule, the subcapsular areas, and the arterial adventitia. The percentage of positive-stained area (pixels/total area) is measured. Values from all consecutive images for each biopsy are averaged.

4 Notes

1. Transfer the section onto "polylysine-coated" slides (generally homemade) or slides suitable for immunohistochemistry (customized). Before starting immunohistochemistry, be sure that all tissue sections are dry enough. As quality of tissue is critical for a fruitful experiment, damaged tissues have to be discarded. Use optical microscope to assure that sections include both glomerular and tubular-interstitium areas.
2. It is possible to leave sections for more than 15 min in xylene without compromising subsequent steps.
3. Be careful while preparing buffers. Sodium citrate buffer (10 mM sodium citrate, pH 6.0): 41 ml citric acid (10.5 g acid citric in 500 ml distilled water), 9 ml sodium citrate (14.7 g sodium citrate in 500 ml distilled water), 450 ml distilled water. Mix to dissolve. Adjust pH to 6.0 with 1 N HCl. Store at +4 °C for longer storage. EDTA (pH = 8): 3.72 g EDTA, 1,000 ml distilled water. Mix o dissolve. Adjust pH to 8.0 with 1 N NaOH. Store at room temperature for longer storage.
4. Check your tissue sections after this step. A pressure cooker is more aggressive than microwave. Thus, use it only if your first experiment by microwave fails. Slides need to stay immersed in buffer at boiling. Pay attention while preparing citrate or EDTA buffer and check pH before use.
5. Homemade or customized PBS. Important: do not leave sections dry; they have to remain humidified always.
6. Be careful to incubate sections in the dark. Seven minutes of incubation may be enough. No agitation required.
7. Choose carefully your blocking buffer. Incubate sections in normal serum-species same as secondary antibodies. For example, if your primary antibody is rabbit and your secondary antibody is goat anti-rabbit, goat normal serum block should be used. For CD8 staining use protein block serum free (Dako) for 10 min at room temperature.
8. Use your primary antibody after dilution in blocking buffer (the same buffer used in the step before). It is more specific than dilution in PBS (washing buffer). Check the datasheet to

assure that your primary antibody is suitable for IHC, especially for paraffin-embedded sections. Some antibodies may require overnight incubation: low temperature (+4 °C) is needed for longer incubation time. For CD8 staining use CD8 antibody mouse monoclonal (Dako) ready to use for 10 min at room temperature. Negative controls are obtained by incubating serial sections with the blocking solution and then omitting the primary antibody. Keep slides protected from light during incubation.

9. For CD8 staining use EnVision G|2 System AP rabbit mouse (Dako, K5355): add 100 μl of Link for 30 min, rinse the slides in wash buffer, add 100 μl of Ap Enzyme for 30 min, and rinse the slides again in wash buffer (Fig. 1).
10. Prepare DAB solution freshly before use: 0.05 % DAB-0.01 % H_2O_2 in PBS. DAB is a suspected carcinogen, so handle with care. For CD8 staining, add 100 Fast Red substrate solution with levamisole to the sections to reveal the color of antibody staining. Allow the color development for <5 min until the desired color intensity is reached. The reaction can be visualized by a red precipitate. To stop the chromogenic reaction, rinse the slides in distilled water.
11. Mayer's hematoxylin allows to visualize nuclei. Diligently wash slides.
12. Negative controls are obtained incubating serial sections with the blocking solution and then the control irrelevant antibody. Two independent observers blinded to the origin of the slides have to observe the entire region of biopsies by optical light microscopy.
13. The number of CD8+ interstitial cells should be measured at high power (400×) field on the entire cortical region of biopsies, while the number of CD8+ glomerular cells should be counted in all glomeruli/sections by two independent observers blinded to the origin of the slides.
14. Prior to perform double labeling, test each primary antibodies individually and set the appropriate dilution. You can perform a single IF.
15. Permeabilization helps you to detect intracellular proteins (e.g., transcription factors such as T-bet, nuclear proteins). Check your datasheet to decide whether or not to perform this step. Follow faithfully the incubation time damages to the biopsies affect tissues.
16. If the two primary antibodies are two different species (first antibody is rabbit and the second is mouse), you can prepare a mix of the two antibodies (and then you should prepare a mix of its respective secondary antibodies for the subsequent step).

Otherwise, you should incubate sections in first primary antibody and its secondary antibody (FITC-conjugated) and, after a second incubation in blocking buffer, you should incubate sections in second primary antibody and its secondary antibody (TRITC-conjugated).

References

1. Strehlau J, Pavlakis M, Lipman M et al (1997) Quantitative detection of immune activation transcripts as a diagnostic tool in kidney transplantation. Proc Natl Acad Sci U S A 94:695–700
2. Lipman ML, Stevens AC, Strom TB (1994) Heightened intragraft CTL gene expression in acutely rejecting renal allografts. J Immunol 152:5120–5127
3. Kummer JA, Wever PC, Kamp AM (1995) Expression of granzyme A and B proteins by cytotoxic lymphocytes involved in acute renal allograft rejection. Kidney Int 47:70–77
4. Lipman ML1, Shen Y, Jeffery JR, Gough J, McKenna RM, Grimm PC, Rush DN (1998) Immune-activation gene expression in clinically stable renal allograft biopsies: molecular evidence for subclinical rejection. Transplantation 27;66(12):1673–1681
5. Hoffmann SC, Hale DA, Kleiner DE, Mannon RB, Kampen RL, Jacobson LM, Cendales LC, Swanson SJ, Becker BN, Kirk AD (2005) Functionally significant renal allograft rejection is defined by transcriptional criteria. Am J Transplant 5:573–581
6. Bromley SK, Mempel TR, Luster AD (2008) Orchestrating the orchestrators: chemokines in control of T cell traffic. Nat Immunol 9: 970–980
7. Campanella GS, Grimm J, Manice LA et al (2006) Oligomerization of CXCL10 is necessary for endothelial cell presentation and in vivo activity. J Immunol 177:6991–6998
8. Qin S, Rottman JB, Myers P et al (1998) The chemokine receptors CXCR3 and CCR5 mark subsets of T cells associated with certain inflammatory reactions. J Clin Invest 101:746–754
9. Menke J, Zeller GC, Kikawada E et al (2008) CXCL9, but not CXCL10, promotes CXCR3-dependent immune-mediated kidney disease. J Am Soc Nephrol 19:1177–1189
10. Steinmetz OM, Turner JE, Paust HJ et al (2009) CXCR3 mediates renal Th1 and Th17 immune response in murine lupus nephritis. J Immunol 183:4693–4704

Index

A

Elena Ranieri (ed.), *Cytotoxic T-Cells: Methods and Protocols*, Methods in Molecular Biology, vol. 1186,
DOI 10.1007/978-1-4939-1158-5, © Springer Science+Business Media New York 2014

D

E

F

G

H

V

W

X

Z